Vitamin K
and
Vitamin K-Dependent Proteins:
Analytical, Physiological, and Clinical Aspects

Edited by

Martin J. Shearer, Ph.D. and **M. J. Seghatchian, Ph.D.**

Haematology Department
Guy's Hospital
London, England

Department of Quality Assurance
National Blood Transfusion Center
London, England

CRC Press
Boca Raton   Ann Arbor   London   Tokyo

Library of Congress Cataloging-in-Publication Data

Vitamin K and vitamin K-dependent proteins: analytical,
  physiological, and clinical aspects/edited by M.J. Shearer and
  M.J. Seghatchian.
      p.   cm.
  Includes bibliographical references and index.
  ISBN 0-8493-6423-X
    1. Vitamin K-dependent proteins.   2. Vitamin K.   I. Shearer, M.
J.   II. Seghatchian, M. J.
  QP552.V58V55   1993
  612.3'99--dc20   92-36184
                                                                                      CIP

FOREWORD

Within the past decade, rapid progress in analytical methods has led to the increasing application of specific techniques for measuring vitamin K and its metabolites in biological fluids. Already such methods are providing new insights into the status and physiology of vitamin K in health and disease. In parallel, new methods and concepts have been applied to the assay of the vitamin K-dependent procoagulant and anticoagulant factors, enabling workers to meet the multiple challenges of improved sensitivity, specificity, precision, and accuracy and giving them the ability to differentiate between native, activated, intermediate complexes and non-functional abnormal forms. Such modern coagulation tests are central to our understanding of hemostasis and the changes that may occur in various pathophysiological states or diseases. Accordingly, major advances in the molecular and functional patterns of hypercoagulability and congenital deficiencies of the vitamin K-dependent clotting factors have been made. The association of malignant disease with hemostatic disturbances is also becoming progressively understood. Newer discoveries have been made on the involvement of various components of the hemostatic systems in the pathogenesis of tumor growth, expansion and metastases, providing planning, therapeutic measures, prevention, and counterattack on related bleeding and thrombotic complications. Recently, much clinical interest has also been shown in the new radioimmunoassays of activation peptides as well as abnormal prothrombin and the bone protein osteocalcin, which are providing sensitive markers of vitamin K deficiency and/or liver and bone diseases. Significant advances have also been made in our understanding of vitamin K deficiency in the newborn, in antibiotic-induced hypoprothrombinemia and the mechanism of action of coumarin anticoagulants.

With rapid progress and increasing specialization, there has been a natural tendency for individual laboratories to become expert in one area, either involving measurements and studies of vitamin K, vitamin K-dependent clotting factors, or other vitamin K-dependent proteins. A major objective of this book is, therefore, to bring together in one volume the experts in these three interrelated fields to review state-of-the-art techniques. Leading scientists and clinical experts will provide an overview of how these techniques have increased our knowledge in particular clinical areas. To ensure clarity of exposition and to allow the reader to extract quickly the essential core information — but at the same time provide sufficient detail to enable an in-depth understanding of the development and application of the techniques within each area — emphasis is placed on new technologies used. This approach is intended to have broad appeal, not only to research workers actively engaged in these fields, but to clinicians, medical technologists, and teachers in higher education. The scope of these presentations is wide. The editors hope that views presented and opinions expressed in this multidisciplinary book will stimulate new ideas and concepts in clinicians involved in the rapidly developing field of hemostasis.

Martin J. Shearer and M. J. Seghatchian

THE EDITORS

Martin J. Shearer, Ph.D., is Principal Biochemist in the Department of Haematology at Guy's Hospital, London and Head of the department's research laboratory in the Clinical Science Laboratories where he also serves as Deputy Director.

After graduating with a B.Sc. in biochemistry from Liverpool University in 1966, Dr. Shearer took a research assistantship to establish a new research laboratory in the Department of Haematology, Guy's Hospital, devoted to the study of vitamin K metabolism in the human, an interest that has continued to this day. In 1973 he was awarded the degree of Ph.D. from the University of London. There followed a postdoctoral appointment until he took the post of Senior Biochemist in 1974 and his present post in 1983.

Dr. Shearer is a member of several learned societies including The Nutrition Society, The Chromatographic Society, The New York Academy of Sciences, and The International Society on Thrombosis and Hemostasis.

Dr. Shearer has been the recipient of several research grants from the Medical Research Council and from private industry. He has given invited lectures at many International Conferences in the U.K., The Netherlands, Germany, U.S.A., Korea, and Japan, and is the author of more than 100 papers or book chapters. He has also served as an expert on government committees for the U.K. Department of Health — from 1988 to 1991 to consider dietary reference values (vitamins) for the Committee on Medical Aspects of Food Policy and in 1992 to consider vitamin K prophylaxis in infancy for the Department of Health/British Paediatric Association Expert Committee. In 1990 he served as a scientific advisor to The Pasteur Institute, Lyon, France.

In recent years, Dr. Shearer's major research interest has been to explore and to develop new, sensitive chromatographic methods for the measurement of the very low tissue concentrations of vitamin K. His laboratory has been at the forefront of this research; the techniques thus developed are being used to obtain a greater understanding of the human biochemistry and nutriture of vitamin K. The research has a strong clinical bias and is directed towards specific pathophysiological problems such as the causes and prevention of vitamin K deficiency in the newborn period. In all these studies Dr. Shearer has enjoyed a fruitful collaboration with a variety of groups and research workers in the U.K., Europe, and the U.S.A.

M. J. Seghatchian, Ph.D., is the Principal Clinical Scientist in charge of the Quality Assurance Laboratory at the North London Blood Transfusion Centre and Honorary Lecturer at Guy's Hospital Medical and Dental School. His basic training is in chemistry, specializing in radiation chemistry/polymerization at CNRS, Orsay, France. Dr. Seghatchian obtained his doctorate in physical chemistry in 1964 from the University of Paris, France. He also obtained a Ph.D. in medical biochemistry from the University of London, in 1972, following postdoctoral studies at Guy's Hospital on the application of radioisotopes in medicine and spectroscopic techniques in drug enzyme interactions.

Since 1973, Dr. Seghatchian's interests have focused on the regulatory control and standardization aspects of the hemostatic components of blood, originating the integrated system of quality assurance at North London Blood Transfusion Centre. As a visiting scientist, he worked for several years at the National Institute for Biological Standards and Control and the MRC Epidemiology and Medical Care Unit at Northwick Park Hospital, on the standardization/automation of coagulation assays and methodological aspects of hypercoagulability. He has pioneered the chromogenic assay of factors VIII/VII and developed a new electrophoretic method for the characterization of native and altered forms of factor VIII/vWF, Protein C/Protein C-inhibitor complexes and thrombogenic components of prothrombin complexes. In the capacity of visiting scientist, he has collaborated with several leading scientists and clinicians in Sweden, France, Italy, U.S.A., Canada, and South America on the molecular abnormalities of hemostatic proteins, inhibitors of proteolytic enzymes, and heparin-induced thrombocytopenia. He has also acted as a WHO expert consultant on coagulation for Mediterranean countries.

Dr. Seghatchian's current research interests include characterization of the activity states of the hemostatic components implicated in hemapheresis procedures and hypercoagulability with particular reference to clinical and methodological aspects of platelet interaction with vitamin K-dependent proteins, factors VIII/vWF and vWF fragments. He has recently been active in the development of simple screening tests for platelet morphological/functional integrity using automated cell counters and assessing platelet activation/release reaction by microplate and flow cytometry techniques.

Dr. Seghatchian is currently an editor of the journals *Transfusion Science* and *Thrombosis Research*. He has co-edited a two-volume publication on *Factor VIII/vWF* (CRC Press, 1990) and *Quality Assurance in Transfusion Medicine* (CRC Press, 1993). He also acts as referee and an editorial advisory member for CRC Press publications. He has published more than 200 scientific papers and abstracts, and has delivered more than 40 guest lectures at national and international meetings. He is a founding member of both the British Society of Blood Transfusion and the British Society of Haemostasis and Thrombosis and a member of several international societies.

CONTRIBUTORS

Catherine Boyer-Neumann, M.D.
Department of Hematology
Hopital Antoine Béclère
Clamart, France

J. L. Francis, Ph.D.
University Department of
  Haematology
General Hospital
Southampton, United Kingdom

A. Ghirardini, M.D.
Department of Human Biopathology
Section of Hematology
University of Rome
Rome, Italy

Caren M. Gundberg, Ph.D.
Department of Orthopedics and
  Rehabilitation
Yale University School of Medicine
New Haven, Connecticut

Yacoob Haroon, Ph.D.
Hoffmann-LaRoche, Inc.
Nutley, New Jersey

John Patrick Hart, Ph.D.
Faculty of Applied Sciences
University of the West of England
Bristol, United Kingdom

William E. Hathaway, M.D.
Professor Emeritus
Department of Pediatrics
University of Colorado
  School of Medicine
Denver, Colorado

A. Iacopino, M.D.
Thrombosis Center
Department of Human Biopathology
Section of Hematology
University of Rome
Rome, Italy

Marjo H. J. Knapen
Department of Biochemistry
University of Limburg
Maastricht, The Netherlands

Marie-Jo Larrieu, M.D.
Department of Hematology
Hopital Antoine Béclère
Clamart, France

Guglielmo Mariani
Department of Human Biopathology
Section of Hematology
University of Rome
Rome, Italy

M. Papacchini, Ph.D.
Department of Human Biopathology
University of Rome
Rome, Italy

B. Kevin Park
Department of Pharmacology and
  Therapeutics
The University of Liverpool
Liverpool, United Kindgom

Hans Prydz, Ph.D.
The Biotechnology Center of Oslo
University of Oslo
Oslo, Norway

M. J. Seghatchian, Ph.D.
Department of Quality Assurance
National Blood Transfusion Center
London, England

Martin J. Shearer, M.D.
Haematology Department
Guy's Hospital
London, England

John W. Suttie, Ph.D.
Department of Biochemistry
College of Agricultural and Life
  Sciences
University of Wisconsin-Madison
Madison, Wisconsin

Cees Vermeer, Ph.D.
Department of Biochemistry
University of Limburg
Maastricht, The Netherlands

Rüdiger von Kries, Ph.D.
Children's Hospital
Heinrich Heine University
Düsseldorf, Germany

Mark J. Winn, Ph.D.
Department of Pharmacology and
  Therapeutics
The University of Liverpool
Liverpool, United Kingdom

Martine Wolf, M.D.
Department of Hematology
Hopital Antoine Béclère
Clamart, France

TABLE OF CONTENTS

INTRODUCTION

AN OVERVIEW OF VITAMIN K AND VITAMIN K-DEPENDENT PROTEINS

The topic of vitamin K and vitamin K-dependent proteins spans a wide spectrum of academic disciplines within the biological and physicochemical sciences and includes such specialities as biochemistry, clinical medicine, nutrition, pharmacology, and molecular biology. Beginning with the discovery of vitamin K by Henrik Dam in the 1930s and the independent discoveries of the first of its dependent proteins (prothrombin) and the "cattle poison" (dicumarol), which turned out to be both the first vitamin K antagonist and the first oral anticoagulant drug, a major research area has been created in the field of hemostasis. From the 1950s to the 1970s much attention was focused on the role in hemostasis of just four proteins, prothrombin (factor II), factor VII, factor IX and factor X which collectively became known as the vitamin K-dependent clotting factors. Although it was realized earlier that vitamin K was required for the expression of the biological activity of these four factors, it was not until 1974 that the molecular role of vitamin K became clear when it was discovered that vitamin K promoted a unique post translational modification in prothrombin whereby specific glutamic acid (Glu) residues were converted to γ-carboxyglutamic acid (Gla) residues. At about the same time the field of hemostasis was further enriched and enlivened by the discovery of two other vitamin K-dependent proteins (proteins C and S) which in contrast to the procoagulant role of the classical vitamin K-dependent clotting factors were found to possess anticoagulant properties. Subsequent studies have revealed the remarkable complexity and feedback control of hemostasis in which the role of the vitamin K-dependent proteins provides an excellent illustration of the growing appreciation of the interplay between circulating and endothelial cell components.

In the 1970s and 1980s we witnessed the discovery of a diverse group of vitamin K-dependent proteins which had no connection with blood coagulation. Of these, the best known and characterized protein is the bone protein osteocalcin (also known as bone Gla protein, BGP) though its precise biological role remains relatively obscure. In retrospect, the discovery of these non-coagulation Gla-containing proteins provided a unified concept of the biological role of vitamin K in protein biosynthesis and perhaps in calcium homeostasis.

In so far as new advances in any scientific speciality are driven by the introduction of new technologies and techniques, the same is true for the fields which encompass the vitamin K and vitamin K-dependent proteins. For example, in the field of hemostasis, new methods and concepts have been developed for the assays of the vitamin K-dependent coagulation proteins (including the important question of the accurate assessment of their activity states) which have enabled investigators to meet the multiple challenges of improved sensitivity, specificity, and precision. For example, using newly introduced assays for activation peptides, intermediate complexes and enzyme-inhibitor complexes, it is now possible to differentiate between native and activated forms, intermediate complexes and non-functional forms. Such modern diagnostic approaches are central to our understanding of hemostasis and the changes that may occur in various physiological and pathophysiological states.

In parallel to the methodological advances of coagulation assays there have been startling advances in molecular biology which, in the context of this volume, are increasing our understanding of the congenital deficiencies of vitamin K-dependent proteins. For example, by pinpointing congenital defects at the molecular level it is now possible to carry out "structure vs. function" studies in which specific molecular defects in the variant protein can be related to the information given by functional assays and thence to the clinical expression of the defect. Although still in their infancy, further studies of abnormal variants based on this structure vs. function approach will also undoubtedly help our understanding of the normal biochemical function of the vitamin K-dependent proteins. At the more practical clinical level, molecular biological techniques have vastly improved the power of detection (including antenatal diagnosis) of carriers of hereditary coagulation disorders involving the vitamin K-dependent coagulation proteins. In this respect, two valuable techniques are those of linkage analysis utilizing the restriction fragment length polymorphisms (RFLPs) and the polymerase chain reaction (PCR) combined with direct sequencing to analyse the amplified DNA fragments. The rapid progress in this field is illustrated by the fact that almost 400 hemophilia B (factor IX) gene defects have been recorded of which over 200 comprise unique mutations. The techniques of molecular biology are also applicable to the detection and characterization of hereditary defects associated with the vitamin K-anticoagulant proteins C and S. Individuals with functional defects or deficiencies of these proteins will, of course, tend to present with thrombophilia as opposed to hemophilia.

The arrival of recombinant technology has led to much research being directed into the commercial production of recombinant vitamin K-dependent proteins which can be used for replacement therapy in hereditary deficiencies or, for example in the case of recombinant factor VII, for the treatment of patients with inhibitors to factor VIII (e.g., as in patients with hemophilia A who develop antibodies in response to factor VIII therapy). These new developments have also shown that the concept of gene therapy for hemophilia is an achievable goal. The objective of such therapy is to introduce a normal gene into the cells of individuals whose body contains cells with an abnormal (mutant) copy of the gene (e.g. factor IX gene in hemophilia B). Before contemplating such a venture, it was nevertheless essential that the structure and fine detail of the normal gene copies were fully established. Having achieved this in the mid-1980s, efforts have been directed to clarify the clinical consequences of possible fluctuating levels of synthesis which in certain cases may result in hypercoagulability or bleeding. Hence further "fine-tuning" studies are required before gene therapy can be finally introduced as an effective therapy in humans. Fortunately, suitable animal models exist for conducting preclinical trials, making gene therapy a near future reality as an inexpensive and long-term "cure" for both developed and developing countries who do not currently have access to concentrates of vitamin K-dependent clotting factors. Concerns about the safety of using a disabled carrier virus have nevertheless been expressed. The most effective strategies and selection of receptor cells also require additional work; cells of the endothelial lining to blood vessels, of skin and of smooth muscle are amongst options, each having some points in favour and some against.

In the field of vitamin K itself, the last decade has seen rapid progress in the development of analytical methods which can be applied to the specific and sensitive measurement of vitamin K and its metabolites in biological fluids and tissues. So far, vitamin K, with its extreme lipophilic character, has proved resistant to immunochemical assay and the ability to measure the naturally low concentrations in most tissues has only proved possible since the advent of new technologies based on the technique of high-performance liquid chromatography (HPLC). Apart from the general advances in the technology and equipment of HPLC (e.g., silica-based microparticulate packing materials, reliable solvent delivery systems and sensitive in-line detectors), the most recent advances which are featured in this volume have stemmed from the favorable chemistry of vitamin K allowing its sensitive detection by electrochemical or fluorometric measurements. Such is the power of these techniques that femtomolar amounts of the K vitamins can be readily detected with a high specificity which is more easily validated than techniques with a comparable sensitivity (e.g., immunoassays). These methods are already proving invaluable for the study of nutritional aspects of vitamin K in health and disease, leading to important advances in our ability to assess vitamin K status from measurements of plasma and liver concentrations of the many molecular forms of vitamin K. In parallel, sensitive immunoassays for undercarboxylated (des-γ-carboxy) forms of prothrombin (PIVKA, *proteins induced by vitamin K absence or antagonism*) have been introduced which offer an alternative approach to assessing subclinical vitamin K deficiency. Such assays have been recently extended to the assessment of undercarboxylated forms of osteocalcin. The acquisition of these techniques may be regarded as particularly apposite in view of certain recent clinical developments, which have seen, for example, a worldwide resurgence of a potentially fatal syndrome known as the "hemorrhagic disease of the newborn". This syndrome is due to vitamin K deficiency, often of no known cause, which presents soon after birth or in the first few weeks after birth. The late onset form of the syndrome peaking at the fourth to sixth week of life is still a leading, worldwide cause of intracranial hemorrhage in infants of this age and often results in death or permanent disability.

With the discovery in 1974 of the role of vitamin K as a cofactor for the conversion of Glu-residues to Gla-residues, the way became open to search for other vitamin K-dependent proteins, either by assaying for the carboxylase enzyme responsible for γ-glutamyl carboxylation or by isolating the product of action of vitamin K, namely Gla. Within a short time, vitamin K-dependent activities had been detected in a wide variety of tissues such as bone, kidney, placenta, pancreas, spleen and lung. The vitamin K-dependent protein, osteocalcin, has proved of interest for a variety of reasons. Firstly, despite being one of the most abundant proteins of the human body, its precise physiological role has remained elusive. Secondly, as a product of the osteoblast, its presence in the serum attracted clinical interest as a possible marker of bone formation. In the last decade, the assay of serum osteocalcin by radioimmunoassay has gone from research tool to an established clinical test for monitoring osteoblast activity. Assays for the measurement of free Gla excreted in the urine are less widely used but have proved valuable in several research contexts as an index of the turnover of all the Gla-containing proteins.

A more recent development is the measurement of the hydroxylapatite binding capacity of osteocalcin as a measure of the Gla content of the protein, and perhaps, as another subclinical marker of vitamin K deficiency. Some tantalizing clinical studies have raised the question of whether the vitamin K status of an individual can influence normal bone metabolism or can influence the progression of bone disease. For example, in a group of postmenopausal women who were given a supplementary daily dose of 1 mg of vitamin K (phylloquinone), both the total serum osteocalcin and the hydroxylapatite binding capacity of osteocalcin increased. Although there is some evidence that vitamin K administration may also decrease urinary calcium excretion in certain patients, many questions remain to be answered before any beneficial claims of vitamin K supplementation can be made with respect to the reduction of bone mineral loss in diseases such as osteoporosis. Another unexpected recent discovery is that protein S, a vitamin K-dependent protein until now associated only with a hemostatic role, is also synthesized and secreted by osteoblasts. The parallel clinical reports of an association of osteopenia in some patients with protein S-deficiency has raised the intriguing possibility that protein S may have two independent roles, one already well established as a natural anticoagulant cofactor of protein C involved in modulating both coagulation and fibrinolysis, and another role in maintaining normal bone turnover and bone mass. Whatever else, these unexpected findings have stimulated an increased interest and new research into the possible role of vitamin K and vitamin K-dependent proteins in bone physiology.

It is pertinent here to reflect on the contribution to this field, both clinically and experimentally, which has been made by the coumarin group of vitamin K antagonists. Today, the story of how the naturally occurring poison, dicumarol (which caused the hemorrhagic disease in cattle called "sweet clover disease") became the first clinically used oral anticoagulant drug and later, how another synthetic coumarin congener (warfarin) evolved from being the world's most successful rat poison to an equally successful human drug seems bizarre indeed. Even Karl Link, whose laboratory isolated and characterized dicumarol, was surprised when in 1941, the clinicians "snatched the cow poison" from his laboratory for clinical trials. For many years the more potent anticoagulant warfarin, one of the many coumarin vitamin K antagonists synthesized by Link's laboratory, had been considered too toxic for human use but, at Link's suggestion, had become a revolutionary, "multiple dose" rodenticide. In 1951, however, there was another twist to this bizarre story when a U.S. Army trainee took a deliberate overdose of warfarin rat poison. As recorded by Link, the trainee's attempt "to shuffle off this mortal coil" was unsuccessful and he admitted himself to the hospital, where his "fully developed hemorrhagic sweet clover disease" was promptly reversed by blood transfusion and large doses of vitamin K. This incident served as a catalyst, and after careful clinical trails warfarin was introduced into clinical practice where it has stayed to this day. Forty years on, we can reflect on the universal acceptance of warfarin (and similar coumarin compounds) as antithrombotic drugs and wonder at its unpromising beginnings. There is however another aspect of the coumarin antagonists which is well represented throughout the pages of this volume. This is their value to the scientist to whom they have offered a powerful tool for investigating the mechanism of action and metabolism of vitamin K, and the role of the vitamin K-dependent proteins in the physiological processes in which they may be involved, e.g., hemostasis and bone metabolism. Two prominent examples of how coumarin anticoagulants have contributed to major discoveries in this field come from the use of anticoagulated animal models. Firstly, the dicumarol-treated bovine model enabled the ready isolation of the abnormal (anticoagulant-induced) prothrombin molecules from plasma and the characterization of their structural deficiency which eventually led to the discovery of γ-carboxyglutamic acid as a vitamin K-dependent amino acid residue of prothrombin. Secondly, the warfarin-treated rat model enabled the identification of the liver metabolite, vitamin K epoxide leading to the deduction of the existence of a metabolic cycle of vitamin K (the vitamin K-vitamin K epoxide cycle) which was closely linked to vitamin K-dependent γ-carboxylation. In this volume, the reader will find many examples of how coumarin vitamin K antagonists continue to make an impact in many different areas of investigation. Some examples are their use in investigating:

- The biochemical role of the vitamin K-dependent procoagulants and anticoagulants in hemostasis, and how such knowledge contributes to improved therapeutic control of conventional anticoagulant therapy and sometimes opens up new treatment strategies (e.g., the possible use of low dose warfarin during surgery or to reduce the risk associated with raised factor VII coagulant activity in ischemic heart disease).
- The biochemical role of vitamin K-dependent proteins in malignancy.
- The metabolism and function of osteocalcin in bone.

As in other branches of science, rapid progress in the field of vitamin K and vitamin K-dependent proteins has led to an increased diversification of interest and inevitably an increased specialization with individuals or groups tending to concentrate on one of three main areas either involving studies of vitamin K itself, the vitamin K-dependent blood coagulation proteins or the non-coagulation vitamin K-dependent proteins. A major objective of this book, therefore, is to bring together in the same volume experts in these three different but interrelated fields to review the state of the art in their respective specialities.

The key aims of the book are:

1. To integrate the diversity of research and interest of several disciplines relating to the chemistry, analysis, physiology, genetics and clinical aspects of vitamin K and vitamin K-dependent proteins.

2. To provide state-of-the-art information of specific analytical methods which are required in each field of study:

    a) in the field of hemostasis, the assays of vitamin K-dependent pro-coagulant and anticoagulant proteins with special emphasis on the specificity for the species being measured (e.g., native, activated, partially cleaved/metabolised or complexed forms);

    b) in the field of analytical chemistry, the measurement of K vitamins and the application of these techniques to nutritional contexts (e.g., the relationship of tissue measurements to the assessment of vitamin K status);

    c) in the fields of bone research and clinical diagnosis, the measurements of serum osteocalcin and urinary γ-carboxyglutamic acid

3. To review and emphasize the pivotal regulatory roles played by vitamin K-dependent proteins, in maintaining the hemostatic balance between procoagulant and anticoagulant processes and the importance of the endothelium to this homeostasis. A common theme is the assessment, origin and treatment of hypercoaguable states involving the vitamin K-dependent proteins.

4. To review current knowledge relating to the nature, diagnosis and treatment of congenital deficiencies of vitamin K-dependent coagulation factors. Special emphasis is placed on the rapid advances being made in this field by the application of molecular biological techniques.

5. To review the role of vitamin K-dependent proteins in malignancy, including the synthesis by tumors of vitamin K-dependent proteins, their role in metastasis and the possible antimetastatic effects of coumarin anticoagulants.

6. To review clinical and nutritional/biochemical aspects relating to "idiopathic" deficiency states of vitamin K or to induced vitamin K deficiency states. Topics covered include the history, diagnosis, etiology and prevention of vitamin K deficiency in the newborn; the biochemical

mechanism and clinical importance of antibiotic-induced deficiency; and pharmacological concepts of the nature of coumarin antagonism in relation to vitamin K metabolism.

7. To review the physiology of non-coagulation vitamin K-dependent proteins in the human. Topics covered include the role of osteocalcin in bone metabolism, the diagnostic significance of serum osteocalcin assays and the possible importance of vitamin K status and/or antagonism to bone metabolism.

We hope that our integrated approach makes this book a useful, if not an indispensable, reference for both those who are interested in obtaining a grasp of current progress in such a multidisciplinary field and for those who are interested in obtaining detailed information in their topics of interest.

The editors wish to thank the many colleagues and individuals who have contributed articles and shared their original experiences, findings, and opinions, bringing, us state-of-the-art information, combined with technical details.

Specials that are also due to our co-workers, relevant secretarial groups, and the CRC Press staff who did work hard for the success of this venture.

Martin J. Shearer and M. J. Seghatchian

Chapter 1

CHANGES IN THE ACTIVITY STATES OF VITAMIN K-DEPENDENT PROTEINS IN HYPERCOAGULABILITY: SOME CONCEPTUAL AND METHOLOGICAL ASPECTS

M. J. Seghatchian

TABLE OF CONTENTS

I. INTRODUCTION

The establishment of an objective association between a clinical manifestation of a hemostatic abnormality and the laboratory measurement of the observed phenomenon is often a complex stepwise process comprising: (1) the conceptual definition of the phenomenon on the basis of accurate family history taking; (2) the provision of accurate methods for the measurement of activity or function; and (3) the effective translation of the basic laboratory findings on the activity state of the various components of the hemostatic system into the clinical decision making.

The conceptual relationship between the changes in the activity state of vitamin K-dependent clotting proteins in hypercoagulable states is a very good example of such an approach where continuous efforts are being made to accurately translate the causal/effect relationships between the triggering or initiation mechanisms and the possible clinical outcome, using more and more sophisticated biochemical and immunological procedures.

Today, a better understanding of the often complex pathophysiological hemostatic abnormalities can be achieved mainly through the methodological diversification and the "integrated" laboratory approaches, using a comprehensive panel of accurate techniques.

Furthermore, only through the application of the population-based epidemiological studies new correlations can be established between the subclinical/clinical manifestation or incoherence in measurements, where often it is difficult to make a distinction between, e.g., dysfunction, abnormality in synthesis, and/or abnormality in metabolism, all of which may produce a similar clinical outcome.

In this article, after a brief outline of general mechanisms of blood coagulation activation/inhibition, with particular relevance to "bioamplification, bioinactivation, and bioattenuation" processes, the current laboratory approaches for assessing changes in the activity state of some vitamin K-dependent proteins are described. The importance of epidemiological studies on hypercoagulability is illustrated by providing specific examples in some areas of work related to the activity states of factor VII and protein C, which have been carried out by the author in collaboration with staffs of the Epidemiology and Medical Care Unit at Northwick Park Hospital, Harrow, England.

II. VITAMIN K-DEPENDENT PROTEINS AND BIOAMPLIFICATION, BIOINACTIVATION, AND BIOATTENUATION PROCESSES

The coagulation process is an extremely complex regulatory mechanism, operating at three levels, namely initiation, propagation, and termination at a given site (space) and time with an amazing biochemical accuracy. Figure 1

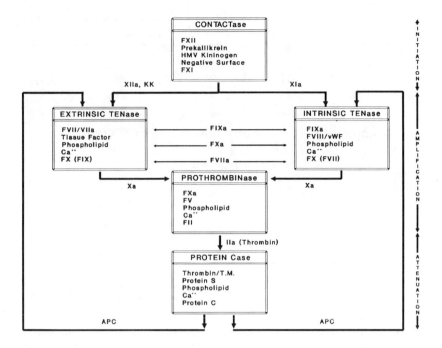

FIGURE 1. The schematic representation of vitamin K-dependent proteins in the bioamplification and bioattenuation of the blood coagulation process, based on the putative formation of intermediate membrane bound complexes. (Modified from Mann, K.G., *The Biochemistry of Coagulation in Clinics for Laboratory Medicine,* Vol. 4, WB Sanders, Philadelphia, 1984.), referred to here as the membrane associated enzyme complexes (MAEC).

The subcomponents of each intermediate complex consists of one native and one active vitamin K-dependent protein as substrate and enzyme. The active forms, produced by limited proteolysis are denoted by subscript a. More than 70% of the activated enzymes remain bound to the surface and are protected from plasma proteolytic inhibitors. Only the thrombin (IIa) is the leaving enzyme from the surface to react with the appropriate cofactors for improved hemostatic effectiveness. This fine "tuning" of events ensure that the coagulation is not ordinarily propagated beyond the site of injury in the physiological milieu.

shows the schematic representation of five components of upstream and downstream control of coagulation, for details see References 1 through 10.

The most striking feature of the coagulation process, is perhaps, the formation of the membrane-associated enzyme complex(es)[5,7] (MAEC) at the site of injury, comprising at least two vitamin K-dependent proteins one acting as an enzyme and the other as a substrate where platelet membrane phospholipids play a pivotal role in recruitment, localization and amplification processes (Figures 2 and 3).

The formation of the MAEC appears to be essential for at least two reasons. First, vitamin K-dependent proteins circulate in plasma in relatively low concentrations in their zymogen forms; hence for optimal efficiency a

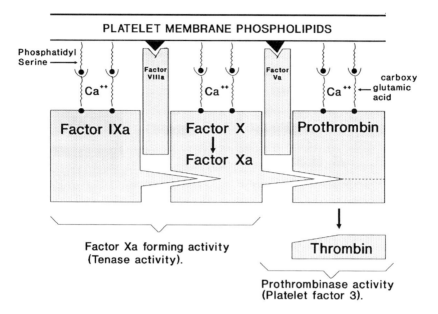

FIGURE 2. The schematic representation of the proposed role of platelet phospholipids (notably phosphotidyl serine) in the amplification of coagulation. The stimulated platelets express not only glycoprotein Ib/IX/V and glycoprotein IIb/IIIa complexes which are receptors of Von Villebrand/factor VIII complexes but also express phosphotidyl serine which interact via calcium ion with both native and activated vitamin K-dependent proteins through their γ-carboxyglutamic acid (Gla) residues.

recruitment process is required to capture and concentrate the relevant sub-components of the MAEC. Second, the amplification process needs to be rapid and a "fine tuning" mechanism is essential to ensure that the process does not propagate, to any great extent, beyond the site of injury. This again emphasizes the importance of localized binding and/or surface-induced conformational changes in the vitamin K-dependent protein to facilitate enzyme-substrate interactions. The above phenomena are applicable to both procoagulant and anticoagulant MAECs which are essential for downstream and upstream modulation of the coagulation process. The endothelial cells (*in vivo*) also play an important role in modulating the outcome of these reactions (Figure 3).

Under laboratory conditions, at least five major intermediate complexes can be identified, which in analogy to the well-accepted terminology for the prothrombinase system,[5-7] have been referred to as contactase, elevenase, extrinsic and intrinsic tenases, prothrombinase, and protein C- and protein Sases. The latter MAEC in contrast to other earlier procoagulant groups is an anticoagulant process, which has been only recently fully characterized.

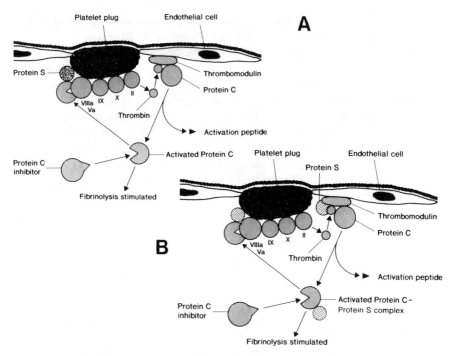

FIGURE 3. The proposed role of stimulated platelets and endothelial cells in promoting the localized procoagulant and anticoagulation effects. Binding to cellular surfaces also protects the activated vitamin K-dependent factors from inhibition by the relevant protease inhibitors. The generated thrombin leave the surface to form clots around the platelet plug and consolidate clots by activating factor XIII. Some thrombin leave to bind to thrombomodulin on endothelium which leads to the release of free protein S from endothelium and the activation of protein C. Activated protein C (APC) is bound via protein S to the platelet plug, neutralizing factor VIIIa and Va cofactor activities hence slowing down the activation process. Excess activated protein C is inhibited by its specific inhibitors. APC also stimulates fibrinolysis via inhibition of TPA inhibitors leading to balanced hemostasis. (B) The rapid rate of clearance of APC *in vivo* ($T^1/_2$ 15 min) is indicative of a surface-bound receptor site or binding to its cofactor protein S and/or complexing with protein C inhibitor (PCI). Whether APC circulates alone or complexed with protein S (the latter is the most effective inhibitor of factors V and VIII) remains to be elucidated. In the light of current experimental findings (see Chapter 6) it is suggested that either a binary, metastable complex (APC-PS) is formed which rapidly modulates the levels of factors V and VIII, or a ternary complex (APC-PS-PCI) is formed which is responsible for the rapid removal of APC. While this hypothesis does not invalidate the concept shown in (A), it provides an alternative pathway which needs further confirmation. In both (A) and (B) free protein may also originate from endothelium cell upon stimulation by thrombin or activated protein C directly or indirectly through tissue plasminogen activator (TPA) and stimulation of fibrinolysis.

A. BIOACTIVATION PROCESS

Under physiological conditions, the blood coagulation process can be triggered in at least three ways. One route is through the exposure of factor XII to negatively charged collagen of the damaged vascular wall, leading to collagen-induced coagulant activity (CICA) or contactase. The stimulation of platelets upon adherence to damaged blood vessels can also directly trigger the coagulation process,[11,12] e.g., through elevenase. In the case of injuries, a clot-promoting substance (thromboplastin or so called tissue factor, [TF]) becomes available on the cellular surface, which through the formation of putative ternary complexes[13] of factor VIIa/TF/IXa or VIIa/TF/Xa directly influences factor Xa generation. The formation of such complexes puts in doubt the separate roles of the intrinsic and extrinsic bioamplification processes of blood coagulation.

In addition to catalytic enhancement, the surface binding also protects activated vitamin K-dependent proteins from inhibition by a host of physiological inhibitors (bioinactivators) and/or specific antibodies. For example, due to its steric relationship, factor IXa (on the surface of activated platelets) and factor Xa (in complex with factor Va/phospholipids) are completely protected from the inhibition by antithrombin III (AT III).

The extent of cleavage of coagulation proteins also differs to a large degree at each stage of the coagulation process. For example, at the initiation stages, in the formation of factor XIIa or factor VIIa only a single peptide bond is cleaved in the molecules and no activation peptide is released. During the activation of factor XI, which consists of two identical polypeptide chains connected by a disulfide bridge, two active centers are formed, whereas when factors IX or X are activated, a peptide bond is cleaved in the carboxy terminal region and activation peptides with molecular weights of 9 kDa and 18 kDa, respectively, are liberated. Finally, in the case of the conversion of prothrombin to thrombin, apart from the cleavage of two NH_2-terminal peptide segments, an intrachain peptide bond is cleaved whereupon the molecular weight of prothrombin is approximately halved.[7]

In addition, at the initiation and propagation stages of the coagulation process, approximately 70% of surface bound vitamin K-dependent protein remains attached to phospholipids by the mediation of calcium. In contrast, in the terminal stage, during the transformation of prothrombin to thrombin, the peptide chain containing the γ-carboxyglutamic acid (Gla) groups is removed. Consequently, the generated enzyme (thrombin), in contrast to generated VIIa, IXa, and Xa, is liberated from the surface, and then either exerts its action in the free state on various other substrates or subsequently binds to new surface sites such as fibrin and/or thrombomodulin where it remains protected from inhibition by one of the major inhibitors of the proteolytic enzyme, AT-III molecules.

Several remarks are pertinent in relation to the properties of the free and membrane-associated enzyme complexes. First, although in the laboratory, the free forms of activated vitamin-K dependent proteins (VIIa, IXa, and Xa) are able to generate thrombin from prothrombin, the catalytic rate of these reactions at the physiological circulating concentrations of substrates and enzymes are almost negligible.[6] On the surfaces, however, particularly in the presence of calcium, phospholipids, and the cofactor, an extremely potent biochemical amplification takes place, increasing the turnover rate of thrombin generation by some 300,000-fold.[6]

Second, the relative contribution of various alternative modes of activation should be taken into account. For example, in comparing the relative contribution of TF/VIIa and factor XIa in the activation of factor IX, Bajaj[11] provided kinetic data favoring the TF/VIIa activation process (about tenfold higher), whereas based on the catalytic efficiency (K_{Cat}/K_m) and considering that the plasmatic concentration of factor VII is approximately sixfold lower than the plasma concentration of factor XI (60 nM) the activation of factor X by factor X1a would potentially predominant. This would hold unless a ternary complex(es) of VIIa/TF/1Xa comprizing two active serine protease is formed.

A third consideration is the contribution of the native vs. the activated cofactors. For example, although the procofactor of prothrombinase factor V can be converted to active cofactor (Va), by the action of either factor Xa or thrombin (IIa), the Xa-induced activation of factor V is reportedly inefficient (turnover rate 0.004 mol thrombin/mol/min) as compared to the activation by IIa (turnover rate 1200 mol thrombin/mol/min).[12-15]

Similarly, in the interaction between the components of contactase, which lead to both direct or indirect activation of factor VII and factor IX, surfaces appear to provide an effective "fine tuning" amplification mechanism improving not only the catalytic activity[15] but also modulating various defense systems for maintaining the hemostatic balance.

B. BIOINACTIVATION PROPERTIES OF SERPINS

Although release of prothrombin activation peptides and the formation of fibrin to repair the damaged vascular wall may be sufficient to regulate further activation of the blood coagulation process, the multistep expression of the coagulation process *in vivo* is nevertheless influenced in the intermediate stages by the presence of a range of protease inhibitors specifically acting at different levels of the propagation of the coagulation process.[16] The majority of these inhibitors, referred to as "serpins", are broad spectrum serine-protease inhibitors.

The properties of the six major proteinase inhibitors together with the two more specific inhibitors of factor VIIa (extrinsic pathway inhibitor — EPI)[17] and activated protein C (APC) are grouped in Table 1. The EPI is currently called a tissue factor pathway inhibition (TFPI). In the presence of heparin, however, the reaction rates of AT III increases by four orders of magnitude with the rate of inactivation of thrombin 1.7×10^9 mol/min. The inactivation rate of factors Xa and IXa, the two most important enzymes of the intrinsic pathway, is also enhanced by one order of magnitude in the presence of heparin.

It is noteworthy that factor VIIa when bound to thromboplastin escapes from the inhibition by AT III. Similarly, thrombin bound to thrombomodulin

TABLE 1
Plasma Serine Proteinase Inhibitors

Target Enzymes	Enzyme inhibitors							
	AT III	Hep CII	C_1E	α_1AT	α_2M	α_2AP	PCI	EPI
FIIa	+	+	−	+	+	+	+	−
FVIIa/TF	?	−	−	−	−	−	−	+
FIXa	+	−	−	−	−	−	−	−
FXa	+	+	−	+	+	+	+	+
FXIa	+	−	+	+	−	+	+	−
FXIIa	+	−	+	−	−	+	−	−
kk	+	−	+	−	+	−	+	−
APC	−	−	+	+	−	+	+	−
TPA	−	−	−	−	−	−	+	−
Plasmin	+	−	+	−	+	+	−	−

Note: The main inhibitors of 10 major serine proteases with their neutralizing capacity for several enzymes. A slight variation in the concentration or structure produces gross haemorrhagic or thrombotic events. Clinical evidence, however, suggests that major thrombotic risk is mainly present when AT III, or proteins C and S are low or abnormal.

The most common inhibitor of activated vitamin K-dependent proteins is antithrombin III (AT III) which circulates with a concentration of 0.2 mg/ml. Almost all active procoagulant enzymes of the clotting process (XIIa, XIa, 1Xa, Xa, and IIa) are inhibited by AT III. It should be noted that AT III by itself is a poor inhibitor of the activated factors, having a second order rate constant of 4×10^5 mol/min for factor Xa or thrombin and 3×10^4 mol/min for IXa requiring approximately 2 h for effective neutralization of the enzymes. ATIII = antithrombin III; HepCII = heparin cofactor II; C_1E = C_1 esterase; α_1AT = α_1 antitrypsin; α_2M = α_2 macroglobulin; PCI = protein C inhibitor; EPI = extrinsic pathway inhibitor (also called time factor pathway inhibitor, TFPI or lipoprotein associated coagulation inhibitor, LAC1); FIIa = thrombin; FVIIa/TF = factor VIIa/tissue factor; KK = kallikrein; APC = activated protein C; TPA = tissue plasminogen activator.

is protected from the inhibitory effect of AT III. Furthermore, the circulating half-life of functionally active forms of serine proteases is determined by the rate of formation of the enzyme-inhibitor complexes, the concentration of each inhibitor, and their structural fitness. The binding strength is characterized by the *association* constant of the enzyme and the inhibitor, ranging from 10^7 to 10^{13} mol/min. This is several orders of magnitude higher than the *activation* constant of serine proteases of the coagulation process for their relevant substrates. In spite of the fact that there are large excesses of effective proteinase inhibitors in the blood, the clotting process still takes place. One explanation for this anomaly is that the reactions of the clotting process take place with greater probability on the surface of platelets. It is documented[16] that when factors X1a, 1Xa, and Xa are on the platelet surface they are protected from the inhibitory effect of AT III, possibly by steric hindrance and/or an altered kinetic constant.

It should be noted, that normal hemostasis is governed by a series of interrelated mechanisms involving humoral, cellular, and biochemical components of platelets, fibrinolytic and other defense systems, all having specific roles in hemostasis. The precise mode of action of these important regulatory processes is outside the scope of the present discussion but it should be noted that inhibitors of one system (i.e., tissue plasminogen activator inhibitor, TPA-I) can have a potent influence on the activity of another process. Similarly, the release of some components from platelets (such as Pf4) can contribute to the *in vivo* protection by neutralizing the small amount of circulating heparin in plasma, rendering it possible for the clotting process to take place at a faster rate at the injury site. Of course the abilities of the vascular endothelial cells and the liver to rapidly clear from circulation the activated clotting factors and/or their intermediates, also are of significant importance in the regulatory mechanism.

Finally it is now well established that patients with either inherited deficiencies or abnormalities of the major inhibitors are at risk for thrombosis. For example, the total prevalence for inherited thrombosis due to AT-III deficiency is higher (1 in 75,000) than that of congenital defects associated with a bleeding disorder (1 in 200,000). This suggests that AT III has a particular role in the pathophysiological mechanism of hemostasis and that slight diminution in its concentration (i.e., below 80% of reference plasma) might produce an abnormal hemostatic event.

C. BIOATTENUATION COMPONENTS

Recently a new regulatory pathway of anticoagulation was rediscovered, where protein C and its cofactor protein S have been shown to play pivotal roles in maintaining the hemostatic balance (Figure 3). The protein C bioattenuation process is also surface dependent, with the surface contributing not only to the catalytic efficiency of the anticoagulation process by increasing the reaction rate between the triggering enzyme complex (thrombin-thrombomodulin), but also protecting thrombin from the inhibition by AT III and other nonspecific inhibitors. In view of the nature of the membrane-associated activity in the bioattenuation pathway, a slight disturbance in the protein C can upset the hemostatic balance, predisposing to thrombotic events often with fatal consequence.

Like the procoagulant MAEC, the protein C anticoagulant MAEC also consists of four well-characterized subcomponents for optimal efficiency. These include: thrombin in complex with thrombomodulin as the major activator (enzyme); protein S on the surface of platelets secreted from endothelium as an essential cofactor; calcium ions as a ligand binder; and protein C as the substrate. The generated APC then proteolytically inactivates factors VIIIa and Va, the two most important cofactors of tenase and prothrombinase, hence bringing the bioamplification process to a halt. The APC activity is regulated, in turn, by two major serine-protease inhibitors (PCI and α-1-antitrypsin) by formation of 1:1 enzyme-inhibitor complexes. APC is also inhibited by C_1 esterase and α-2 antiplasmin as indicated in Table 1. The halflife of APC is very short (about 15 min).

It has been suggested that inflammation reduces the effectiveness of the anticoagulant pathway in several ways. One way is by increasing the level of C4b binding protein (C4bBp), which neutralizes the functional activity of protein S. Inflammation also reduces endothelium thrombomodulin expression, hence providing a link between mediators of both inflammation and coagulation processes.

III. NEW APPROACHES TO THE ASSESSMENT OF HYPERCOAGULABILITY

There has been considerable difficulty in establishing, with certainty, markers which enable clinicians to detect activation of the coagulation process while at the same time discriminating between normal physiological variations. Some of the observed variations seem to be more related to heterogeneity in both patient and normal population groups, rather than to the specificity of the molecular markers. In fact, the recent improvement in the precision of newer assays appear not to be associated with improved detection of hypercoagulability.

Despite the above problems, the newer assays such as measurement of activation fragments of IXa, Xa, and F1 + 2 together with protease/protease inhibitor complexes have provided a clearer biochemical definition of hypercoagulability. The full diagnostic potential of these assays however can only be established when more carefully controlled clinical studies have been carried out, e.g., by comparing different groups of patients with similar symptoms and translation of this information into improved strategies of diagnosis and treatment as well as evaluating the prevalence, onset, and time course of hypercoagulability.

A. ESSENTIAL REQUIREMENTS OF MOLECULAR MARKERS
The key requirements of any useful molecular marker are:

1.   Its level should not be artifactually altered (i.e., by either venepuncture or processing and storage prior to assay). This problem is particularly acute when assays are subjected to more general usage than in the expert laboratory during their development.

2.   Its rate of clearance from circulation should be neither too fast nor too slow. The rate of clearance is often related to molecular size of the marker. The lower the molecular size of the marker, the faster it clears from the circulation and it, therefore, may not reflect the true level of activation. On the other hand, the high molecular-weight markers are cleared more slowly and may reflect a cumulative effect of the activation of the coagulation process. Fibrinopeptide A (FPA), the marker of

thrombin generation (which is known to be extremely sensitive to artifacts from venepuncture and to inadequate handling of samples before testing) is a very good example of a marker with a short halflife; it clears within 3 min. In contrast, the D-dimer or fibrin fragment E, which persist beyond 8 h, limits its usefulness as a marker to certain special cases only.

3.   Its suitability with reference to the changes in molecular forms, the extent of activation, and temporal position of the marker in the activation process are key. For example, some markers such as factor Xa bind to other components of plasma such as phospholipid and circulate for a longer period because the phospholipids protect the enzyme from the effect of various inhibitors.

4.   Its assay should be both sensitive and specific. Sensitivity is related to the lower limit of detection required for a positive diagnosis (compared to a control group), whereas specificity is related to the ability of the marker to distinguish patients of risk (i.e., the percentage of negative diagnoses should be low). The markers of early proteolytic events usually provide more appropriate information than those of later events. For example, to evaluate thrombin activity several assays have been designed which are either based on the direct determination of thrombin (by synthetic peptides[18] or the release of FPA[19]) or based on the indirect quantitation of the soluble fibrin generated in plasma (using precipitation techniques with either protamine or ethanol followed by N-terminal analysis or gel filtration[20]).

Recently, methods have been designed based either on the ability of soluble fibrin to potentiate tissue plasminogen activator (T-PA)[21] or to use a monoclonal antibody against a synthetically manufactured hexapeptide (Gly-Pro-Arg-Val-Val-Glu) which corresponds to the N-terminal of the alpha chains of fibrin.[22-24] In clinical studies, however, because of the multifunctional activities of thrombin the above markers are only used in conjunction with each other including molecular markers of the platelet release reaction[25-30] such as β-thromboglobulin and platelet factor 4.

Unfortunately, both of the above platelet-released markers are sensitive to collection and processing artifacts which limit their usefulness. One area in which the measurement of FPA and Pf4 levels has been shown to be useful is the objective monitoring of heparin during extracorporeal circulation.[31-34] The platelet release markers currently measured in conjunction with FPA had other activation peptides of vitamin K-clotting peptide proteins, such as factor IX, factor X, and prothrombin activation peptides.

B. ACTIVATION PEPTIDES OF PROTHROMBIN AND HYPERCOAGULABILITY

The cleavage of prothrombin by tenase complexes is known to be associated[35] with the release of an activation peptide (fragment 1 + 2 [F1 + 2]) by two different pathways leading either to the formation of an intermediate zymogen, prethrombin 2 (Pr2), or a meizothrombin, another intermediate product of the reaction which is capable of converting fibrinogen to fibrin, but, with a reduced catalytic efficiency as compared to thrombin. Meizothrombin, is subsequently converted to thrombin, releasing F1 + 2 in a second stage.

Immunoassays for the measurement of F1 + 2 and Pr2 as well as thrombin-antithrombin (TAT) have been developed and applied to normal and patient populations in various pathophysiological states.[36-40] More recently protein C, and factors 1X and X peptides have been used in conjunction with F1 + 2 to discriminate the abnormality in the protein C, extrinsic (VIIa) and intrinsic contact pathways, but their usage is still limited to specialized laboratories. These areas of molecular-marker applications are covered by Bauer et al.[41-44] Briefly, the levels of F1 + 2 and Pr2 in a normal population have been found to be 1.97 to 97 nM and 0.184 to 0.8 nM, respectively.[41] Furthermore, elevated F1 + 2, greater or equal to 2.9 nM have been shown in patients with disseminated intravascular coagulation (DIC), leukemia and deep venous thrombosis (DVT).[41,44] For a better characterization of primary and secondary hypercoagulability the levels of F1 + 2 and Pr2 should be evaluated in conjunction with TAT, FPA, and other activation peptides.

C. ACTIVATION PEPTIDE OF PROTEIN C AND HYPERCOAGULABLE STATES

Once thrombin has been released from prothombinase it is able to act on various substrates, such as fibrinogen, factors VIII and V, factor XIII and protein C, etc., before becoming inhibited by its physiological inhibitor AT III to form irreversible complexes of TAT or modified AT III (MAT).

The anticoagulant effect due to protein C activation is only initiated by removal of a decapeptide from the N-terminal end of the heavy chain of protein C.[40] A radioimmunoassay for the protein C activation peptide, which effectively measures the activity of the thrombin-thrombomodulin complex has been developed. The levels of these peptides in the normal population have been reported to be 6.47 ± 2.39 pmol.[40]

In contrast to secondary hypercoagulable states where elevated factor levels or their increased activation may account for a higher overall procoagulant activity, primary hypercoagulation is associated with abnormally low functional activities of two vitamin K-dependent proteins, protein C and protein S.[41] In these patients, hypercoagulability is therefore due to an inbalance between the coagulation process (involving tenase and prothrombinase), the anticoagulant process (protein C-ase/protein Sase) and antithrombin abnormality, leading to the same outcome through different mechanisms.

Bauer et al.[41,42,45] using 3 important markers of terminal outcome (F1 + 2, FPA, and protein peptide (PCP) in asymptomatic individuals with congenital deficiency of protein C found that there was no significant correlation between

F1 + 2 and PCP. Comparative analysis of the same group of patients but receiving warfarin anticoagulation therapy showed a marked suppression of F1 + 2 levels (which reflected in the PT ratio), whereas FPA and PCP were not significantly different from the levels of these markers in the stable anticoagulant. Based on similar findings it is indicated that F1 + 2 is the most appropriate marker for determining the minimum dose of warfarin as prophylaxis against DVT.[45,46]

Another potential marker of hypercoagulability, such as that found in the early stage of oral anticoagulation is the change in the activity state of protein C and the formation of intermediate complexes, as identified by crossed immunoelectrophoresis.[47,48] These procedures, however, require a stringent standardization program if they are to become useful diagnostic procedures in a routine laboratory.

IV. FUTURE TRENDS

It is well known that hypercoagulability leading to thrombotic complications constitutes a significant clinical problem in many pathophysiological states. On the other hand, despite the well-established etiological factors, the prevalence of hypercoagulability in the general population is still confused as is the clinical management with anticoagulants with respect to both type and duration of treatment.

The clinical conditions or risk factors often associated with hypercoagulability leading to thrombotic complications include polycythemia (benign or malignant), thrombocytosis, lupus anticoagulant, anticardiolipin antibodies, elevated T-PA inhibitor type I, elevated level factor VII, (and possibly other procoagulant vitamin K-dependent proteins), and acquired congenital deficiencies of AT III, protein C, protein S, heparin cofactor II, plasminogen, T-PA, fibrinogen, lipoprotein, and endothelial-cell abnormalities.

Despite these associations the relative prevalence of each of these acquired or hereditary defects and disorders in the general population still remains unknown. Based on the results of the management in 100 consecutive patients, Bick et al.[49] recently concluded that if careful clinical assessment (complete history, review of symptoms, and physical examination) is combined with an astute laboratory assessment (complete blood count, routine biochemistry as well as routine and less common tests for blood protein defects associated with hypercoagulability and thrombophilia) then the etiology of deep vein thrombosis can be clearly defined in about 80% of patients.

Using this combined approach it appeared that 47% of patients have a plasma defect that is known to be associated with hypercoagulability. The plasma defects were more commonly acquired than congenital and their prevalences in descending order of probability were: anticardiolipin antibodies, AT III deficiency, protein S deficiency, lupus anticoagulant protein C deficiency, and T-PA deficiency. In the future assays for these defects will become an essential part of the initial hypercoagulability screening panel in patients presenting with clinically unexplained venous thrombosis. Other tests consisting of functional fibrinogen, plasminogen, heparin cofactor II, and PA1-I, the nature of elevated factor VII and factor XII as well as changes in the activation states of pro- and anticoagulant proteins should only be considered as a secondary panel of tests.

The underlying mechanisms involved in triggering a prethrombotic state remains a major scientific challenge requiring a broad spectrum of assays for a better characterization and assessment of the activation states of each components involved.[50-52] In this respect, there has been a resurgence of interest to characterize the activity state in relation to hypercoagulability using both specific- and broad-spectrum molecular markers. These markers are currently being applied to various pathophysiological activation of hemostasis with promising results.[49-53] More development work is required to ascertain the involvement of the endothelial cells in each case. The issue of cause or effect in hypercoagulability remains an unresolved problem and has been addressed in recent publications (see References 54–63).

ACKNOWLEDGMENTS

The author wishes to express his sincere thanks to Usha Mistray and to Vivian Sproule for their assistance in typing this manuscript.

REFERENCES

1. **Davie, E. W. and Fujikawa, K.,** Basic mechanisms in blood coagulation, *Annu. Rev. Biochem.,* 44, 799, 1975.
2. **Ogston, D. and Bennett, B.,** *Haemostasis; Biochemistry, physiology and pathology,* John Wiley & Sons, London, 1977.
3. **Davie, E. W., Fujikawa, K., Kurachi, K., and Kisiel, W.,** The role of serine proteases in the blood coagulation cascade, *Adv. Enzymol.,* 48, 277, 1979.
4. **Elodi, S. and Elodi, P.,** Surface-governed molecular regulation of blood coagulation, *Molec. Aspects Med.,* 16, 291, 1983.
5. **Mann, K. G.,** Membrane-bound enzyme complexes in blood coagulation, in *Progress in Hemostasis and Thrombosis,* Spaet, T. H., Ed., Grune & Stratton, Orlando, FL, 1984.
6. **Mann, K. G., Tracy, P. B., Krishnaswamy, S. Jenny, R. J., Odegaard, B. H., and Nesheim, M. F.,** Platelet and coagulation, in *Thrombosis and Haemostasis,* Verstraete, M., Vermylen, J., Lijnen, R., and Arnout, T., Eds., Leuven University Press, Belgium, 1987, 505.
7. **Rosing, J., Tans, G., and Govers, R.,** The role of phospholipids and factor Va in the prothrombinase complex, *J. Biol. Chem.,* 255, 274, 1980.
8. **Nesheim, M. E., Tracy, R. P., and Mann, K. G.,** "Clotspeed", A computer simulation of the functional properties of prothrombinase, *J. Biol. Chem.,* 259, 1447, 1984.
9. **Griep, M. A., Fujikawa, K., and Nelsest ven, G. L.,** Binding and activation properties of human FXII, prekallikrein and derived peptides with lipid vesicles, *Biochemistry,* 24, 4124, 1985.

10. **Shimada, T., Sugo, T., Kato, H. Y., Yoshida, K., and Iwanaga, S.,** Activation of factor XII and prekallikrein with polysaccharide surfaces and sulphatides: comparison with Kaolin-mediated activation, *J. Biochem.,* 97, 429, 1985.

11. **Bajaj, S. P.,** Co-operative Ca^{++} binding to human factor X1a. Effect of Ca^{++} on the kinetic parameters of the activation of FIX by factor X1a, *J. Biol. Chem.,* 257, 4127, 1982.

12. **Soons, H., Janssen-Clasessen, T., Hemker, C., and Tans, G.,** The effect of the platelets in the activation of factor 1X, *Blood,* 68, 140, 1986.

13. **Silverberg, S. A., Nemerson, Y., and Zur, M.,** Kinetics of the activation of bovine coagulation factor X by components of the extrinsic pathway, *J. Biol. Chem.,* 252, 8481, 1977.

14. **Foster, V. W., Nesheim, M. E., and Mann, K. G.,** The factor Xa catalysed activation of factor V, *J. Biol. Chem.,* 258, 13,970, 1983.

15. **Berrettini, M., Lamoule, B., and Griffin, J. H.,** Initiation of coagulation and relationships between intrinsic and extrinsic coagulation pathways, in *Thrombosis and Haemostasis,* Verstraete, M., Vermylen, J., Lijnen, R., and Arnaut, T., Eds., Leuven University Press, Belgium, 1987, 473.

16. **Carrell, R. W., Christey, P. B., and Boswell, D. R.,** Serpins: antithrombin and other inhibitors of coagulation and fibrinolysis, in *Thrombosis and Haemostasis,* Verstraete, M., Vermylen, J., Lijnen, R., and Arnaut, T., Eds., Leuven University Press, Belgium, 1987, 1.

17. **Broze, G. J., Warren, L. A., Giard, J. J., and Miletich, J. P.,** Isolation of the lipoprotein associated coagulation inhibitor produced by Hep G_2 cells using bovine fXa affinity chromatography, *Thromb. Res.,* 48, 253, 1987.

18. **Seghatchian, M. J.,** Enzymology of thrombin: purification, characterisation, surface binding, stability, unitage and standardization, in *Thrombin,* Machovich, R., Ed., CRC Press, Boca Raton, FL, 1984, 1.

19. **Fareed, J., Bick, R. L., Squillaci, G., Walenga, J. M., Bermes, E. W., Jr.,** Molecular markers of hemostasis disorders. Implications in the diagnosis and therapeutic management of thrombotic and bleeding, *Clin. Chem.,* 29, 1641, 1983.

20. **Lane, D. A.,** Fibrinogen derivatives in plasma, *Br. J. Haematol.,* 47, 329, 1981.

21. **Wiman, B. and Ranby, M.,** Determination of soluble fibrin in plasma by a rapid and quantitative spectrophotometric assay, *Thromb. Haemostasis,* 55, 189, 1986.

22. **Scheefers-Borchel, U., Muller-Berghaus, G., Fughe, P., Eberle, R., and Heimburger, N.,** Discrimination between fibrin and fibrinogen by a monoclonal antibody against a synthetic peptide, *Proc. Natl. Acad. Sci. U.S.A.,* 82, 7091, 1985.

23. **Muller-Berghaus, G., Scheefers-Borchel, U., Fughe, P., Eberle, R., and Heimburger, N.,** Detection of fibrin in plasma by a monoclonal antibody against the aminoterminus of the alpha-chain of fibrin, *Scand. J. Clin. Lab. Invest.,* 45 (Suppl. 178), 145, 1985.

24. **Scheefers-Borchel, U. and Muller-Berghaus, G.,** Determination of soluble fibrin in plasma by a monoclonal fibrin-specific antibody, in *Fibrinogen and Its Derivatives,* Muller-Berghaus, G., Ed., Elsevier, Amsterdam, 1986, 261.

25. **Nichols, A. B., Owen, J., and Kaplan, K. L., Fibrinopeptide A,** platelet factor 4 and beta-thromboglobulin in coronary heart disease, *Blood,* 60, 650, 1982.

26. **Borok, Z., Weitz, J., Owen, J., Auerbach, M., and Nossel, H. L.,** Fibrinogen proteolysis and platelet and α-granule release in preeclampsia/eclampsia, *Blood,* 63, 525, 1984.

27. **Douglas, J. T., Lowe, G. D. O., Forges, C. D., and Prentice, C. R. M.,** Plasma fibrinopeptide A and beta-thromboglobulin in patients with chest pain, *Thromb. and Haemostasis,* 50, 541, 1983.

28. **Ireland, H., Lane, D. A., Wolff, S., and Foadi, M.,** In vivo platelet release in myeloproliferative disorders, *Thromb. Haemostasis,* 48, 41, 1982.

29. **Johnson, H., Orinius, E., and Paul, C.,** 1979 Fibrinopeptide A (FPA) in patients with acute myocardial infarction, *Thromb. Res.,* 16, 255, 1979.
30. **Cocheri, S., Mannucci, P. M., and Palareti, G.,** Significance of plasma fibrinopeptide A and high molecular weight fibrinogen in patients with liver cirrhosis, *Br. J. Haematol.,* 52, 503, 1982.
31. **Ireland, H., Lane, D. A., and Curtis, J. R.,** Objective assessment of heparin requirements for haemodialysis in humans, *J. Lab. Clin. Med.,* 103, 643, 1984.
32. **Ireland, H., Lane, D. A., Flynn, A., Anastassiades, E., and Curtis, J. R.,** The anticoagulant effect of heparinoid Org 10172 during haemodialysis: an objective assessment, *Thromb. Haemostasis,* 55, 271, 1986.
33. **Lane, D. A., Ireland, H., Flynn, A., Anastassiades, E., and Curtis, J. R.,** Haemodialysis with low MW heparin: dosage requirements for the elimination of extracorporeal fibrin formation, *Nephrol. Dialys. Transplant.,* 1, 179, 1986.
34. **Ireland, H., Lane, D. A., Flynn, A., Pegrum, A. C., and Curtis, J. R.,** Low molecular weight heparin in haemodialysis for chronic renal failure: dose finding study of CY222, *Thromb. Haemostasis,* 59: 240 1988
35. **Rosing, J. and Tans, G.,** Meizothrombin a major product of factor Xa-catalyzed prothrombin activation, *Thromb. Haemostasis,* 60, 355, 1988.
36. **Lau, H. K., Rosenberg, J. S., Beeler, D. L., and Rosenberg, R. D.,** The isolation and characterization of a specific antibody population directed against the thrombin-antithrombin complex, *J. Biol. Chem.,* 254, 8751, 1979.
37. **Conway, E. M., Lau, H. K. F., Bauer, K. A., and Rosenberg, R. D.,** Development of a radioimmunoassay for quantitating prethrombin 2 in human plasma, *J. Lab. Clin. Med.,* 110, 567, 1987.
38. **Lau, H. K. and Rosenberg, R. D.,** The isolation and characterization of a specific antibody directed against the thrombin-antithrombin complex, *J. Biol. Chem.,* 255, 5885, 1980.
39. **Pelzer, H., Schwarz, A., and Heimburger, N.,** Determination of human thrombin-antithrombin III complex in plasma with an enzyme-linked immunosorbent assay, *Thromb. Haemostasis,* 59, 101, 1988.
40. **Esmon, C. T.,** Protein C: biochemistry, physiology and clinical implications, *Blood,* 62, 1155, 1983.
41. **Bauer, K. A., Kass, B. L., Beeler, D. L., and Rosenberg, R. D.,** Detection of protein C activation in humans, *Blood,* 74, 2033, 1984.
42. **Bauer, K. A. and Rosenberg, R. D.,** The pathophysiology of the prethrombotic state in humans: insights gained from studies using markers of hemostatic activation, *Blood,* 70, 343, 1987.
43. **Bauer, K. A., Goodman, T. L., Kass, B. L., and Rosenberg, R. D.,** Asymptomatic patients with congenital antithrombin deficiency, *J. Clin. Invest.,* 76, 826, 1985.
44. **Bauer, K. A., Broekmans, A. W., and Bertina, R. M. et al.,** Hemostatic enzyme generation in the blood of patients with hereditary protein C deficiency, *Blood,* 71, 1418, 1988.
45. **Conway, E. M., Bauer, K. A., Barzegar, S., and Rosenberg, R. D.,** Suppression of hemostatic system activation by oral anticoagulants in the blood of patients with thrombotic diatheses, *J. Clin. Invest.,* 80, 1535, 1987.
46. **Boisclair, M. D., Ireland, H., and Lane, D. A.,** Assessment of hypercoagulable states by measurement of activation, fragments and peptides, *Blood Rev.,* 4, 25, 1990.
47. **Seghatchian, M. J. and Stirling, Y.,** A comparative analysis of protein C in normal and warfarinized plasmas, *Thromb. Haemostasis,* 54, 143, 1985.
48. **Stirling, Y. and Seghatchian, M. J.,** Further studies on the heterogeneity of protein C in normal and warfarinized plasmas, evaluated by crossed immunoelectropheresis, *Br. J. Haematol.,* 71 (Suppl. 1), 34, 1989.

49. **Bick, R. L., Jacway, J., and Baker, W. F.**, Deep vein thrombosis: prevalence of etiologic factors and results of management in 100 consecutive patients, *Seminars in Thromb. Haemostasis,* 18, 269, 1992.
50. **Fareed, J., Baker, W. H., Walenga, J. M., and Messmore, H. L.**, Molecular markers of pathophysiological activation of haemostasis: current perspective and future trends, in *Thrombosis and Hemorrhagic Diseases,* Ultin, O. N. and Vinazzer, H., Eds., Gozlem, Turkey, 1986, 83.
51. **Vinazzer, H.**, The alteration of AT III, protein C, and other natural inhibitors in eiterosclerosis and thromboembolism, in *Thrombosis Hemorrhagic and Diseases,* Ultin, O.N. and Vinazzer, H., Eds., Gozlom, Turkey, 1986, 6.
52. **Schafer, A. I.**, The hypercoagulable states, *Ann. Intern. Med.,* 102, 814, 1985.
53. **Lechner, K.**, Lupus anticoagulants and thrombosis, in *Thrombosis and Haemostasis,* Verstraete, M., Vermylens, Lijnen, R., and Arnout, J., Eds., Leuven University Press, Belgium, 525, 1987.
54. **Mitropoulos, K. A., Martin, J. C., Reeves, B., and Esnouf, M. P.**, The activation of the contact phase of coagulation by physiologic surfaces in plasma: the effect of large negatively charged liposomal vesicles, *Blood,* 73, 1525–1533. 1989.
55. **Miller, G. J., Cruickshank, J. K., Ellis, L. J., Thompson, R. L., Wilkes, H. C., Stirling, Y., Mitropoulos, K. A., Allison, J. V., Fox, T. E., and Walker, A. O.**, Fat consumption and factor VII coagulant activity in middle-aged men. An association between a dietary and thrombogenic coronary risk factor, *Atherosclerosis,* 78, 19–24, 1989.
56. **Meade, T. W., Dyer, S., Howarth, D. J., Imeson, J. D., and Stirling, Y.**, Antithrombin III and procoagulant activity: sex diferences and effects of the menopause, *Br. J. Haematol.,* 74, 77–81, 1990.
57. **Mitropoulos, K. A., Martin, J. C., Burgess, A. I., Esnouf, M. P., Stirling, Y., and Howarth, D. J.**, The increased rate of activation of factor XII in late pregnancy can contribute to the increased reactivity of factor VII, *Thromb. Res.,* 63, 349–355, 1990.
58. **Miller, G. J., Wilkes, H. C., Meade, T. W., Bauer, K. A., Barzegar, S., and Rosenberg, R. D.**, Haemostatic changes that constitute the hypercoagulable state, *Lancet,* 338, 1079, 1991.
59. **Meade, T. W., Miller, G. J., and Rosenberg, R. D.**, Characteristics associated with the risk of arterial thrombosis and the prethrombotic state, in *Thrombosis in Cardiovascular Disorders,* Fuster, V. and Verstraete, M., Eds., W.B. Saunders Co., 1992, 79–97.
60. **Esnouf, M. P., Mitropoulos, K. A., and Burgess, A. I.**, The relation of hyperlipidaemia to the hypercoagulable state, In *Thrombosis and Update,* Serneri, G. N. N., Gensini, G. F., Abbate, R., and Pisco, D., Scientific Press, 1992, 715–729.
61. **Miller, G. J. and Meade, T. W.**, Hypercoagulability, in *Thrombosis Embolism and Bleeding,* Butchart, E. G., Bodnar, E., Eds., ICR Publishers, 1992, 81–92.
62. **Meade, T. W.**, Atheroma and thrombosis in cardiovascular disease: separate or complementary? in *Coronary Heart Disease Epidemiology.,* Marmot, M. and Elliott, P., Oxford University Press, 1992, 287–297.
63. **Meade, T. W.**, Low intensity oral anticoagulation, in *Thrombosis and its Management,* Poller, L. and Thompson, J. M., Eds., Churchill Livingstone, 1992, 84–97.

Chapter 2

THE EXPLOITATION OF THE ELECTROCHEMICAL PROPERTIES OF K VITAMINS FOR THEIR SENSITIVE MEASUREMENT IN TISSUES

John Patrick Hart

TABLE OF CONTENTS

I. INTRODUCTION

In recent years electrochemical techniques of analysis have advanced considerably when compared to classical direct current (DC) polarography. Although the poor detection limit (about 0.1 mM) of the traditional DC polarographic technique has severely limited its use as an analytical method of measurement, a variety of polarographic/voltammetric waveforms have now been introduced which can discriminate the unwanted capacitative current from the required faradaic current, e.g., normal pulse and differential pulse waveforms; such methods allow submicromolar concentrations to be determined. Stripping voltammetry, which involves preconcentration of the analyte at the working electrode prior to the voltammetric measurement, has extended the limits of detection for some species to the subnanomolar level. Perhaps one of the most powerful analytical techniques to emerge in recent years has been high-performance liquid chromatography (HPLC) with electrochemical detection (HPLC-ECD). This technique has been applied to the determination of a number of biologically important compounds and allowed, in some instances, picomolar concentrations to be determined in body fluids. The general principles of polarographic, voltammetric, and HPLC-ECD techniques, especially as they pertain to the analysis of compounds of biological significance have recently been reviewed[1-6] and will not be discussed further here.

There is a perceived and increasing need for sensitive, selective, and reliable methods for the analysis of K vitamins and their derivatives. Such analyses are assuming greater importance, for example, in the nutritional field as well as in clinical chemistry and research.[7,8] However, these determinations may present difficult analytical problems for a variety of reasons. For example, the assay of K vitamins in blood may be subject to interferences from both structurally similar vitamers or from the presence of other naturally occurring compounds. In addition, the low endogenous levels put considerable constraints on both the sensitivity and selectivity of potential analytical procedures.[9]

Electroanalytical techniques have been used to overcome some of the analytical problems involved in measuring the K vitamins and it is one of the intentions in this chapter to describe examples where such methods have been applied. The chapter consists of two main sections. The first part describes the electrochemical behavior of the K vitamins; the second discusses the exploitation of this behavior for the analysis of these compounds.

II. ELECTROCHEMICAL BEHAVIOR OF K VITAMINS

Vitamin K_1 (II, phylloquinone), K_2 (III, menaquinone group) and K_3 (I, menadione) all contain the electroactive 1,4-naphthoquinone moiety (Figure 1) and therefore the electrochemical behavior of these substances is quite similar.

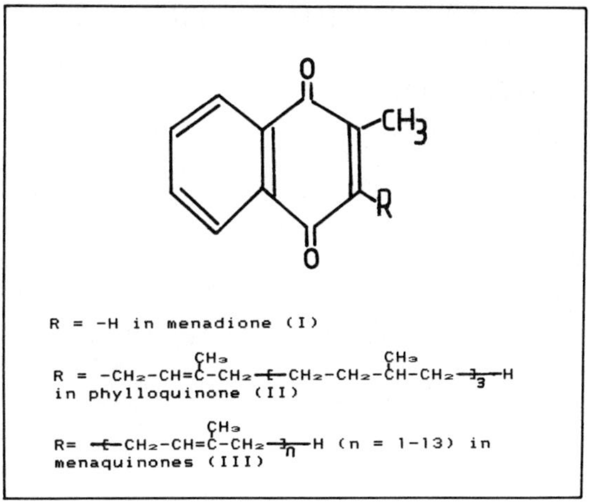

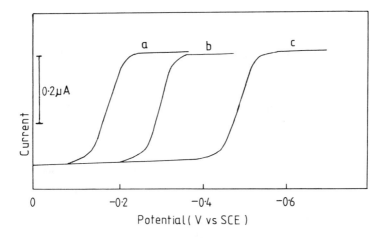

FIGURE 1. Structural formulas of the major forms of vitamin K.

FIGURE 2. Sampled DC polarograms of phylloquinone dissolved in Britton-Robinson buffers containing 90% ethanol; the apparent pH values were: (a) 4.8; (b) 6.7; (c) 9.8.

This author[10] has investigated the electrochemical reduction of phylloquinone over a wide pH range using sampled DC polarography; the supporting electrolytes consisted of 0.1 M sulfuric acid and Britton-Robinson buffers pH 2 to 11 containing 90% ethanol. The concentration of the vitamin was 1.09 × 10⁻⁴ M. Figure 2 shows several typical polarograms obtained for the vitamin. As may be seen, under these conditions one well-defined pH-dependent wave was obtained which became more negative with increasing pH.

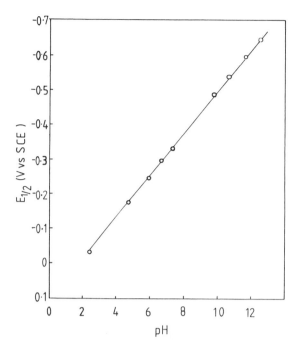

FIGURE 3.   Variation of $E_{1/2}$ with apparent pH for phylloquinone.

The number of electrons (n) transferred in the reduction, throughout the pH range studied, was determined from the equation[11]

$$n = \frac{0.0564}{E_{1/4} - E_{3/4}} \tag{1}$$

where $E_{3/4}$ and $E_{1/4}$ are the potentials measured at three quarters and one quarter of the limiting diffusion current value; the latter is usually denoted as i_d and is measured from the foot of the wave to the plateau. The value of n for the vitamin was constant and calculated to be 2 electrons.

The number of protons (m) involved in the reduction process was found from the equation[3]

$$dE_{1/2}/dpH = 0.059 \, m/n \tag{2}$$

where $E_{1/2}$ is the potential measured at half the i_d value. The value of $dE_{1/2}/dpH$ was determined from the slope of the $E_{1/2}$ vs. pH plot (Figure 3) and was found to be 0.060 mV/pH unit. Therefore, it could be calculated that 2 protons were consumed in the reduction.

Vire and Patriarche[12,13] have also investigated the electrochemical behavior of phylloquinone (II) by DC, alternating current (AC) and differential pulse polarography (DPP) using 85% methanolic acetate buffers. One well-defined cathodic peak or wave was obtained in acid or neutral solutions when the vitamin concentration was 5×10^{-4} M. These electrochemical signals were found to shift to more negative potentials when the pH was increased, but there was a change in the slope of the $E_{1/2}$ vs. pH plot at about pH 7. In addition, when the pH of the supporting electrolyte was adjusted to a value of 9.6, both AC and DP polarograms exhibited two peaks which the authors suggested may have resulted from the adsorption of phylloquinone at the surface of the mercury electrode. Further investigations of this adsorption phenomenon were carried out by Hart and Catterall[14] using cyclic voltammetry at a hanging mercury drop electrode (HMDE). To do this phylloquinone was solubilized at concentrations of 4 μM in acetate buffers (pH 6.0) containing either ethanol or methanol at concentrations of either 70 or 90% and the voltammogram obtained at scan rates of between 10 and 100 mV/s. The cyclic voltammograms obtained on these four solutions using a scan rate of 100 mV/s is shown in Figure 4. The presence of adsorption at the electrode is clearly indicated by the triangular symmetry of the peaks obtained when the vitamin was dissolved in 70% alcoholic solutions. The magnitude of the peak currents indicated that adsorption was greatest in the 70% methanolic solution. It should be noted that the cyclic voltammograms also indicated that the reduction was reversible and that the reduced form of the vitamin was also adsorbed. Further evidence of adsorption was obtained by plotting $i_p/cv^{1/2}$ vs. $v^{1/2}$ (where i_p is the peak current in μA, c is the vitamin concentration in mmol/l, v is the scan rate in mV/s). As shown in Figure 5, the graphs of both cathodic and anodic scans showed an increase in current function with increasing scan rate. This suggests that both the oxidized and reduced forms of the vitamin are adsorbed at the mercury electrode although the decreased slopes in solutions containing 90% methanol or ethanol suggested that this adsorption was quite weak in solutions containing high concentrations of alcohols.

The investigations discussed above strongly suggest that phylloquinone undergoes a reversible 2 e^-, 2 H^+ reduction to produce the corresponding hydroquinone (Figure 6). In addition, the vitamin has also been shown to undergo adsorption at the mercury electrode. The results reported[12,14] suggest that the extent of adsorption is dependent on several factors: these include the concentration and type of alcohol used in the supporting electrolyte and the pH of the buffer.

The electrochemical behavior of a vitamin K_2 compound (menaquinone-4) was studied by Takamura and Hayakawa[15] using DC and AC polarography and cyclic voltammetry at a HMDE. These authors reported that only one diffusion-controlled DC polarographic wave was observed in a solution containing 10^{-4} M of the vitamin dissolved in 70% methanolic acetate buffer pH 4.8 and containing 0.2 M sodium perchlorate. The proposed mechanism of reduction of the naphthoquinone moiety was the same as that shown in

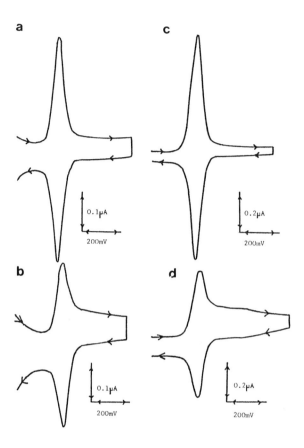

FIGURE 4. Cyclic voltammograms for acetate-buffered 4 μM phylloquinone solutions: (a) 70% ethanol; (b) 90% ethanol; (c) 70% methanol; (d) 90% methanol. Initial potential -0.1 V, scan rate 100 mV/s. (From Hart, J. P. and Catterall, A., *Anal. Chim. Acta,* 128, 245, 1981. With permission.)

Figure 7 for phylloquinone, i.e., a two-electron, two-proton reversible reduction to produce the corresponding hydroquinone. In addition, it was reported that the AC polarograms showed three cathodic peaks, two of which were associated with adsorption behavior. Further evidence of adsorption was obtained from plots of mercury drop-time vs. applied potential. These showed an inflection in the region 0 V to -0.5 V in the presence of the vitamin but this was absent in supporting electrolyte only. Conclusive evidence for adsorption was then obtained by cyclic voltammetry in similar studies to those described above for phylloquinone.[14] It was concluded that menaquinone-4 was adsorbed at mercury via the long isoprenoid side chain.

The nature of the electrochemical reduction process for menadione (vitamin K_3) has been investigated by Patriarche and Lingane[16] using DC

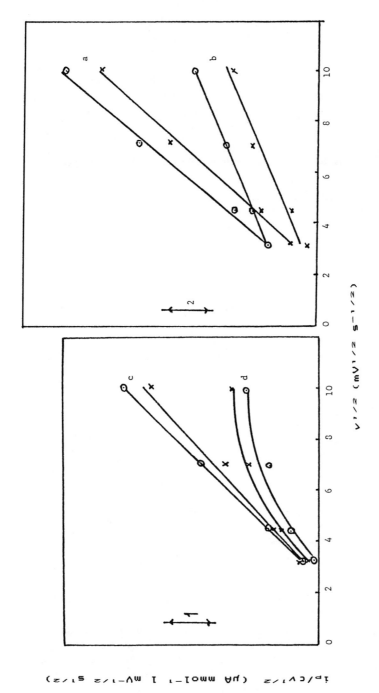

FIGURE 5. Graphs of $i_p/cv^{1/2}$ vs. $v^{1/2}$ for acetate-buffered 4 μM phylloquinone solutions; (a) 70% ethanol; (b) 90% ethanol; (c) 70% methanol; (d) 90% methanol; (○) Cathodic scan; (×) anodic scan. (From Hart, J. P. and Catterall, A., *Anal. Chim. Acta*, 128, 245, 1981. With permission.)

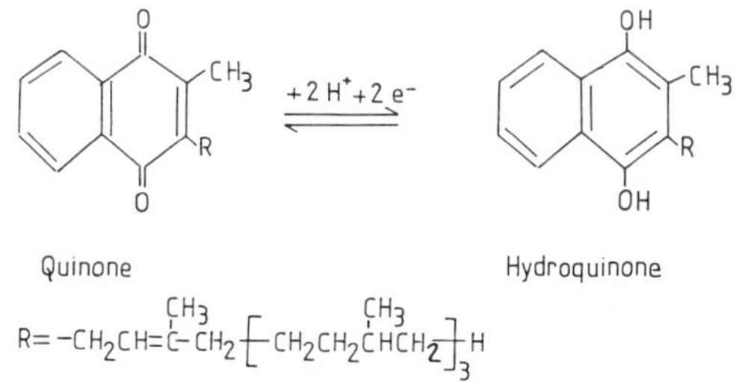

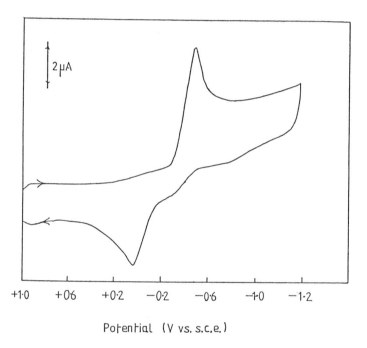

FIGURE 6. Mechanism of reduction of phylloquinone in aqueous buffers containing alcohols.

FIGURE 7. Cyclic voltammogram of 0.1 m*M* phylloquinone in methanol-0.05 *M* acetate buffer, pH 3.0 (95:5, v/v) using a planar glassy-carbon electrode. Initial potential, + 1.0 V; scan rate, 20 mV/s. (From Hart, J. P. et al., *Analyst,* 109, 477, 1984. With permission.)

polarography and cyclic voltammetry at a HMDE with supporting electrolytes of phosphate, or acetate buffers, containing 3 to 10% methanol. From Equation 1 it was calculated that 2 electrons were involved in the reduction process. The product of reduction was the corresponding hydroquinone. This process was stated to be quasi-reversible since the difference between the cathodic and anodic cyclic voltammetric peaks was greater than the theoretical value (i.e., > 59/n mV). Subsequent electrochemical studies by Vire and Patriarche[12] indicated that adsorption of menadione occurred at the mercury electrode at pH 7. However, Takamura and Hayakawa[15] carried out cyclic voltammetric studies on menadione in 70% methanolic acetate buffer, pH 4.8 and reported that the reduction was simply diffusion controlled with no indication of adsorption. Therefore, it would appear that the concentration of alcohol and pH of the buffer may play an important role in the adsorption of vitamin K_3 at the mercury surface: as discussed earlier this was also found for phylloquinone.

The electrochemical characteristics of phylloquinone and menadione have also been investigated at carbon electrodes. Hart et al.[17] carried out cyclic voltammetry on phylloquinone using a glassy carbon electrode in a supporting electrolyte containing methanol 0.05 M acetate buffer, pH 3.0 (95:5, v/v). As shown in Figure 7 one cathodic peak was obtained on the cathodic scan which is consistent with a 2 e^-, 2 H^+ reduction of the quinone to the hydroquinone; the reverse scan also showed one anodic peak which was due to the reoxidation of the vitamin back to the quinone. However, the separation between the cathodic and anodic peaks was clearly greater than 59/n mV which indicates that the process is quasi-reversible. In addition, the product but not the reactant was found to undergo adsorption at the glassy carbon electrode. In contrast, phylloquinone was reported to produce two reduction peaks using thin-layer voltammetry at a carbon electrode.[18] It was concluded that the first peak was due to a 1 e^-, 1 H^+ reduction to the semiquinone and the second to a further 1 e^-, 1 H^+ transfer producing the hydroquinone. However, in the same study the authors reported that menadione was reduced in a reversible 2 e^-, 2 H^+ reaction to the hydroquinone.

Cauquis and Marbach[19] have investigated the electrochemical reactions occurring for menadione at a platinum electrode in acetonitrile containing 0.1 M tetraethylammonium perchlorate. In neutral, nonbuffered solution, cyclic voltammetry showed two peaks on both the forward and the reverse scans. This indicated a stepwise reduction to the dianion:

$$Q \xrightarrow{\ e^-\ } Q^- \xrightarrow{\ e^-\ } Q^{2-}$$

where Q is menadione.

In the presence of water, a different mechanism was found to operate:

$$Q \xrightarrow{\ e^-\ } Q^-$$
$$\downarrow H^+$$
$$QH^{\cdot} \xrightarrow{\ e^-\ } OH^-$$

In the same investigation the authors reported that in the presence of strong acids a different mechanism occurred:

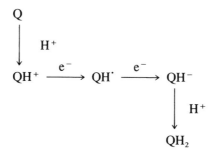

The nature of the electrochemical reduction for menadione bisulfite (IV), which is a synthetic vitamin K_3 compound, has been studied by Vire and Patriarche.[20] They postulated that the reduction mechanism was different to that for menadione due to the loss of conjugation at the 1, 2, 3, and 4 positions. The polarographic behavior of menadione bisulfite was demonstrated to be pH dependent and to be rather complex. In neutral solution (pH 7) two DC waves were reported and the mechanism of reduction was that shown in Figure 8. In strong acid solution the second wave was found to merge with the first which resulted in one wave with increased magnitude. At high pH values the polarographic behavior became even more complex due to the degradation of the compound to produce menadione by simple cleavage at the 2 position. A detailed study of the degradation of menadione bisulfite was carried out by Vire et al.[21] using DC, AC, and DP polarography. In this investigation a total of eight different polarographic signals were observed which corresponded to the reduction of eight different compounds.

The electrochemical oxidation of vitamin K_5 (V) (4-amino-2-methyl-1-naphthol hydrochloride) was investigated by Takamura and Watanabe[22] using DC and AC polarography. The DC polarogram obtained at pH 3.3 showed two well-defined anodic waves; the first was stated to be the result of oxidation to produce the corresponding quinoimine (Figure 9). The second anodic wave was apparently due to the formation of mercurous chloride which formed a deposit on the mercury electrode, the chloride being supplied through dissociation of the vitamin.

III. ELECTROANALYSIS OF K VITAMINS

A. METHODS INVOLVING POLAROGRAPHIC AND VOLTAMMETRIC TECHNIQUES

Hart and Catterall[23] have carried out detailed studies to find the optimum conditions for the determination of low levels of phylloquinone by DPP. In this investigation the effect of ionic strength, concentration of ethanol, and

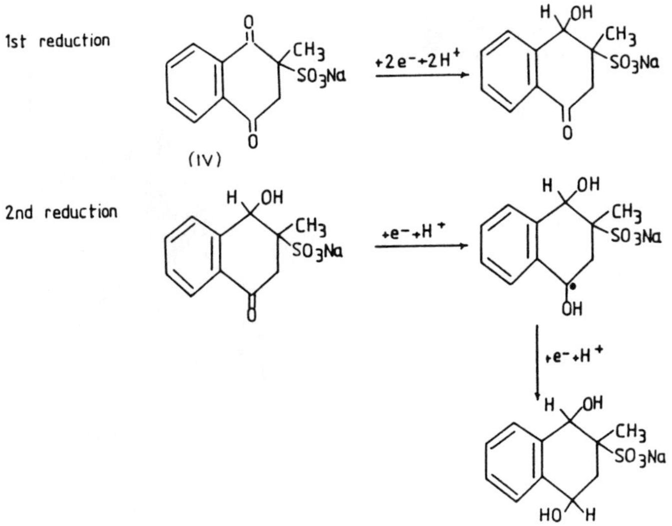

FIGURE 8. Mechanism of reduction of menadione-sodium bisulfite in neutral solution.

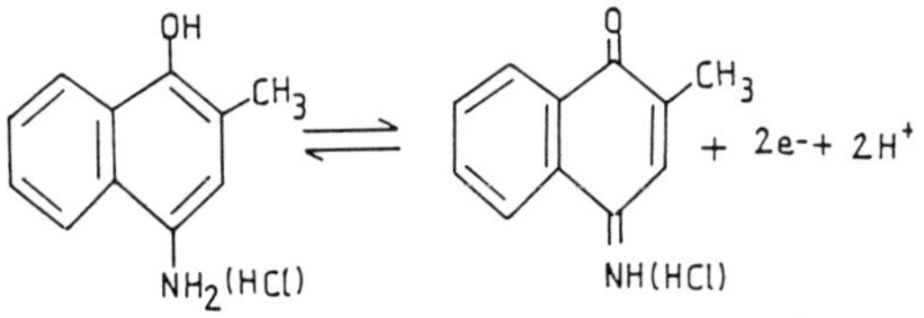

FIGURE 9. Mechanism of oxidation of vitamin K_5.

the pH of acetate buffers on the DPP peaks was examined. It was shown that the peak current measured at -0.36 V vs. the saturated calomel electrode (SCE) was proportional to the concentration of phylloquinone over the range 0.26 to 1.5 μM when the supporting electrolyte was ethanol -0.05 M acetate buffer, pH 6.0 (9:1, v/v). The same authors[24] subsequently employed this technique to follow the plasma clearance rates of phylloquinone in human subjects after an intravenous injection of 20 mg of the vitamin. For plasma measurements, the vitamin was first extracted with chloroform/methanol and DPP carried out after first dissolving the chloroform-soluble residue in the above supporting electrolyte. The polarogram exhibited a peak at -0.58 V vs. the SCE which was due to the reduction of the vitamin. The shift in potential of the peak current from that given by the pure vitamin (-0.36 V) was considered to be caused by the coextracted lipid material. However this effect on the peak potential did not interfere with the quantitative determination of the vitamin in plasma extracts and the sensitivity of the method was suitable

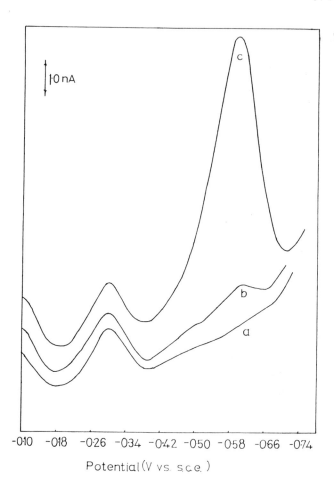

FIGURE 10. Differential pulse polarograms of: (a) control plasma (2 ml); (b) plasma (2 ml) spiked with 412 ng of phylloquinone; (c) plasma (2 ml) spiked with 6.18 μg of phylloquinone. (From Hart, J. P. et al., *Anal. Chim. Acta,* 144, 267, 1982. With permission.)

for the assay of amounts down to 200 ng/ml of plasma. There was no interference from other naturally occurring substances (Figure 10).

Other workers have also considered the possibility of using DPP for the measurement of low concentrations of phylloquinone, although they did not actually apply the technique to studies on biological matrices.[12,25]

The DPP technique was also used by this author and colleagues in some studies concerned with the analysis and the stability of menadione and its bisulfite derivative in plasma.[2] Since initial DPP studies on menadione bisulfite, dissolved in various acidic buffers (pH 0 to 5.0), revealed that the largest and best-defined signal occurred in 1-*N* sulfuric acid, this medium

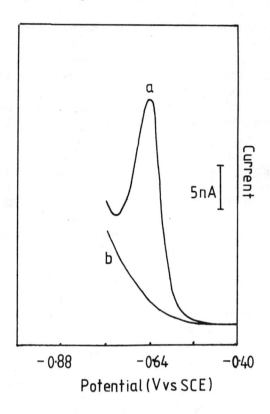

FIGURE 11. Differential pulse polarograms of: (a) menadione bisulfite in plasma per 1 *N* sulfuric acid (1:1); (b) control plasma per 1 *N* sulfuric acid (1:1).

was chosen for subsequent studies. In order to evaluate this method for plasma analysis, menadione bisulfite was spiked into a plasma sample (2.5 ml) to which 5-*N* sulfuric acid and distilled water were then added to produce a final concentration of 1-*N* sulfuric acid. To prevent foaming during deaeration, 0.1 ml of *n*-octanol was added to the solution. Under these conditions a well-defined DPP peak was obtained (Figure 11) and concentrations down to 230 ng/ml of plasma could be readily measured. Using this procedure the stability of menadione bisulfite in plasma at 37°C was examined. Samples were spiked with identical amounts of the vitamin and then DPP was carried out at timed intervals. It was shown that the polarographic current decreased rapidly and after 30 min no DPP peak could be detected. This indicated that the vitamin was being degraded to a species which was not polarographically active in the range of potentials investigated. One possibility was that menadione was being produced from menadione bisulfite through simple cleavage of the bisulfite group. This was actually shown to occur by spiking the bisulfite compound into plasma at 37°C and then performing the method of Hart et al.[24] Unfortunately, the recovery of menadione by this method of analysis was found to be poor. This appeared to be related to the instability of menadione at 60°C and also to its lability in the supporting electrolyte used. The recovery of menadione from plasma was greatly improved when the extraction procedure and supporting electrolyte were suitably modified. The extraction solvent used was diethyl ether (peroxide-free) and this was added to plasma which had been adjusted to pH 6.0 with phosphate buffer. After shaking and centrifuging, the solvent was evaporated to dryness at 25°C under nitrogen. The residue was then dissolved in a supporting electrolyte of ethanol -0.05 M acetate buffer, pH 3.0 (9:1, v/v). Under these conditions a well-defined DPP peak was obtained at -0.5 V (vs. SCE) and the recovery of menadione from plasma was 90% when added in concentrations ranging from 250 to 1000 ng/ml.

In a related study, it was of interest to ascertain whether menadione existed in the ''free'' state in plasma after storing at 37°C. To do this, plasma samples were spiked with menadione and incubated for various times before assaying by the modified DPP method. It was discovered that the peak at -0.5 V decreased rapidly with a half-life time of disappearance of about 28 min. These results were in agreement with those of Scudi and Buhs[26] who, using a colorimetric method involving cysteine, also showed that free menadione disappeared rapidly from plasma. These authors indicated that menadione reacted with plasma proteins. Therefore, in our polarographic studies it would seem that either the menadione-plasma complex was not polarographically active, or that this complex was not extracted into ether.

Akman et al.[27] have developed a polarographic method which appears to be capable of measuring menadione in spiked plasma samples and in plasma following an oral dose of menadiol diphosphate.[27] In this study a solvent extraction step was carried out with diethyl ether and the plasma phase was frozen before transferring the ether to a separate vessel. This procedure was repeated, the ether extracts combined and calcium chloride added. After separating off the calcium chloride the ether was evaporated to dryness and the residue dissolved in buffer. When this was submitted to DPP, a peak for menadione was obtained at -0.28 V. This was then used to determine the plasma levels of the vitamin following oral doses. It would be of interest to evaluate this method on spiked plasma samples incubated at 37°C for various times as discussed above; this may throw some light on the possible menadione-protein interactions previously observed.[2,26]

Investigations involving differential pulse voltammetry at a HMDE have indicated that this approach is more sensitive than DPP for the analysis of phylloquinone.[14] The limit of detection for phylloquinone was 10 ng/ml in a supporting electrolyte containing 60% methanolic acetate buffer. This increased sensitivity appeared to be the result of adsorption of the vitamin onto the HMDE. However, it should be added that these determinations were performed in supporting electrolyte only. In order to apply this to the mea-

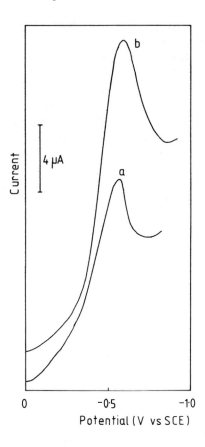

FIGURE 12.   Linear sweep voltammograms of phylloquinone (10^{-5} M) in 50% ethanol, 0.05 M acetate buffer, pH 5.0 (1:1, v/v) after accumulating at a carbon-paste electrode for: (a) 1 min with stirring and 30 s quiescence; (b) 5 min with stirring and 30 s quiescence. Scan rate 20 mV/s; initial potential 0.0 V.

surement of phylloquinone in plasma it would be necessary to purify plasma extracts after the solvent extraction step.

Another voltammetric approach to phylloquinone analysis which may prove to be useful involves the use of carbon paste electrodes.[28] Preliminary results have indicated that the vitamin can be preconcentrated at the carbon paste electrode from ethanolic solutions. This was carried out at open circuit with stirring; the magnitude of the current produced and its increase with time as the vitamin accumulated at the electrode was encouraging (Figure 12). The voltammetric measurement may be carried out in the same supporting electrolyte or after transferring the electrode to a different solution; this is known as medium exchange.[6] The latter method should eliminate any interferences from plasma compounds which remain in solution and which give peaks close to phylloquinone. Further investigations are currently being carried out with this technique.

B. METHODS INVOLVING HIGH-PERFORMANCE LIQUID
CHROMATOGRAPHY WITH ELECTROCHEMICAL
DETECTION (HPLC-ECD) OR ELECTROCHEMICAL
DERIVATIZATION

The search for a sensitive, selective analytical method for the determination of normal and subnormal endogenous levels of vitamin K compounds in plasma has been of interest to workers in a variety of biomedical fields. However, these determinations are difficult because of the low levels present and also because interference may occur from other plasma constituents.

One of the first studies to indicate that HPLC-ECD may be an appropriate technique for such analysis was reported by Ikenoya et al.[29] In this study phylloquinone was extracted from rat plasma with hexane following the administration of an oral dose of 1 mg/kg body weight. The extracted lipid residue was then dissolved in isopropyl alcohol for injection onto an octadecylsilyl (C-18) reversed-phase column. The mobile phase consisted of sodium perchlorate/perchloric acid dissolved in ethanol-methanol (6:4, v/v) and the vitamin was detected at a potential of -0.3 V (vs. Ag/AgC1). The authors stated that the minimum detection limit was 100 pg.

Hart et al.[17] carried out detailed electrochemical studies to optimize the HPLC-ECD conditions for the determination of endogenous phylloquinone levels in human plasma. The detector consisted of a thin-layer cell containing a glassy carbon working electrode which was operated in the reductive mode. Phylloquinone was separated from 10 ml of plasma by solvent extraction with hexane after flocculation of proteins with ethanol. The plasma extract was further purified by sorbent extraction on silica cartridges followed by normal-phase HPLC. HPLC-ECD was then carried out on a reversed-phase (C-8) column with a mobile phase containing methanol -0.05 M acetate buffer, pH 3.0 (95:5, v/v) and an applied potential of -1.0 V (vs. Ag/AgC1). The detection limit was found to be about 500 pg which was suitable for the determination of normal circulating levels of phylloquinone (range, 0.08 to 1.24 ng/ml). The sensitivity of this reductive electrochemical method was shown to be about three times greater than a UV-detection method which had been developed earlier by one of the authors of this group.[30] An important finding was that this reductive electrochemical method gave plasma values in the same range as the UV method and that there was a good correlation between both methods when compared directly.

Ueno and Suttie[31] also investigated reductive mode HPLC-ECD for the determination of phylloquinone in human serum. These workers also used a glassy carbon electrode but the HPLC conditions were based on those used by Ikenoya et al.[29] with a C-18 column and a mobile phase of sodium perchlorate/perchloric acid in methanol–ethanol–water (37:57:8, by volume) The signal to noise ratio was optimized at a potential of -0.275 V which was near to the half-wave potential of the hydrodynamic voltammogram. Despite this sacrifice in potential sensitivity, the method was shown to be capable of detecting serum levels down to a concentration of 300 pg/ml when 1.5 ml of serum was extracted. However, the mean endogenous concentration of phylloquinone in normal adults determined by this method was about 1 ng/ml which was about double that found by Hart et al.[17] using the reductive HPLC-ECD method outlined above.

The disadvantages of all these reductive HPLC-ECD methods for measuring low endogenous serum concentrations of phylloquinone are chiefly those associated with the coreduction of interfering compounds. For example, the simultaneous reduction of oxygen at the detector electrode means that low background currents and acceptable baseline drift could only be achieved by meticulous attention to deaeration procedures. This problem, however, may be entirely overcome by employing a detector with a dual-electrode cell with the electrodes arranged in series. In this configuration the reversible redox couple exhibited by certain compounds (e.g., quinones) may be exploited such that the product of a reduction reaction formed at the first electrode can be detected downstream at a second electrode by reoxidation at a much lower working potential than by using reduction alone. The feasibility of this approach to the detection of vitamin K compounds was first shown by Haroon et al.[32] using a dual-electrode cell containing porous graphite electrodes in series. The principle of the redox technique as applied to K vitamins is therefore to reduce the quinone moiety at the upstream (generator) electrode and to reoxidize the hydroquinone (quinol) product at the downstream (detector) electrode. The electrolysis current generated by the reoxidation step is detected and recorded as a chromatographic peak. As described by Haroon et al.[32] the method was shown to be capable of the sensitive detection of phylloquinone, menaquinones, and other vitamin K compounds. The minimum detectable amount for phylloquinone was about 100 pg while preliminary experiments suggested that the method would be suitable for detecting phylloquinone in tissue matrices such as serum and liver.[32]

More detailed studies with the aim of using redox mode HPLC-ECD for the reliable and sensitive measurement of both normal and depressed plasma concentrations of phylloquinone were carried out by Hart et al.[33] using the electrochemical instrumentation as Haroon et al.[32] but using the same methanolic acetate buffers that had been successfully used for their earlier reductive HPLC-ECD method.[17] A major aim was to improve the sensitivity sufficiently to allow the volume of plasma required for the phylloquinone assay to be reduced to 3 ml or less. In order to find the optimal potentials which needed to be applied to each of the two electrodes in series HPLC-ECD, hydrodynamic voltammetry was performed. This was done in two stages. In the first stage, the potential of the upstream electrode was kept constant at a suitably negative value to reduce the quinone to the hydroquinone and the peak heights given by the same injected amount of phylloquinone were determined while varying the potential at the downstream electrode. Next, the latter was held constant at a suitably positive potential to reoxidize the hydroquinone, and the first

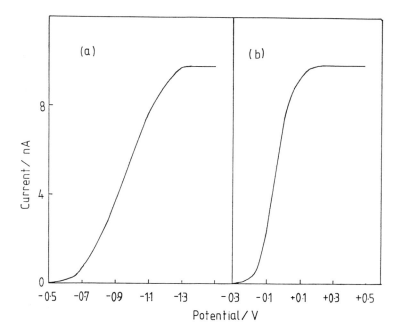

FIGURE 13. (a) Cathodic hydrodynamic voltammogram for 1-ng injections of phylloquinone
with the downstream electrode held constant at +0.2 V; and (b) anodic hydrodynamic voltammogram for 1-ng injections of phylloquinone with the upstream electrode held constant at −1.3
V. (From Hart, J. P., Shearer, M., and McCarthy, P. T., *Analyst*, 110, 1181, 1985. With
permission.)

electrode potential was varied. The resulting hydrodynamic voltammograms
are shown in Figure 13. From these it was concluded that the most suitable
potentials for the analysis of phylloquinone by HPLC-ECD were −1.3 V at
electrode 1, and +0.2 V at electrode 2. However, it was found more beneficial
to use a potential of 0 V at electrode 2 because this reduced interference from
coextracted material. There are several advantages of the redox approach. A
major advantage is that there is no need to deaerate the mobile phase because
oxygen products do not interfere at the detector electrode and this greatly
improves the signal to noise ratios compared to HPLC-ECD in the reductive
mode. A second improvement in the sensitivity comes from the coulometric
cell design and the greater surface area of the porous graphite electrodes
compared to the thin-layer cell and glassy carbon working electrode used in
the earlier method.[17] This means that a much greater proportion of phylloquinone in the mobile phase is electrolyzed during its passage through the
porous graphite electrodes than occurs at the surface of the glassy carbon
electrode. The overall effect of using a cell containing dual, porous, graphite
electrodes in series, and operated in the redox mode, was to increase the
sensitivity of the method by an order of magnitude.[33] This method was also

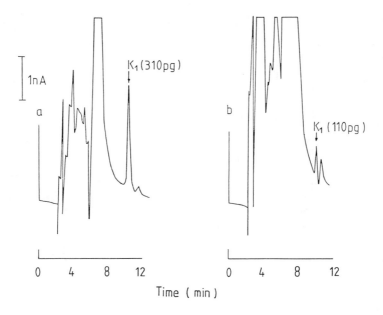

FIGURE 14. Chromatograms of plasma samples obtained by HPLC-ECD in the redox mode for: (a) a normal subject (endogenous concentration of 240 pg/ml in plasma); (b) a patient with osteoporosis and fractured neck of the femur (endogenous concentration of 60 pg/ml in plasma). (From Hart, J. P., Shearer, M. J., and McCarthy, P. T., *Analyst*, 110, 1181, 1985. With permission.)

found to be about 30 times more sensitive than a method using UV detection after HPLC.[30]

The HPLC-ECD method using redox mode detection was first applied to the determination of plasma phylloquinone in normal subjects and in patients suffering from osteoporosis. Figure 14 shows some typical chromatograms. Clearly, in both cases well-defined peaks were obtained; the injected volumes were equivalent to only 1.3 and 1.8 ml of plasma, respectively. This method has been successfully applied to the measurement of *depressed* circulating phylloquinone levels in osteoporotic patients with subcapital[34] and trochanteric[35] fractures of the femur, as well as spinal crush fractures.[36,37] In further studies this redox method was used to determine circulating levels in patients with traumatic fractures including femur, ankle, and humerus;[38] the levels were followed over various periods of time during fracture healing. With some adaptations,[39,40] such as the addition of 0.1 mM EDTA and recycling the mobile phase (found to aid baseline stability and prolong sensitivity) the same method has been used by Shearer and colleagues to measure plasma levels of phylloquinone in a variety of clinical and nutritional studies.[41-43] Another adaptation for plasma assays was the use of an internal standardized calibration procedure (with menaquinone-6 as the internal standard) in place of the external calibration procedure of the original method. Both methods of calibra-

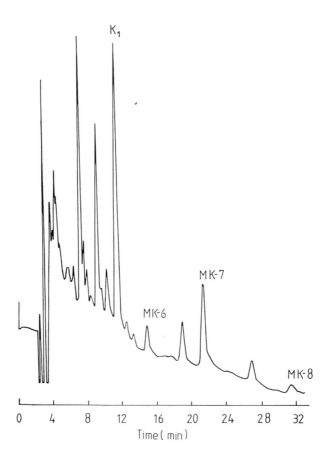

FIGURE 15.   Redox-mode HPLC-ECD chromatogram of a plasma sample taken from a patient with hypertriglyceridemia.

tion provide a similar range of values for plasma phylloquinone in a normal population.

The original collaborating groups in London (at Guy's Hospital and the Kennedy Institute of Rheumatology) have also demonstrated the feasibility of using HPLC-ECD in the redox mode to detect and measure concentrations of menaquinones in both plasma[42,44] and liver tissues.[42] A chromatogram showing the analysis of K vitamins in a plasma sample from a patient with hypertriglyceridemia is shown in Figure 15. Such patients have elevated levels of K vitamins and the detection of peaks putatively identified as menaquinones 6, 7, and 8 is readily seen. In normal subjects menaquinone 6 is undetectable but peaks with the same retention times as menaquinones 7 and 8 are usually measurable.[44]

The series dual-electrode approach to electrochemical analyses of K vitamins has also been investigated by other workers. Notably Langenberg et al.[45] compared the same dual-electrode coulometric detector as in the studies described above to a system containing a coulometric generator electrode (upstream electrode) and an amperometric detector electrode (downstream electrode). The authors indicated that the latter system was slightly superior in terms of selectivity, but had a somewhat lower limit of detection (280 pg) than that given by the system in which both cells were of coulometric design (150 pg). Neither of these methods were apparently applied to plasma samples but the same authors[45] also reported a novel use of the dual-electrode coulometric detector for the post-column derivitization of K vitamins to produce, by electrochemical reduction, their hydroquinone forms which could be detected on line by a fluorescence detector. The dual electrodes were operated at a potential of -0.4 V while the mobile phase contained 0.03 M sodium perchlorate dissolved in methanol–water (95:5, v/v). Under these conditions the limit of detection was about 25 pg. For the determination of plasma phylloquinone levels an aliquot of 1 ml of plasma was extracted with isopropanol–hexane mixtures: after evaporation of the hexane phase, the residue was dissolved in 1 ml of methanol and 50 μl were injected onto the reversed-phase column. The concentration found in plasma from a fasting subject was 2.3 ng/ml. This is somewhat higher than found by other workers and may be due to the lack of a clean-up step prior to chromatography.

With its high sensitivity the electrofluorometric detection system also allows the determination of phylloquinone in foods containing high amounts of the vitamin without recourse to the clean-up stages of chromatography normally needed for techniques based on HPLC with UV detection. Thus Langenberg et al.[7,46] analyzed the phylloquinone content of vegetables after extraction with isopropanol–hexane mixtures. An aliquot of the hexane phase could then be analyzed directly after reconstitution in methanol.

Kusube et al.[47] have also used electrofluorometric detection, following HPLC, for the determination of phylloquinone and a K_2 vitamer (menaquinone-4) in rat plasma. In this study, the mobile phase consisted of sodium perchlorate/perchloric acid dissolved in acetonitrile-isopropanol (9:1, v/v) and this was deaerated with argon. The column was a reversed-phase octadecylsilyl column, the electrochemical reactor consisted of carbon cloth working electrodes and the potential was set at a value of -1.4 V. The fluorometric excitation and emmission wavelengths were set at 330 and 430 nm, respectively. It was shown that both phylloquinone and menaquinone-4 could be detected in plasma following oral or intravenous dosing with these compounds; control plasma samples, however, did not show chromatographic peaks for these two K vitamins. The limits of detection were 1 ng for both compounds. The authors suggested that the electrochemical derivatization method was simpler than a method involving fluorescence detection following post-column chemical reduction.[48]

Another innovative use of electrofluorometric detection, introduced by Langenberg and Tjaden,[49] is the determination of phylloquinone epoxide, a metabolite of phylloquinone which is known to be released into the circulation

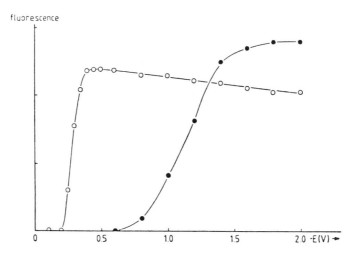

FIGURE 16. Relationship between the fluorescence intensity and the potentials applied to the electrodes of the electrochemical cell for phylloquinone (○) and phylloquinone epoxide (●). (From Langenberg, J. P. and Tjaden, U. R., *J. Chromatogr.*, 289, 377, 1984. With permission.)

after anticoagulant therapy with coumarin or indanedione drugs. In order to electrochemically reduce the epoxide, a commercial polarographic analyzer was used which allowed the necessary large negative potential to be set at the working electrode. Figure 16 shows the hydrodynamic voltammogram obtained for the epoxide derivative of phylloquinone as well as for phylloquinone itself. From these results the authors selected -1.8 V as being suitable for the simultaneous determination of these compounds. It was said that the product of reduction was probably the 1,4-hydroquinone derivative, i.e., the same product that is obtained after reduction of phylloquinone. Using this method, Langenberg and Tjaden showed that it was possible to measure phylloquinone epoxide in human plasma (9.6 ng/ml) 14 h after an oral dose of 10 mg of phylloquinone. In addition, it was possible to measure this metabolite at endogenous levels in patients receiving treatment with coumarin vitamin K antagonists. Figure 17 shows the chromatogram obtained from such a patient where the epoxide concentration was 0.92 ng/ml plasma; in a total of ten patients on anticoagulation therapy the values ranged from 150 pg/ml to 1.2 ng/ml. The authors did not find circulating epoxide levels in normal untreated subjects and suggested that this was probably below their limit of detection, i.e., 120 pg/ml. On the other hand, using a method based on the same electrofluorimetric detection principle but with apparently greater sensitivity, Hirauchi et al.[50] recently reported that endogenous concentrations of the epoxide in normal fasting subjects ranged from 50 to 170 pg/ml with slightly higher levels being found in the post-prandial state.

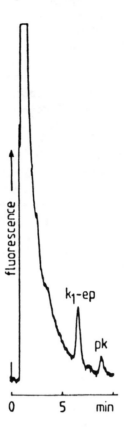

FIGURE 17. Extract of plasma of a patient under anticoagulant therapy with the coumarin drug phenprocoumon. Peaks indicated are phylloquinone epoxide (k_1-ep, 0.92 ng/ml) and phylloquinone (pk, 0.28 ng/ml). Applied potential -1.8 V. (From Langenberg, J. P. and Tjaden, U. R., *J. Chromatogr.*, 289, 377, 1984. With permission.)

IV. CONCLUSION

In this chapter the electrochemical properties of vitamin K compounds have been described. These reactions are mainly reduction/oxidation processes which occur at mercury electrodes; however, some discussion of the reactions occurring at carbon and platinum electrodes has also been included. The exploitation of this behavior for the electroanalysis of the K vitamins in biological material has been illustrated with examples which indicate the wide variety of electrochemical techniques that may be used for quantitative measurements of the K vitamins.

DPP has been applied to pharmacokinetic studies involving phylloquinone in plasma following an intravenous injection. Similar investigations have been carried out on vitamin K_3 after an oral dose. These studies required fairly straightforward solvent extraction steps to separate the vitamins from plasma and micromolar levels could be monitored. It may be possible to improve detection limits for phylloquinone using adsorption stripping voltammetry at a HMDE; however, further clean-up of the extract would probably be necessary. In preliminary studies carbon paste electrodes have also shown promise for the adsorption stripping voltammetric analysis of phylloquinone. This latter technique may prove fruitful in situations where the use of mercury is undesirable. These methods have involved the differential pulse or linear sweep waveforms but future applications may involve a relatively new technique known as large amplitude square wave voltammetry[51] which appears to improve the sensitivity over that of the differential-pulse waveform.

The determination of endogenous concentrations of phylloquinone in plasma has been successfully carried out using LCEC. Although measurements of normal circulating levels have been achieved by amperometric reduction at a thin-layer glassy carbon electrode, a much improved response and stability has been obtained using a dual-electrode coulometric cell operated in the redox mode. Electrofluorimetric detection methods in which the electrochemical detector serves as a post-column reactor for the generation of the fluorescent hydroquinone form of the vitamin also possess the required sensitivity and selectivity for the measurement of normal and subnormal concentrations of phylloquinone in plasma.

Menaquinones show similar voltammetric properties to phylloquinone and the detection of members of this series of K vitamins has been achieved using dual-electrode coulometric detectors either by straight electrochemical detection in the redox mode or by electrofluorimetric detection (i.e., coulometric reduction coupled to fluorimetric detection). The detection of the much lower concentrations of menaquinones in plasma is more difficult but measurements of menaquinones 7 and 8 have been reported using the dual-electrode redox method.

The utility of the electrofluorimetric method for the measurement of phylloquinone epoxide has been demonstrated. This technique seems especially suitable for the measurement of plasma levels of the epoxide of phylloquinone metabolite which is released into the blood as a consequence of the inhibitory effects of coumarin or indanedione antagonists on vitamin-K metabolism in the liver. Besides the well known clinical role of oral anticoagulants, new congeners have been developed which are powerful rodenticides. The detection of this epoxide metabolite by the electrofluorimetric method is currently showing promise as a toxicological screen for the presence of anticoagulant residues in the body (see Chapter 14). It may also be possible to measure phylloquinone epoxide using dual series HPLC-ECD under the appropriate solution conditions and applied potentials.

An impressive feature of modern developments in the electrochemical or electrofluorimetric detection of K vitamins is the continuing improvements being made in sensitivity. Thus two recent reports from the same laboratory[50,52] show that with fine tuning, the electrofluorimetric method is capable of tissue detection limits for K vitamins in the range of 30 to 50 pg/ml and 40 to 80 pg/g when extracting 1 ml of plasma[50] and 1 g of liver,[52] respectively. Under optimum conditions, the dual-electrode, coulometric electrochemical method[33] with recent refinements[39,40] is also capable of detection limits of this order.[52] With continuing improvements in instrumentation, even lower limits of detection should be achievable.

Until now, electrochemically based measurements of vitamin K have been mainly applied to clinical investigations in relation to coagulation problems and bone disease. In the future, it seems likely that other areas of biomedicine such as nutrition and epidemiology will require vitamin K analyses and that the advanced electroanalytical techniques described in this chapter will continue to find an application for the sensitive and specific measurement of the variety of chemical forms which together comprise the vitamin K group of compounds.

REFERENCES

1. **Bond, A. M.,** *Modern Polarographic Techniques in Analytical Chemistry,* Marcel Dekker, New York, 1980.
2. **Hart, J. P.,** Polarography and its application to the determination of low levels of vitamins and coenzymes, in *Investigative Microtechniques in Medicine and Biology,* Vol. 1, Bitensky, L. and Chayen, J., Eds., Marcel Dekker, New York, 1985, 199.
3. **Fleet, B. and Fouzda, N. B.,** Unit processes in organic voltammetric analysis-II, determination, in *Polarography of Molecules of Biological Significance,* Smyth, W. F., Ed., Academic Press, London, 1979, 37.
4. **Hanekamp, H. B., Bos, P., and Frei, R. W.,** Electrochemical detectors in flowing liquid systems: an assessment of their use, *Trends Anal. Chem.,* 1, 135, 1892.
5. **Kissinger, P. T. and Heineman, W. R., Eds.,** *Laboratory Techniques in Electroanalytical Chemistry,* Marcel Dekker, New York, 1984.
6. **Wang, J.,** Adsorptive stripping voltammetry, *Int. Lab.,* 15, 68, 1985.
7. **Langenberg, J. P.,** Bioanalysis of ultratrace levels of K vitamins using electroflourometric detection in HPLC, Ph.D. thesis, Leiden State University, Leiden, Netherlands, 1985.
8. **McCarthy, P. T.,** Assay of vitamin K_1 (phylloquinone) and vitamins K_2 (menaquinones) in human liver and plasma by high-performance liquid chromatography with electrochemical detection, Ph.D. thesis, University of London, U.K., 1988.
9. **Hart, J. P.,** Applications of modern electroanalytical techniques in clinical chemistry, in *Electrochemistry Sensors and Analysis, Analytical Chemistry Symposia Series,* Vol. 25, Smyth, M. R. and Vos, J. G., Eds., Elsevier, Amsterdam, 1986, 355.
10. **Hart, J. P.,** Unpublished data, 1979.
11. **Jordan, J. and Stalica, N. R.,** Polarography and other voltammetric techniques, in *Handbook of Analytical Chemistry.* Meites, L., Ed., McGraw-Hill, New York, 1963, 39.

12. **Vire, J. C. and Patriarche, G. J.,** Electrochemical study of 1,4-naphthoquinone and K-series vitamins, II. Vitamins K_1 and K_3, *Analysis,* 6, 395, 1978.

13. **Patriarche, G. J. and Vire, J. C.,** Electroanalytical applications in pharmacy and pharmacology, in *Electroanalysis in Hygiene, Environmental, Clinical and Pharmaceutical Chemistry,* Smyth, W. F., Ed., Elsevier, Amsterdam, 1980, 209.

14. **Hart, J. P. and Catterall, A.,** Electrosorption of vitamin K_1 at mercury and its determination at submicrogram levels by differential pulse voltammetry at a hanging mercury electrode, *Anal. Chim. Acta,* 128, 245, 1981.

15. **Takamura, K. and Hayakawa, Y.,** Electrosorption of vitamin K_2 studied by cyclic voltammetry in aqueous methanol, *J. Electroanal. Chem.,* 49, 133, 1974.

16. **Patriarche, G. J. and Lingane, J. J.,** Electrochemical characteristics of 2-methyl-1,4-naphthoquinone (vitamin K_3), a coulometric micromethod of determination, *Anal. Chim. Acta,* 49, 241, 1970.

17. **Hart, J. P., Shearer, M. J., McCarthy, P. T., and Rahim, S.,** Voltammetric behavior of phylloquinone (vitamin K_1) at a glassy-carbon electrode and determination of the vitamin in plasma using high-performance liquid chromatography with electrochemical detection, *Analyst,* 109, 477, 1984.

18. **Ksenzhek, O. S., Petrova, S. A., Kolodyazhnyi, M. V., and Oleinik, S. V.,** Redox properties of K group vitamins, *Bioelectrochem. Bioenerg.,* 4, 335, 1977.

19. **Cauquis, G. and Marbach, G.,** The redox behavior of biological quinones and its relation with the mitochondrial respiratory chain, *Experientia Suppl.,* 18, 205, 1971.

20. **Vire, J. C. and Patriarche, G. J.,** Electrochemical study of 1,4-naphthoquinone and K vitamins, III. Vitamin K_3 sodium bisulphite, *Analysis,* 7, 144, 1979.

21. **Vire, J. C., Patriarche, G. J., and Christian, G. D.,** Electrochemical study of the degradation of vitamin K_3 and vitamin K_3-bisulphite, *Anal. Chem.,* 51, 752, 1979.

22. **Takamura, K. and Watanabe, F.,** Polarographic studies of the oxidation of vitamin K_5 in aqueous solution, *Anal. Biochem.,* 74, 512, 1976.

23. **Hart, J. P. and Catterall, A.,** Polarographic analysis of some quinones of clinical significance, in *Electroanalysis in Hygiene, Environmental, Clinical and Pharmaceutical Chemistry, Analytical Chemistry Symposia Series,* Vol. 2, Smyth, W. F., Ed., Elsevier, Amsterdam, 1980, 145.

24. **Hart, J. P., Nahir, A. M., Chayen, J., and Catterall, A.,** Determination of vitamin K_1 in plasma by differential pulse polarography and its possible clinical application, *Anal. Chim. Acta,* 144, 267, 1982.

25. **Lindquist, J. and Farroha, S. M.,** Application of differential pulse polarography to the assay of vitamins, *Analyst,* 100, 377, 1975.

26. **Scudi, J. V. and Buhs, R. P.,** Reactions of 2-methyl-1,4-naphthoquinone with whole blood and plasma studied by means of a rapid colorimetric method, *J. Biol. Chem.,* 144, 599, 1942.

27. **Akman, S. A., Kusu, F., Takamura, K., Chlebowski, R., and Block, J.,** Differential pulse polarographic determination of plasma menadione [menaphthone], *Anal. Biochem.,* 14, 488, 1984.

28. **Hart, J. P., Blackmore, P., Morgan, I., Taylor, G., and Wring, S. A.,** Unpublished data, 1988.

29. **Ikenoya, S., Abe, K., Tsuda, T., Yamano, Y., Hiroshima, O., Ohmae, M., and Kawabe, K.,** Electrochemical detector for high-performance liquid chromatography, II. Determination of tocopherols, ubiquinones and phylloquinone in blood, *Chem. Pharm. Bull.,* 27, 1237, 1979.

30. **Shearer, M. J., Barkhan, P., Rahim, S., and Stimmler, L.,** Plasma vitamin K_1 in mothers and their newborn babies, *Lancet,* 2, 460, 1982.

31. **Ueno, T. and Suttie, J. W.,** High-pressure liquid chromatographic-reductive electrochemical detection analysis of serum *trans*-phylloquinone, *Anal. Biochem.,* 133, 62, 1983.

32. **Haroon, Y., Schubert, C. A. W., and Hauschka, P. V.,** Liquid chromatographic dual electrode detection system for vitamin K compounds, *J. Chromatogr. Sci.,* 22, 89, 1984.

33. **Hart, J. P., Shearer, M. J., and McCarthy, P. T.,** Enhanced sensitivity for the determination of endogenous phylloquinone (vitamin K_1) in plasma using high-performance liquid chromatography with dual-electrode electrochemical detection, *Analyst,* 110, 1181, 1985.

34. **Hart, J. P., Catterall, A., Dodds, R. A., Klenerman, L., Shearer, M. J., Bitensky, L., and Chayen, J.,** Circulating vitamin K_1 levels in fractured neck of femur, *Lancet,* 2, 283, 1984.

35. **Klenerman, L., Ferris, B., and Hart, J. P.,** Vitamin K_1 levels in proximal femoral fractures, Brief report, *J. Bone Joint Surg.,* 70-B, 286, 1988.

36. **Hart, J. P., Shearer, M. J., Klenerman, L., Reeve, J., Sambrook, P. N., Dodds, R. A., Bitensky, L., and Chayen, J.,** Electrochemical detection of depressed circulating levels of vitamin K_1 in osteoporosis, *J. Endocrinol. Metab.,* 60, 1268, 1985.

37. **Hart, J. P., Yaakub, R., Shearer, M. J., Klenerman, L., Catterall, A., Reeve, J., Sambrook, P. N., Bitensky, L., and Chayen, J.,** Depressed circulating vitamin K_1 levels in osteoporotic patients, *Clin. Sci.,* 68, 29P, 1985.

38. **Bitensky, L., Hart, J. P., Catterall, A., Hodges, S. J., Pilkington, M. J., and Chayen, J.,** Circulating vitamin K_1 levels in patients with fractures, *J. Bone Joint Surg.,* 70-B, 663, 1988.

39. **Shearer, M. J.,** *Vitamins, in HPLC of Small Molecules: A Practical Approach,* Lim, C. K., Ed., IRL Press, Oxford, 1986, 157.

40. **Shearer, M. J.,** Measurement of plasma phylloquinone (vitamin K_1), in *Laboratory Haematology: An Account of Laboratory Techniques,* Chanarin, I., Ed., Churchill-Livingstone, Edinburgh, 1989, 339.

41. **Shearer, M. J., Bechtold, H., Andrassy, K., Koderisch, J., McCarthy, P. T., Trenk, D., Jähnchen, E., and Ritz, E.,** Mechanism of cephalosporin-induced hypoprothrombinemia: relation to cephalosporin side chain, vitamin K metabolism and vitamin K status, *J. Clin. Pharmacol.,* 28, 88, 1988.

42. **Shearer, M. J., McCarthy, P. T., Crampton, O. E., and Mattock, M. B.,** The assessment of human vitamin status from tissue measurements, in *Current Advances in Vitamin K Research,* Suttie, J. W., Ed., Elsevier, New York, 1988, 437.

43. **Cohen, H., Scott, S. D., Mackie, I. J., Shearer, M., Bax, R., Karran, S. J. and Machin, S. J.,** The development of hypoprothrombinaemia following antibiotic therapy in malnourished patients with low serum vitamin K_1 levels, *Br. J. Haematol.,* 68, 63, 1988.

44. **Hodges, S. J., Pilkington, M. J., Shearer, M. J., Bitensky, L., and Chayen, J.,** Age-related changes in the circulating levels of congeners of vitamin K_2, menaquinone-7 and menaquinone-8, *Clin. Sci.,* 78, 63, 1990.

45. **Langenberg, J. P. and Tjaden, U. R.,** Determination of (endogenous) vitamin K_1 in human plasma by reversed-phase high-performance liquid chromatography using fluorometric detection after post column electrochemical reduction: comparison with ultraviolet, single and dual electrochemical detection, *J. Chromatogr.,* 305, 61, 1984.

46. **Langenberg, J. P., Tjaden, U. R., De Vogel, E. M., and Langerak, D. I.,** Determination of phylloquinone in raw and processed vegetables using reversed-phase HPLC with electrofluorometric detection, *Acta Aliment,* 15, 187, 1986.

47. **Kusube, K., Abe, K., Hiroshima, O., Ishiguro, Y., Ishikawa, S., and Hoshida, H.,** Determination of vitamin K analogues by high performance liquid chromatography with electrochemical detection, *Chem. Pharm. Bull.,* 32, 179, 1984.

48. **Abe, K., Hiroshima, O., Ishibashi, K., Ohmae, M., Kawabe, K., and Katsui, G.,** Fluorometric determination of phylloquinone and menaquinone-4 in biological materials using high-performance liquid chromatography, *Yakugaku Zasshi,* 99, 192, 1979.

49. **Langenberg, J. P. and Tjaden, U. R.,** Improved method for the determination of vitamin K_1 epoxide in human plasma with electrofluorimetric reaction detection, *J. Chromatogr.,* 289, 377, 1984.

50. **Hirauchi, K., Sakano, T., Nagaoka, T., and Morimoto, A.,** Simultaneous determination of vitamin K_1, vitamin K_1, 2,3-epoxide and menaquinone-4 in human plasma by high-performance liquid chromatography with fluorimetric detection, *J. Chromatogr.,* 430, 21, 1988.

51. **Osteryoung, J. G. and Osteryoung, R. A.,** Square wave voltammetry, *Anal. Chem.,* 57, 101(A), 1985.

52. **Hirauchi, K., Sakano, T., Notsumoto, S., Nagaoka, T., Morimoto, A., Fujimoto, K., Sachiko, M., and Suzuki, Y.,** Measurement of K vitamins in animal tissues by high-performance liquid chromatography with fluorimetric detection, *J. Chromatogr.,* 497, 131, 1989.

Chapter 3

REACTION DETECTION METHODS FOR K VITAMINS AND THEIR 2'3'-EPOXY METABOLITE IN LIQUID CHROMATOGRAPHY

Yacoob Haroon

TABLE OF CONTENTS

I. INTRODUCTION

The measurement of K vitamins in complex biological matrices has proved to be difficult and has presented severe challenges to most conventional physicochemical methods of analysis. The generally low concentrations of K vitamins in animal tissues and fluids and their instability towards alkali precludes the use of saponification to remove bulk lipids. These problems have been compounded by the existence in animal tissues of multiple forms of K vitamins, namely phylloquinone (vitamin K_1) and menaquinones 4 through 15 (vitamins K_2) (Figure 1).

Between the late 1960's and the early 1970's, Matschiner's group developed physicochemical methods for the isolation, characterization, and measurement of K vitamins in animal tissues.[1] These techniques generally required extracting large quantities of animal tissues with acetone, light petroleum, or ether. The addition of a tracer amount of radioactive vitamin K after the extraction procedure, was found to be a valuable aid in following the purification and also for estimating the recovery of vitamin K. After extraction, an initial conventional chromatographic step on silicic acid was employed to obtain bulk separation of nonpolar lipids in liver samples.[2] Further purification of the lipid extract obtained after silicic acid chromatography was achieved by reversed-phase procedures, either on thin-layers or columns.[1-3] Even after these multistage fractionations of lipid extracts, by conventional chromatographic procedures, it was not possible to resolve K vitamins from contaminating lipids in liver samples.

In attempting to overcome these difficulties, Matschiner's group introduced new techniques for the resolution of K vitamins using argentation chromatography; this mode of chromatography was found to be particularly useful for the identification of partially saturated menaquinones.[4] Despite these chromatographic advances, Matschiner[1] concluded that "there remains the obstacles of excessive amounts of lipids or low concentrations of vitamin K in initial extracts and small amounts of persistent contaminants in the later stages of chromatography." A further advance came when Matschiner[1] described the use of Claisen's alkali for the purification of K vitamins from biological sources. The principles of this technique are that reduced forms (hydroquinones) of natural K vitamins may be extracted into Claisen's alkali (35% KOH in aqueous methanol) and then recovered into organic solvents after oxidation to the quinone. When this technique was applied to the isolation of K vitamins from a biological matrix, more than 99% of associated contaminating lipids could be removed with an overall recovery for vitamin K of 50 to 70%. The major advantage of introducing the Claisen's alkali step in the multistage purification procedure was that it permitted the fractionation step on reversed-phase columns to be omitted.[5] In addition, the use of the Claisen's alkali step also facilitated the isolation of K vitamins from

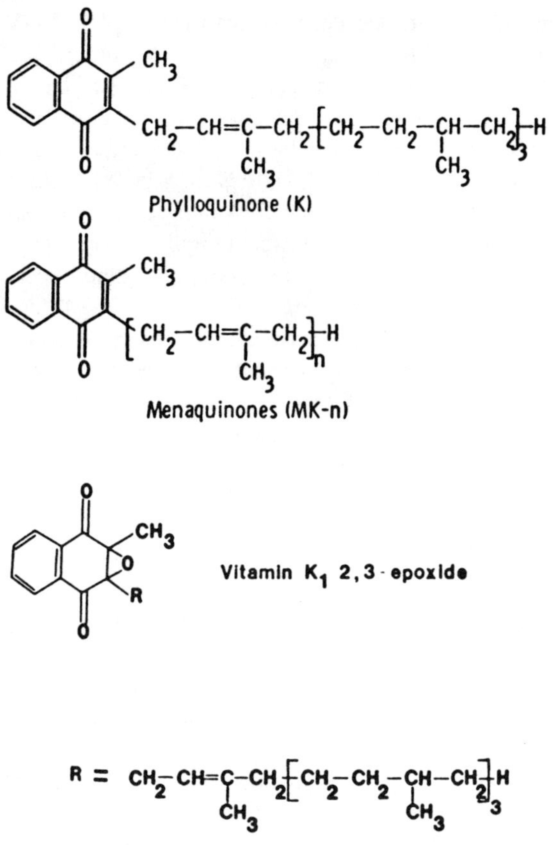

FIGURE 1. Structural formulas phylloquinone (vitamin K_1), menaquinones (vitamins K_2) and phylloquinone (vitamin K_1) 2,3-epoxide.

significantly smaller quantities of starting material than was possible using purely chromatographic procedures.[1]

It will be apparent from this short account, and perhaps not surprising, that the facility for making routine measurements of K vitamins in clinical and nutritional samples, had to await the development of chromatographic methods with direct detection capabilities. During the last decade or so, high-performance liquid chromatography (HPLC) has played a major role in the analysis of K vitamins.[6-9] The application of HPLC has made possible the first direct measurements of vitamin K, mainly phylloquinone, in a wide variety of biological samples.[10-19] Also, in combination with highly selective and sensitive detection modes, HPLC has facilitated the measurement of phylloquinone on semimicro- and micro-scales.[9-26]

A characteristic of the majority of the early liquid chromatographic assay procedures for phylloquinone, which were developed in the late 1970's and

the earlier part of the next decade, was that they employed UV-spectropho-
tometric detectors.[10-13,16,17] The principles of photometric detection are well
known and its application to the detection of K vitamins has been reviewed
elsewhere.[6-8] The limitation of UV detection is its relative lack of selectivity
and sensitivity. In order to overcome these problems, most investigators found
it was necessary to process large quantities of material (e.g., 5 to 10 ml of
plasma and 10 to 15 ml of milk) to detect K_1 concentrations between 0.5 and
2.0 ng/ml. A common experience was that phylloquinone could not be measured in biological materials by a single column method because the chromatographic peak of K_1 is always masked by other UV-absorbing contaminants. It has, therefore, been necessary to increase the selectivity for the
separation of these impurities by using two stages of HPLC in which the
principles of separation are different.[9-18] Nevertheless, the stability of UV
detectors is excellent and in combination with multistage purification procedures reliable results can be obtained.[6-9]

During the late 1970's, interesting developments were beginning to emerge
from the research laboratories of the Eisai Company of Japan with regard to
their methods for the assay of phylloquinone in biological samples based on
fluorometric detection[14] and electrochemical detection (ECD).[15] For both electrochemical and fluorometric detection a well-known oxidation-reduction or
redox property of K vitamins (quinone) to form vitamin K hydroquinones
was explored. The first combined HPLC-ECD measurement of phylloquinone
used reductive mode detection with cells based on thin-layer designs (amperometric) and containing a glassy-carbon working electrode. The principle
of this method is as follows. When a sufficiently negative potential is applied
to a glassy-carbon electrode over which vitamin K is flowing, the quinone
moiety is reduced to the hydroquinone and the flow of electrons from the
electrode can be measured as current. The magnitude of the current observed
by the detector is proportional to the amount of vitamin K electrolyzed at the
electrode surface. With amperometric detectors, a small fraction, usually 2
to 5% of the analyte is reduced (see also Chapter 2).

Although other groups[20,21] have also developed HPLC-ECD methodologies for phylloquinone based on the reduction of the quinone to the hydroquinone, reductive mode ECD has several practical disadvantages. One of
these is the need to remove oxygen from the mobile phase, liquid chromatograph, and sample. The relatively large negative potentials (0.8 to 1.2 V)
required to reduce phylloquinone also reduces oxygen at the electrode surface
and therefore, the oxygen reduction current interferes with the detection of
the vitamin leading to high background currents, detector noise and baseline
drift. Additionally, a general problem of HPLC-ECD, especially using electrodes based on a thin-layer design, is the passivation of the electrode surface
leading to loss of sensitivity. Although the sensitivity of detection for phylloquinone by HPLC-ECD in the reductive mode (at a glassy-carbon electrode)

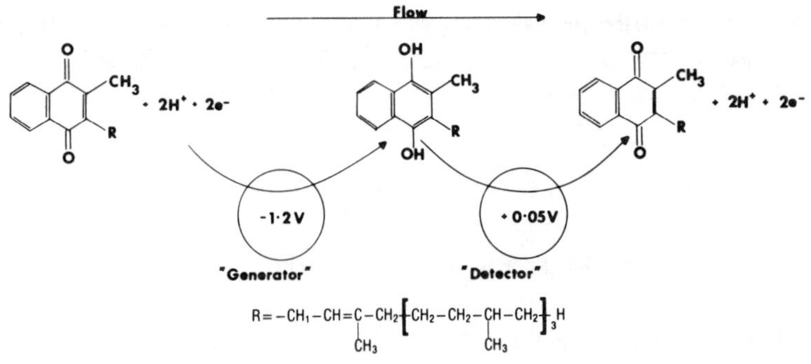

FIGURE 2. Schematic diagram of redox ECD for phylloquinone.

is about 2.5 to 3 times greater than UV detection,[21] its practical utility for assays in biological material is limited.

The development of a redox ECD method[22] for vitamin K reduces interference from the reduction of oxygen. In this method, the electrochemical detector consists of two electrodes in series (dual electrode cell). Phylloquinone is reduced at the upstream (generator) electrode to the hydroquinone and this product is reoxidized at the downstream (or detector) electrode (Figure 2). Since the reoxidation of vitamin K hydroquinone requires a relatively low oxidation potential at the downstream (detector) electrode, without concomitant oxidation of most other lipids or species (e.g., peroxide or water are the products of oxygen reduction at the generator electrode), the redox mode is considerably more sensitive and selective than reductive-mode HPLC-ECD.[22,23] The sensitivity is also enhanced by the use of "coulometric" cells with a flow-through porous graphite design. Methods based on redox-mode ECD are capable of measuring phylloquinone down to 25 to 50 pg in only 1 to 2 ml aliquots of plasma[23] and milk.[27] Although (redox mode) HPLC-ECD assays for K_1 in biological samples have reduced sample size and detection limits compared to UV-photometric detectors, ECD assays still require two-stages of HPLC before K_1 can be quantitated.[23,27] A more detailed account of HPLC-ECD assays for vitamin K is described elsewhere in this volume (see Chapter 2).

The same laboratory which introduced the electrochemical detection of isoprenoid quinones has also developed methods for detecting K vitamins and the related 2,3-epoxy derivatives based on the fluorescent properties of vitamin K hydroquinones.[14] In this method, K vitamins are first separated in their quinone form on C_{18} columns and detected fluorometrically after reacting the column effluent with ethanolic sodium borohydride in a reaction coil connected on-line to the chromatographic column. This was the first application of a chemical post-column reaction detection method for the measurement of K vitamins.

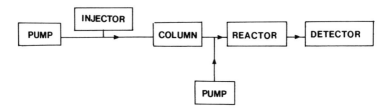

FIGURE 3. Basic features of an HPLC-RD system.

The aim of this chapter is to discuss the present status and future prospects for the analysis of K vitamins using post-column reaction detection (RD) methods in combination with HPLC (HPLC-RD). As will be shown, the application of HPLC-RD methods have opened up new areas of vitamin K studies which were more difficult or impossible using traditional methods of analysis.

II. REACTION DETECTION METHODS FOR K VITAMINS AND RELATED COMPOUNDS

A. BACKGROUND

The K vitamins possess two outstanding physicochemical attributes which make them particularly suited for analysis and detection by HPLC-RD techniques. First, the vitamins can be reduced or degraded with relative ease by electrochemical, chemical, and photochemical means. The reduction reaction leads to the formation of highly fluorescent vitamin K hydroquinones from the nonfluorescent vitamin K quinones. In instances where vitamin K is degraded to products other than the hydroquinone, as in photochemical reactions, the degraded product(s) have also been shown to possess fluorescent properties.[24] Second, the fast reaction kinetics for the formation of these fluorophores (hydroquinones or degraded vitamin K products) is ideally suited for on-line reaction followed by fluorometric detection during HPLC.

The basis of modern RD methods lies, of course, in much older chemistries describing the chemical reactions of the compound(s) of interest; for example, the reactions of K vitamins and related quinones have already been well characterized and documented[28] and need only be adopted and/or modified for HPLC-RD. As mentioned earlier, a major attraction of HPLC-RD to the analysis of K vitamins is to be able to increase the range of fluorometric detection by derivatization methods which convert the vitamin with its originally poor fluorescent properties to compound(s) that can be detected with high fluorometric sensitivities. Besides enhancing the detection of the analyte of interest, RD techniques can also enhance the selectivity of the overall analytical process.

The basic features of a liquid chromatograph equipped with an on-line post-column RD are shown in Figure 3. The mobile phase is pumped through the chromatograph by a pump. After separation of the compounds on the analytical column, they are derivatized in the post-column reactor. The product(s) of the reaction(s) is passed through the appropriate detector and the signal is recorded.

Most reaction detection systems require an additional pump to deliver the derivatizing reagent to the compound eluting from the analytical column. In other more elegant RD systems, the derivatizing reagent is incorporated as part of the mobile phase for HPLC. In these instances, the reaction is initiated in the reactor by temperature, UV light or metal(s).

Several advantages are realized when HPLC and post-column RD techniques are coupled. These are listed below.

1.   Artifact formation plays a minor role in RD methods.
2.   The reaction need not be complete or fully defined. The only requirement is reproducibility.
3.   Different detection principles can be used (UV, ECD, fluorescence).
4.   The compounds are separated in their original form, which allows the adaptation/modification of previously developed chromatographic mobile phases.

Although the rapidly growing number of publications pertaining to post-column RD methods for K vitamins and other compounds by HPLC reflects the growing acceptance of RD techniques, nevertheless, there are certain shortcomings. First, as already mentioned most post-column RD systems for the analysis of K vitamins require an additional pump to deliver the derivatizing reagent to the quinone as it elutes from the analytical column. Second, the optimum mobile phase for the separation of K vitamins is often not the ideal media/conditions for converting vitamin K quinones to fluorescent hydroquinones, or other fluorescent species. In this respect, Abe et al.[14] described the problem of the gradual decomposition of sodium borohydride (reducing reagent) in the semi-aqueous mobile phases (ethanol-water mixtures) used for the separation of K vitamins in their reversed-phase RD system. This problem is further compounded by the formation of hydrogen gas and alkali during the reaction of sodium borohydride with ethanol.

An important consideration for HPLC-RD techniques is the reactor design, because the use of inappropriate reactors will lead to poor reaction kinetics and poor chromatographic resolution. In HPLC-RD of K vitamins, three types of reactors have been used. A brief description of each will be given here. For more detailed information, the reader is referred to another review.[29] Open-tubular reactors are the simplest type and consist of stainless steel or PTFE tubing. The tubing (typically 5 m × 0.5 mm I.D.) is coiled, knitted, or crocheted. Knitting or crocheting is attractive as it decreases band broadening. Open-tubular reactors have been knitted or crocheted around UV lamps to form photochemical reactors for the production of fluorophores of K vitamins.[24,30] In these types of systems, a compromise is required between reactor length, reaction time, and the contribution of the reactor pressure drop (back pressure) to the overall HPLC system. Pressure drop over the reactor increases with decreasing I.D. of the tubing used to form the open-tubular reactor.

Packed-bed reactors have also been developed for HPLC-RD of K vitamins.[31] These reactors consist of glass or stainless steel columns filled with packing material, such as zinc (Zn) metal, which participates in the reaction leading to the formation of vitamin K hydroquinones. Packed bed reactors of this type need to be replenished with the packing material. The frequency of replenishment will depend, among other factors, on the quantity of Zn metal consumed during the reaction with vitamin K and other components. Ideally, packed bed reactors should contain a catalyst or immobilized enzyme that can be used over a long period of time provided no poisoning occurs.

A third type of reactor that should be mentioned is the segmented flow tubular reactor. These reactors are similar to open tubular reactors but the effluent flow through them is segmented by bubbles or immiscible solvent plugs. These types of reactors are useful for slower reaction kinetics such as the formation of K hydroquinones with sodium borohydride.[24]

Although the paper by Abe et al.[14] describing HPLC-RD for K vitamins was published in 1979, 3 years elapsed before another RD system was published in the literature.[24] This delay reflected the initial technical difficulties encountered with the reduction of K vitamins by sodium borohydride in semi-aqueous mobile phases and the relative lack of sensitivity; thus, Abe et al.[14] reported a minimum level of detection for phylloquinone (vitamin K_1) and menaquinone-4 (MK-4) of 400 pg ($\approx$1 pmol), which was similar to that obtained with UV photometric detectors (500 pg). Most of the work relating to HPLC-RD of K vitamins has been published in the past decade or so. The next section reviews the progress that has been made in developing systems for the detection of K vitamins and related compounds using different post-column reactors.

B. POST-COLUMN REACTORS FOR VITAMIN K
1. Electrochemical Reactors

In 1984, two groups demonstrated the usefulness of post-column electrochemical methods for the reduction of K vitamins to their fluorescent hydroquinone derivatives. Both groups employed reversed-phase HPLC systems with similar mobile phases but different column packings (C_8 or C_{18}) and different designs for the post-column reactor. Thus, while Langenberg and Tjaden[25] chose a coulometric electrochemical detector with two porous graphite cells connected in series, the second group, namely Kusube et al.,[26] used carbon cloth electrodes based on the thin-layer design. With semi-aqueous mobile phases of water in methanol containing 0.03 M sodium perchlorate, Langenberg and Tjaden[25] obtained quantitative reduction of K_1 at an applied potential of -0.4 V. Kusube et al.[26] also used sodium perchlorate as the supporting electrolyte for the electroreduction of vitamin K, but this required a potential of -1.4 V. These authors also found that the optimum fluorometric response for K_1 and MK-4, was obtained by the addition of 0.1% perchloric acid to their mobile phase of sodium perchlorate (0.05 M), acetonitrile, and isopropanol. In contrast, Langenberg and Tjaden[25] observed a 50% decrease in fluorometric response for K vitamins after the addition of 0.1% perchloric acid to their mobile phase mixtures of water in methanol.

An interesting finding was the different degree of fluorometric response obtained for similar quantities of K_1, MK-4, and MK-6. The data obtained by Langenberg and Tjaden[25] suggest that equimolar quantities of K_1 and MK-6 produced similar fluorometric responses. The fluorometric response for MK-4 was, however, 30% less than that for K_1. In this respect, there is little information available on the effects, if any, of different substituent groups (at position 3 of the 1,4 naphthoquinone moiety) on the electrochemical reduction and fluorometric detection of K vitamins. It is possible that substituent groups on the parent quinone (Q) may affect both the rate of electrochemical reduction and fluorometric properties of the reduced quinone (QH_2).

The minimum levels of detection reported by Langenberg and Tjaden[25] were between 25 and 50 pg for K_1 depending on the mobile phase. Kusube et al.[26] found a minimum detection limit of about 1 ng for both K_1 and MK-4. Since both groups used similar excitation and emission wavelengths for the detection of K vitamins, these differences probably reflect the different vitamin K reduction efficiencies of their post-column reactors. In addition, the degree of anaerobicity achieved by the two groups also reflected the minimum quantity detected. In fact, a general disadvantage of fluorometric detection for K vitamins in the low picogram range is the necessity of removing oxygen from the HPLC system. In the presence of oxygen, dissolved in the mobile phase (10^{-4} to 10^{-3} M), vitamin K hydroquinone is oxidized back to the (nonfluorescent) parent quinone with the formation of hydrogen peroxide.[32]

$$QH_2 + O_2 \rightarrow Q + H_2O_2 \tag{1}$$

Even when extreme precautions are taken to isolate vitamin K hydroquinones from oxygen during HPLC, by sparging the eluent with helium, oxygen-free air, or reacting oxygen with zinc metal (to scavenge oxygen), the problem of low levels of oxygen permeation via the gaskets employed in commercially available fluorometer cells still remains. In other instances, deoxygenation of the sample to be injected is also required. Oxygen is somewhat retained on reversed-phase columns and elutes as a broad quench peak. Purging of samples then becomes necessary if the analyte of interest elutes in the oxygen elution region of the chromatogram. The removal of oxygen is also a prerequisite for efficient electroreduction of K vitamins. If oxygen is not removed then the reduction of oxygen interferes with the reduction of the vitamin.[22]

Another disadvantage of HPLC-RD methods which use electroreduction to reduce K vitamins is their incompatibility with the highly efficient non-aqueous reversed-phase systems that have traditionally been employed for the separation of these vitamins by HPLC.[35,36] This restriction is imposed by the necessity of having an eluent which can dissolve the supporting electrolyte required for vitamin K electrolysis.[6] Similarly, the detection of highly lipophilic K vitamins after gradient elution would also appear to be limited, though possible. Some preliminary experiments have suggested that gradient elution of K vitamins (MK-4 through -10) is possible during the electrochemical reduction of these vitamins in mobile phase mixtures of methanol and isopropanol containing sodium acetate and zinc chloride. The practical difficulties encountered under these conditions were the fluorometric baseline drift as the concentration of isopropanol was increased and the decreased fluorometric response with increasing isopropanol concentrations.[33]

With the elucidation of electrofluorometric methods for K vitamins by Langenberg and Tjaden[25] and Kusube et al.,[26] other groups[37-41] have also developed similar methods for their detection. These methods differ in the type of electrode (porous graphite or glassy carbon) and chromatographic conditions used for vitamin K reduction and separation, respectively. Apart from their favorable sensitivities, a major reason for the popularity of electrofluorometric methods perhaps stems from the enhanced fluorometric selectivity for detecting the K vitamins in complex clinical and nutritional samples. In developing these and other purely ECD based detection systems, all groups have noted the problem of electrode passivation with consequent loss of sensitivity.

A post-column RD method for K vitamins employing a modified porous graphite electrochemical cell has also been developed. Instead of applying an electrochemical potential to reduce K vitamins, the reaction process is achieved with zinc metal coated onto the surface of a porous graphite electrode.[33] The principle of this method is based on the finding that the K group of vitamins can be reduced to their corresponding hydroquinones (KH_2) with zinc metal and in the presence of zinc ions.

$$Zn \rightarrow Zn^{2+} + 2e^- \tag{2}$$

$$\frac{K_1 + 2H^+ \rightarrow K_1H_2}{Zn + K_1 + 2H^+ \rightarrow Zn^{2+} + K_1H_2} \tag{3}$$

$$\tag{4}$$

The porous graphite electrode is initially modified by reducing zinc ions (added to the mobile phase) onto the surface of the electrode at an applied potential of -0.8 to -1.0 V. The E_o for zinc reduction is -0.762 V. In

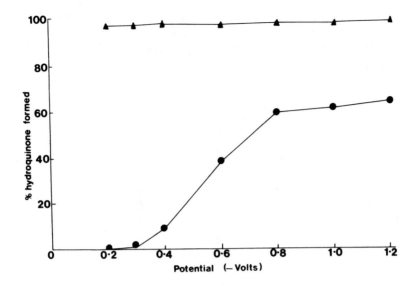

FIGURE 4.   Hydrodynamic voltammogram for K_1 after pre-column electrochemical reduction in the presence ($\blacktriangle — \blacktriangle$) and absence ($\bullet — \bullet$) of zinc metal. Chromatographic conditions: Microsorb C_8; mobile phase, 95% methanol containing aqueous zinc chloride (pH 3.3); 254 nm; flow-rate, 1.0 ml/min.

order to obtain reproducible reduction of K vitamins, it is necessary to apply a reduction potential for about 2 to 4 h such that sufficient zinc is deposited on the surface of the electrode. With electrodes modified in this manner and under anaerobic conditions, vitamin K reduction is possible over a wide range of potentials (0.0 to − 1.2 V). Reduction is also possible when the potentiostat is disconnected from the electrochemical cell.[34] Under these conditions, however, the reduction efficiency tends to decrease over a period of time (200 min) due to consumption of Zn metal during vitamin K reduction.[34] An advantage of Zn-modified electrodes lies in their greater efficiencies for vitamin K reduction compared to purely electrochemical reduction (Figure 4).

2. Solid-Phase Metal Containing Reactors

Although reductions of organic compounds by metals and metal catalysts have been used extensively in organic chemistry,[42,43] their history as post-column reactors in HPLC and vitamin K reduction is relatively recent.

Metal containing reactors are usually simple in design and easy to construct. In most cases, they consist of short stainless steel or glass columns (50 or 30 mm in length and 4.6 or 2.1 mm I.D.) which are packed with the relevant catalyst or metal.

At the present time, two types of metal containing post-column reactors have been developed for vitamin K reduction.[34,44,45] The systems developed by Haroon et al.[31,34,45] consist of columns packed with metallic zinc

(200-mesh) and is based on the reaction of vitamin K with zinc metal in the presence of zinc ions (Reaction 4). A second system developed by Shino[44] exploits the principles of classical catalytic hydrogenation with platinum oxide to achieve vitamin K reduction. During catalytic hydrogenation of K vitamins with platinum oxide, Shino observed that, in addition to hydroquinone formation, reduction of the isoprenoid double bond(s) of the K vitamins also occurred. For example, for K_1 which contains one double bond (C-2′,3′) in the first isoprene unit, catalytic hydrogenation leads to the formation of K_1 hydroquinone with the (C-2′,3′) double bond saturated [K_1 hydroquinone (I-H_2)]. For the MK series of K vitamins where different numbers and degrees of saturation of the isoprenoid units of the side chain are possible, mass spectral data[44] suggest total reduction of all the double bonds in the respective MKs with the formation of hydroquinones of MK-n (H_{2n}). In contrast, Haroon et al.[31,34] observed that the fluorescent product detected after reduction of K_1 by zinc metal was primarily K_1 hydroquinone. The experimental evidence for purely hydroquinone formation was obtained from two different sets of experiments. First, the zinc reducer column was placed in the pre-column mode (between the injector and the analytical column) and K_1 was reacted on-line with zinc metal. After separating the putative generated K_1 hydroquinone peak from the unreacted K_1, it was possible to show that the former had an identical retention time to authentic K_1 hydroquinone. In similar experiments with K_1 (I-H_2), it was found that the retention times of the hydroquinones of K_1 and K_1 (I-H_2) were different. In the second experiment, the putative K_1 hydroquinone peak was collected after chromatography. The K_1 hydroquinone was converted back to K_1 by air oxidation and reinjected into a chromatographic system which contained no zinc reducer column. After separation and UV detection, it was found that the injected compound eluted at the retention time of authentic K_1. This retention time was also different than that of authentic K_1 (I-H_2). These data suggest that the reduction of K_1 with zinc, leads only to the formation of K_1 hydroquinone with the (C-2′,3′) isoprenoid double bond intact (unsaturated).

During the characterization of the zinc reducer column, Haroon et al.[34] have also documented the efficiency of the reduction of phylloquinone by the post-column reactor. It was generally found that about 95% of the injected K_1 quinone could be reduced to the corresponding hydroquinone with mobile phase mixtures of aqueous-methanol containing about 10 mM zinc chloride. The low level of K_1 detected in these experiments is probably formed from the reoxidation of K_1 hydroquinone by oxygen present in the mobile phase. Oxygen is present in air-equilibrated methanol at 2.1 mM and in water at 0.27 mM.[46]

Although it is difficult to compare the reduction efficiencies between the Zn/Zn^{2+} system and the platinum oxide reactor because of the differing chromatographic systems employed, both Shino[44] and Haroon et al.[45] obtained similar minimum levels of detection (about 25 pg) for K_1. In comparing the

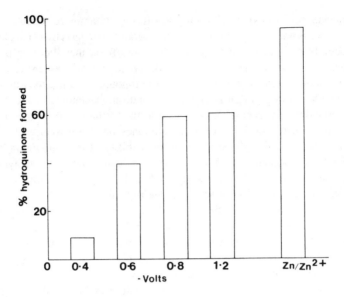

FIGURE 5. Comparison of electrochemical and chemical (Zn) reduction efficiencies for vitamin K_1. For conditions see Figure 4.

efficiencies for K_1 reduction between electroreduction and zinc reduction, Haroon et al.[31,34] found that the Zn/Zn^{2+} system was about 35% more efficient than electroreduction (Figure 5). This difference in reductive efficiencies is reflected in the lower minimum level of K_1 detected with the Zn/Zn^{2+} system (25 pg) compared to electroreduction (50 pg).

The optimal reaction time for both reduction systems (Zn/Zn^{2+} and platinum oxide catalyst) is short (5-20 s) and allows relatively high flow rates to be used without causing a large pressure drop in the reactor. Furthermore, reoxidation of the reduced compounds in the anaerobic conditions is not severe, so the signal does not decrease sharply beyond the optimal reaction time. Haroon et al.[34] have studied the effects of flow-rate on the reduction efficiency of phylloquinone with zinc metal. Flow-rates were varied between 0.5 to 2.0 ml/min to obtain the desired residence times (5 to 20 s) for K_1 in the post-column reactor. During these experiments no significant difference in the reduction efficiency was observed between the higher and lower residence times.

Both zinc metal and platinum oxide require activation prior to use. Shino[44] achieved an initial activation of the platinum oxide catalyst with hydrogen gas in tetrahydrofuran. A second activation step was required by sparging hydrogen gas through the mobile phase and HPLC system for 5 h before use. The activation of zinc metal was achieved *in situ* by passing the HPLC mobile phase containing zinc chloride over the metal for about 1 h. Maximum reduction efficiency was obtained between 1.0 to 10.0 mM zinc chloride.[34]

The precise function(s) of zinc chloride during vitamin K reduction with metallic zinc is not known. A survey of the literature suggests that zinc chloride is frequently used to remove zinc oxide layers from metallic zinc prior to reduction.[42] Layers of zinc oxide tend to deactivate metallic zinc surfaces and cause induction periods in reactions with compounds.[42] Zinc ions may also interact with vitamin K to form ion pairs in solution. Depending on the stability of the ion pairs, the process can also lead to the formation of triple ions. The formation of metal ion pairs of other quinones has been reported.[28] These metal ion pairs are thought to increase the stability of the quinone radical.[28] Stabilized phylloquinone radicals, if formed, can participate in hydrogen abstraction reactions which ultimately leads to hydroquinone formation via a disproportionation reaction of semiquinone radicals.

In the post-column reduction of phylloquinone by zinc, the methanol in the mobile phase serves as the hydrogen atom donor (HAD). When methanol is replaced by a solvent such as acetonitrile, which is not an HAD, hydro-quinone formation is not observed.[33] Since a carbon-hydrogen bond is broken during the abstraction reaction, its strength will influence the efficiency of the reaction. In this respect, isopropanol is a better HAD donor than methanol. Presumably this is a result of a weaker carbon-hydrogen bond.

In developing their respective assays for phylloquinone in biological samples, Haroon et al.[35] and Shino[44] also reported the separation and detection of menaquinones after post-column reduction with zinc metal and platinum oxide catalyst, respectively. Haroon et al.[35] found that a mixture of K_1 and MK-4 through -10 could be separated and detected by a gradient elution system in which the proportion of dichloromethane in methanol was increased linearly during the run. Shino[44] examined the isocratic elution and detection of K_1 and MK-3 through -10 after post-column reduction with platinum oxide catalyst; for MKs he found that there was a gradual decrease in the detection response with increasing side chain length. It is not known if the lower response factors for the more lipophilic MKs is due to the lower reduction efficiencies or to the different fluorometric properties of the hydroquinone forms generated. Decreased response for lipophilic MKs was also observed during gradient elution of MK-4 through -10. Under these conditions, fluo-rescence quenching due to increasing dichloromethane content may be a cause for low response factors for MK-7 through -10 (Figure 6).

3. Wet-Chemical Reactors

The earlier post-column reaction detection techniques which were de-veloped for the reduction of K vitamins employed open-tubular reactors and sodium borohydride[14,24,47] as the reductant. In these methods, the well-known reducing properties of sodium borohydride for quinones is exploited. When vitamin K is reduced with sodium borohydride or its derivatives (e.g., sodium cyanotrihydridoborate; $NaBH_3CN$), the reaction products are vitamin K hy-droquinone and alkali.[48] The major difficulty of using sodium borohydride

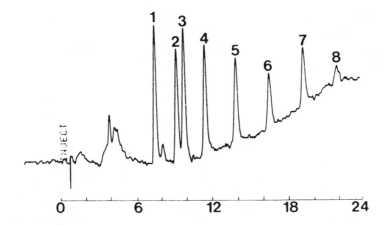

FIGURE 6. Separation of vitamin K compounds (200 pg each) by reversed-phase HPLC on Hypersil C_{18} by gradient elution. Chromatographic conditions: (A) 20% dichloromethane in methanol containing 10 mM zinc chloride; (B), 40% dichloromethane in methanol containing 10 mM zinc chloride and 0.1 M acetic acid-sodium acetate (pH 4.5); (linear gradient) 0 to 100% B in 20 min; (Ex) 248 nm; (Em) 420 nm; (flow-rate) 1.0 ml/min; (peaks) 1 = MK-4, 2 = MK-5, 3 = K_1, 4 through 8 = MK-6 to MK-10, respectively.

as the reductant is its incompatibility with chromatographic mobile phases. Sodium borohydride tends to decompose in methanolic or ethanolic eluents.[14,24] Additionally, mixing irregularities and air bubble formation in the detector did not encourage further development of this type of wet-chemical reactor until 1986. In fact, a general trend observed between 1979 to 1986 was a gradual change from UV modes of detection to ECD methods for the vitamin K group of quinones.

In order to overcome the technical difficulties associated with sodium borohydride-based post-column reactors, Lambert et al.[49-51] developed a post-column reactor employing tetramethylammonium octahydridotriborate, $[(CH_3)_4NB_3H_8]$. This reductant was found to be more stable than sodium borohydride in the methanolic and ethanolic eluents used for the separation of K vitamins. The reactor design was an open-tubular knitted coil of PTFE tubing (5 m × 0.5 mm I.D.) which contained a total volume of 950 μl. After separation, K vitamins are passed into the reactor into which the reductant $[(CH_3)_4NB_3H_8]$ dissolved in methanol is pumped. In their initial studies, Lambert et al.[49,50] employed a flow rate of 0.3 ml/min and a reductant concentration of 600 ng/ml. In the most recent version of this assay, Lambert et al.[51] combined the reductant with the chromatographic mobile phase, thus eliminating the requirement for a second pumping system.

A prerequisite for the reduction of vitamin K with $(CH_3)_4NB_3H_8$ is that the reactor temperature needs to be maintained at a high temperature (80°C);[49,50] indeed, it is this very dependence on a high reaction temperature that enabled the development of the simplified method in which the reductant is added to the mobile phase.[51] An even greater fluorometric response could be obtained by raising the temperature above 80°C or by using higher concentrations of reductant;[49] however, these conditions were found to be unsuitable practically, either because the increased temperature caused boiling of the mobile phase or because the higher reagent concentrations led to crystallization of $(CH_3)_4NB_3H_8$. These data suggest that the reduction of K_1 with $(CH_3)NB_3H_8$ is incomplete. It is quite possible that the reduction of K_1 with complex hydrides, such as $(CH_3)_4NB_3H_8$, may lead to the formation of other ring hydroxylated derivatives in addition to K_1 hydroquinone. For example, lithium aluminum hydride has been shown to reduce menadione (2-methyl-1,4-naphthoquinone) in yields of less than 10% to 1,2,3,4-tetrahydro-1,4-dihydroxy-2-methylnaphthalene and to 1,2,3,4-tetrahydro-4-hydroxy-1-keto-2-methylnaphthalene.[42] If similar products are indeed formed during the reduction of K_1 with $(CH_3)_4NB_3H_8$, then these hydroxylated derivatives may have different fluorometric properties to K_1 hydroquinone.

4. Photochemical Reactors

Although the concept of detecting K vitamins after photodegradation was originally explored by Lefevere et al.,[24] these methods have only recently been developed to any appreciable degree.

Two types of reaction detection methods for phylloquinone have been described using photochemical reactors. These are known as photoreduction fluorescence (PRF)[30] and photocatalytic chemiluminescence (PCCL).[52] The principle of PRF detection of phylloquinone is as follows. After chromatographic separation, phylloquinone is exposed to a UV light source as it passes through an open-tubular knitted/crocheted post-column (PTFE) reactor. During this process, the K_1 molecules are initially excited and then decay and undergo internal conversion to the lowest excited triplet state. It is generally accepted that the lowest triplet states participates in hydrogen abstraction reaction with an HAD (methanol from the mobile phase) leading to the formation of K_1 semiquinone and α-hydroxymethoxy radicals.[53-55] In the final step of this reaction sequence, two semiquinone radicals disproportionate to generate a molecule of K_1 hydroquinone and a molecule of the parent quinone. These reactions are summarized below:

$$Q + hv \rightarrow {}^1Q* \tag{5}$$

$$^1Q* \rightarrow {}^3Q* \tag{6}$$

$$^3Q* + CH_3OH \rightarrow {}^\circ CH_2OH + {}^\circ QH \tag{7}$$

$$^\circ CH_2OH + Q \rightarrow {}^\circ QH + CH_2O \tag{8}$$

$$(2{}^\circ CH_2OH \rightarrow CH_3OH + CH_2O) \tag{9}$$

$$(2°CH_2OH \rightarrow OHCH_2CH_2OH) \qquad (10)$$

$$2°QH \rightarrow Q + QH_2 \qquad (11)$$

Key: $Q = K_1$ quinone; $°QH = K_1$ semiquinone radical; $QH_2 = K_1$ hydroquinone.

Although these reaction schemes are shown with methanol as the HAD, isopropanol or ethanol can also function as HAD substrates. The above photoreduction reactions for K_1 only occur under anaerobic conditions. If oxygen is introduced after K_1 hydroquinone formation is complete, the K_1 hydroquinone will be oxidized to the parent quinone with the production of hydrogen peroxide. Although the major product of K_1 formed during photochemical reaction(s) appears to be K_1 hydroquinone the possibility of other products arising from cyclization and degradation of the phytyl side-chain cannot be excluded.[56] Among the products that can result from the photocyclization reaction of K_1 are a fluorescent naphthochromenol and other rearrangement products.[56-59]

In order to obtain the optimum fluorescence response for K_1 after photoreduction it was necessary to deoxygenate the mobile phase and the sample. In addition, to preserve the integrity of the photoproducts and improve reproducibility, the PTFE reactor needed to be cooled from the heat generated from the light source. A water-filled reactor housing was designed to obtain cooling by circulating ice-cold water around the reactor. The water was also deoxygenated to prevent permeation of oxygen into the reactor.[30]

The principles of PCCL[52] are similar to PRF, except that during PCCL detection the photoreactions are performed in the presence of oxygen. Under these conditions, oxygen reacts with K_1 semiquinones and ultimately leads to the formation of K_1 hydroperoxide (QOOH) and hydrogen peroxide.

$$°QH + O_2 \rightarrow °QOOH \qquad (12)$$

$$2°QOOH \rightarrow 2Q + H_2O_2 + O_2 \qquad (13)$$

As none of these products possesses chemiluminescence (CL), a second reaction is performed which leads to the production of CL. During this reaction, hydrogen peroxide is reacted with peroxyoxalate in the presence of fluorophores such as rubrene. This reaction ultimately leads to the generation of CL. The magnitude of CL is proportional to the hydrogen peroxide generated from K_1 quinone. Details of this CL reaction have been reviewed elsewhere.[60-62]

An interesting feature of PCCL is the catalytic nature of the photooxidation reaction. Since K_1 will cycle through the photooxidation reaction sequence many times during its residence in the photoreactor, each cycle producing hydrogen peroxide, the K_1 signal is "chemically amplified". This is in contrast to PRF where K_1 completes the photoreduction sequence only once.[30,52] In practice, however, a major difference between aerobic (PCCL) and anaerobic (PRF) reaction detection methods for phylloquinone, as developed to date, is the poor sensitivity of PCCL. For example, 25 pg of K_1 could be detected by PRF compared to 35 to 54 ng (depending on the length of the reactor) for PCCL methods.[30,52] This poor CL response toward K_1 may be due to the formation of nonproductive reactions. Products such as cyclic trioxanes and side-chain fragmentation resulting from oxidative cleavage of the C-2′,3′ double bond of the phytyl side-chain may not lead to hydrogen peroxide formation. Photoepoxidation of K_1 to K_1 epoxide may be another factor.[57] The fact that menadione could be detected with high sensitivity, suggests that photocyclization of the phytyl side-chain of K_1 may be a reason for its poor CL response.

C. REACTOR DESIGN, MINIMUM LEVELS OF DETECTION, AND FLUOROMETRIC EXCITATION WAVELENGTH CONSIDERATIONS

Key considerations in choosing the excitation wavelength during fluorometric detection of vitamin K hydroquinones are their spectral distribution and absorptivity over the range of lamp output and the potential for high backgrounds caused by high-absorbing impurities in the solvents. The general class of 2,3-disubstituted 1,4-naphthoquinones, to which K vitamins belong, exhibit a characteristic absorption spectrum with a pair of maxima in the region 240 to 250 nm due to the benzenoid contribution and a similar pair in the region 260 to 270 nm due to the quinonoid contribution. Upon vitamin K reduction, the quinonoid contribution is decreased with the appearance of an intense benzenoid contribution at 248 nm (Figure 7). These reduced forms of K vitamins have been shown to possess two characteristic excitation maxima at 248 and 335 nm.[33,44] This suggests that a low pressure mercury lamp which is a line source and has most of its energy concentrated in the 254-nm region would be an efficient source for K hydroquinone excitation. Unfortunately, most studies to date have used either deuterium or xenon lamps as excitation sources. It is possible that K_1 hydroquinone excitation with mercury lamps will excite different spectral bands to those excited by either deuterium or xenon lamps. This could lead to a greater fluorometric signal intensity, i.e., more photons may be absorbed by K hydroquinone at its strongest band. An added benefit of using a mercury lamp may be the gain in selectivity for detecting K vitamins in complex biological sources as compared to deuterium or xenon sources.

The emission profiles of deuterium lamps begin at about 220 nm and extend with relatively smooth intensity to wavelengths of about 300 nm. The xenon output ranges from between 250 and 600 nm. Both lamps are suitable for the detection of vitamin K and exploit either the 248 (deuterium) or 335 nm (xenon) excitation bands for K hydroquinones. At the present time, there

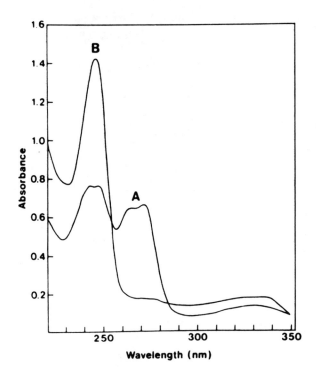

FIGURE 7. Ultraviolet absorption spectra of oxidized (A) and reduced (B) forms of phylloquinone.

is little information relating to the intensities and selectivities of the 248 and 335 nm excitation bands of K hydroquinones. Both excitation wavelengths have been used and similar minimum levels of detection (ca. 25 pg) reported (Table 1).

Apart from their obvious use for detection and quantitation, the two different fluorometric excitation maxima of K hydroquinone can be used as an aid to peak identification. The determination of ratios of the fluorometric response at different specific excitation wavelengths can provide a useful check of peak identification and purity. The application of these techniques as a diagnostic aid to establish peak identity and purity in the assay of phylloquinone and its epoxide metabolite (phylloquinone 2,3-epoxide) has been briefly discussed.[45]

Table 1 summarizes the minimum on-column limits of detection for phylloquinone. The lowest detectable amounts of K_1 were between 25 and 3000 pg depending on the reactor type and reductant. Although widely different chromatographic conditions and reaction schemes have been used, generally, it has been found that those based on photolysis or chemical reduction with platinum oxide catalyst or zinc metal have comparable sensitivities. The minimum amount of K_1 detected with these reactors is about 25 to 30 pg.

TABLE 1
Detection of K Vitamins in HPLC

Reaction scheme	Vitamin K	Reactor	Reagent	Detection limits (pg)	Ex/Em (nm)	Ref.
Chemical	K$_1$, MK-4	OTR[a]	NaBH$_3$	400	320/430	14
	K$_1$, MK-4 K$_1$O, MK-4 epoxide	OTR	NaHSO$_3$- HCl:	2000	320/430	71
			NaBH$_3$CN	3000		
	K$_1$, MK-4, MK-5 to -15	OTR	NaBH$_3$	50 —	320/430	47
	K$_1$	OTR	NaBH$_3$	150	320/420	13
	K$_1$, MK-4	OTR	TMAOB[b]	150	325/430	49
	K$_1$, K$_1$O, MK-4 to -10	Zn	ZnCl$_2$	25 —	248/418	45
	K$_1$, MK-3 to -5	PtO	H$_2$	25	254/430	44
	MK-7, MK-10	PtO	H$_2$	60 150	254/430	44
Electroreduction	K$_1$, K$_1$O	EC[c]	NaClO$_4$	25, 60, respectively	320/420	25
	MK-4, MK-5	EC	NaClO$_4$	NA	320/420	25
	K$_1$, MK-4	EC	NaClO$_4$	1000	330/430	26
	K$_1$	ECD (redox)	Acetate buffer	50	—	23
	K$_1$	ECD (redox)	PO$_4$ buffer	100	—	22
Photo-reduction	K$_1$	OTR	Vitamin C; acetate buffer	150	320/420	24
	K$_1$	OTR	None	30	244/370	30

[a] Open tubular reactors.
[b] Tetramethylammonium octahydridotriborate.
[c] Electrochemical.

Similar detection limits have been obtained by electroreduction followed by fluorometric detection (Table 1).

The open-tubular reactors which use sodium borohydride or its derivatives can detect amounts of K$_1$ down to about 150 pg. A reason for their inferior limit of detection, perhaps lies either in the inability to obtain quantitative reduction of K$_1$ or because of the formation of products other than K$_1$ hydroquinone, with different fluorometric properties.

From the point of view of tissue analyses of phylloquinone, an advantage of highly sensitive assays is that the sample requirement is considerably reduced. For example, using an assay with a detection limit of about 25 to

30 pg, as little as 250 μl of blood plasma or serum can be used to detect normal fasting levels of K_1 of about 500 pg/ml. Hand-in-hand with this improvement has come an increased complexity of the overall chromatographic system. It is, therefore, useful to discuss the advantages and disadvantages of the reactors currently employed for K detection.

Where large number of samples need to be processed, electrofluorometric reactors are perhaps the most difficult and time consuming to operate.[45] A major drawback of these reactors appear to be electrode passivation leading to poor reduction of K_1 and dramatic loss in sensitivity. Electrode passivation is thought to occur via metal and lipid deposits forming on the surface of the electrode.[8] Although electrode passivation by metals can be inhibited by the addition of 0.1 mM EDTA to the mobile phase, the reduction efficiencies eventually decrease to unacceptable levels. On occasions, it is possible to oxidize the metals off the generator electrode surface *in situ* by reversing the electrode polarity ("burn off"). Ultimately, the electrodes have to be removed from the system and washed with 2 M sodium hydroxide (to remove lipids) and with 6 M nitric acid (to remove metals).[8]

The electrochemical reduction of K_1 also suffers from poor reduction efficiencies. When extreme care is taken to remove oxygen from the mobile phase and sample, typical reduction efficiencies for K_1 hydroquinone formation of about 57 to 70% can be achieved.[31,34] Increased efficiency of reduction (95%) is, however, possible when the electrodes are modified by depositing metallic zinc on the surface. Because these zinc-modified electrodes can be operated at considerably lower negative potentials, they appear to be less susceptible to passivation by reduction of metal onto the electrode surface. Even these electrodes eventually fail. This failure is thought to occur, not so much by electrode passivation, but by the consumption of the deposited zinc metal by oxygen in the mobile phase.

$$Zn + O_2 + 2H^+ \rightarrow Zn^{2+} + H_2O_2 \tag{14}$$

$$Zn + H_2O_2 + 2H^+ \rightarrow Zn^{2+} + 2H_2O \tag{15}$$

The open-tubular reactors developed by Lambert et al.,[49-51] though a technical improvement over electroreduction methodologies, require between 1 and 2 ml of blood plasma to assay endogenous levels of K_1. The reduction reaction performed in these open-tubular reactors is carried out at 75 to 80°C. This requirement limits the use of this reactor to mobile phases with high boiling points. Such a limitation, though not particularly serious for measurements of phylloquinone, may present difficulties for the measurement of the more lipophilic menaquinones whose elution from ODS packings usually requires the addition to the mobile phase of nonpolar solvents with low boiling points. To date, the most versatile and relatively trouble-free reactors appear to be those based on metals (platinum oxide or zinc) and the photochemical systems. These reactors seem to reduce K_1 to one major product; the reduction reactions are quantitative allowing for low picogram levels of K_1 hydroquinone to be detected and are more compatible with the nonaqueous mobile phases which allow the most efficient separation and sample dissolution of K vitamins for reversed-phase systems. The platinum oxide catalytic reactor[44] is considerably more durable than reactors based on zinc metal.[31,34] Once the catalyst has been activated and packed into columns, Shino[44] reports a reactor-bed lifetime of up to a year under anaerobic conditions and provided no catalytic poisoning occurs. Under similar conditions, the maximum useful life of the zinc-reducer columns is about 7 d.[31] These columns tend to lose their K_1 reducing capacity long before most of the zinc metal is consumed. The mechanism of the decay in performance seems to be a result of zinc dissolution leading to voids and channeling in the reactor bed. To obtain maximum column life, it is necessary to insert a second zinc column between the injector and the analytical column to scavenge oxygen mainly from the mobile phase. Even under these highly anaerobic conditions, the formation of voids, particularly at the reactor inlet still persists. It is believed that reactor voiding is related to the inherent nature of the reaction of K_1 with metallic zinc, in addition to the dissolution of zinc by its reaction with oxygen. Evidence for the consumption of zinc during K_1 reduction has been obtained from off-line experiments. When K_1 was reacted with zinc metal in the presence of zinc ions, in methanol, it was found that for each mole of K_1 reacted, 1.2 mol of zinc ions was generated.[31]

As previously mentioned, the catalytic hydrogenation of K vitamins with platinum oxide also leads to the saturation of the phytyl-chain double bonds[44] in addition to K_1 hydroquinone formation. This reaction also generates heat, approximately 30 kcal/mol per double bond (hydrogenated).[42] For the reduction of the highly lipophilic MKs, it is possible that the heat of reaction may raise the temperature inside the reactor bed above the critical temperature of the components of the reaction mixture. When one or more components is volatilized, the reactor pressure will also increase. From the chromatographic point of view, high pressure drop in the system will lead to poor peak shape and may also be a cause for the development of voids and channeling in the reactor. If, in fact, volatilization of MKs does occur then peak dilution and/or tailing will be observed during subsequent fluorometric detection.

Although the practicality of performing high-sensitivity gradient elution for K vitamins has been demonstrated for the zinc containing post-column reactor (Figure 6), it is not known if the platinum oxide[44] or photolytic[30] reactors offer similar capabilities. The elegance of the photoreduction system lies in the fact that no reagents or metals are required for the formation of fluorescence derivatives of K_1. These photolytic reactors offer another dimension for the determination of chromatographic peak purities. As each analyte will exhibit a characteristic change in peak intensity when the photoreactor lamp is turned off, it is possible to obtain confirmation of the peak's identity. This "lamp on/off" approach has been used with considerable success in conjunction with photochemical reaction detection systems.[30]

As elucidated previously, a major concern in the fluorometric detection of vitamin K hydroquinones is to reduce oxygen to very low levels. Apart from oxidation of the hydroquinones to quinones, oxygen can also cause fluorescence "quenching". The presence of oxygen can lead to intersystem energy transfer from the excited state of the fluorophore resulting in decreased signal (quenching) through this nonradiative pathway.[63,64] As most open-tubular reactors are constructed with PTFE tubing which is permeable to oxygen, these reactors require to be isolated from oxygen. Various methods have been devised from simple sparging of the mobile phase to immersing the reactor in silicone-oil baths. A more useful strategy is to employ zinc oxygen-scrubber columns as described by MacCrehan and May.[65] These columns are inserted between the injector and analytical column and oxygen removal is obtained *in situ* (Reactions 14 and 15).

III. REACTION DETECTION METHODS FOR PHYLLOQUINONE 2,3-EPOXIDE

A. BACKGROUND

It is now 20 years since Matschiner and co-workers[66] discovered a major metabolite of phylloquinone, namely phylloquinone 2,3-epoxide (K_1O). This metabolite of vitamin K_1 was shown to accumulate in livers of warfarin treated rats[67] and Matschiner's group further proposed that the vitamin K-dependent step in the synthesis of clotting factors is linked to epoxidation of the vitamin.[68]

Further research has established that 4-hydroxycoumarin and indandione anticoagulants such as warfarin and phenindione interfere with the metabolism of vitamin K and inhibit one or more of the microsomal enzymes which first reduce K_1O to K_1 and then K_1 to the hydroquinone (K_1H_2). These reactions normally operate together as part of a metabolic cycle (the vitamin K-epoxide cycle), to supply the KH_2 required by the vitamin K-dependent carboxylase. This microsomal enzyme converts specific glutamate residues in proteins to γ-carboxyglutamic acid (Gla). The enzymology of the vitamin K-epoxide cycle is complex and has been reviewed elsewhere.[69]

In the past decade or so, both clinical and nutritional information for the parent K vitamers (K_1 and MKs) have been increased significantly through the development of HPLC assays capable of detecting the low levels of K vitamins present in biological samples. In contrast, knowledge of the metabolic fate of phylloquinone 2,3-epoxide in various situations has lagged behind that of the parent vitamin; limited information of the disposition and metabolism of the epoxide has derived either from studies which employed radio-labeled phylloquinone 2,3-epoxide or from experiments where large doses of K_1 have been administered in the presence of anticoagulant drugs.[70] Only recently have techniques become available which are capable of measuring the low physiological levels of K_1O in clinically important samples.

As previously described, the detection of low levels of K_1 has proved technically difficult. These difficulties are equally applicable to the measurement of its epoxide metabolite. Additionally, the levels of K_1O in plasma[45] (in the absence of anticoagulant therapy) are considerably lower than K_1 and, therefore, detection methods for K_1O need to be more sensitive and selective. The next section reviews post-column reaction methods for the detection of K_1O and also describes assay methodologies for the simultaneous measurement of K_1 and K_1O in blood plasma.

B. POST-COLUMN REDUCTION OF PHYLLOQUINONE 2,3-EPOXIDE

1. Detection of Standards

Several investigators have detected K_1O fluorometrically after post-column reduction; the methods include reduction with derivatives of sodium borohyhride/HCl mixtures,[71] electrochemical reduction[72] and reduction with zinc metal.[31,34,45] For the electrochemical reduction of K_1O, it was found necessary to modify commercially available detectors such that high negative potentials could be realized. This modification was made by Langenberg and Tjaden[72] by connecting the electrochemical cell to a simple polarograph. Under these conditions the fluorometric peak plateau for K_1O was obtained at -1.75 V. At this potential the response for K_1 was about 20% less than at -0.4 V. Although these data suggest different electrochemical properties for K_1O and K_1, Langenberg and Tjaden suggest that the chromatographic properties of the reduction product of K_1O was similar to that found during vitamin K_1 reduction.

Several years after the publication of Langenberg and Tjaden's manuscript,[72] Haroon et al.[34] made the observation that a fluorometric response for K_1O occurred possibly after reacting the epoxide with zinc metal and in the presence of zinc ions. This observation was initially made during the development of an electrofluorometric assay for K_1 employing zinc modified electrodes.[31] It was later shown that a similar reaction also occurred when the electrochemical cell was replaced with post-column reactors packed with zinc metal (Figure 8).

The currently available data suggest that K_1O is converted to K_1 (reaction 16) followed by a further reduction of the generated K_1 to form K_1 hydroquinone (Reaction 4).

$$K_1O + 2H^+ + 2e^- \longrightarrow K_1 + H_2O \qquad (16)$$

Evidence for this has come from collecting the fluorometric peak which represented K_1O and reinjecting the sample without removal of solvents. After chromatography followed by UV-detection (248 nm) three peaks are usually detected. Two of these peaks correspond to the capacity factors for K_1 and K_1 hydroquinone. The nature of the third peak which eluted at or about the

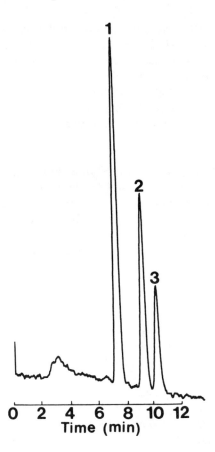

FIGURE 8. Separation of vitamin K compounds by reversed-phase HPLC. Chromatographic conditions: (Mobile phase) 20% dichloromethane in methanol containing 10 mM zinc chloride and 0.1 M acetic acid-sodium acetate (pH 4.5). For other conditions see Figure 6; (peaks) 1 = K_1O, 2 = K_1, 3 = $K_1(I-H_2)$.

column void-volume is not known. This peak is only partially resolved from K_1 hydroquinone and elutes as a broad band compared to K_1 and K_1 hydroquinone. Perhaps this peak represents an intermediate during the air oxidation of K_1 hydroquinone back to K_1. No K_1-epoxide was detected in these experiments. From the peak height ratios of K_1 and K_1 hydroquinone detected, it was found that about 71% of the injected K_1O was converted to K_1 hydroquinone. In other similar experiments when the K_1O peak was reinjected after removal of solvents and air oxidation of the products, a single peak corresponding to K_1 was detected. In the absence of ESR and EPR data these chromatographic results support the conclusion that K_1O is converted to K_1 when reduced with zinc metal/zinc ions.

In comparing the peak heights for equimolar amounts of K_1O and K_1 after reduction with zinc metal, it was found that the response factor for K_1O was considerably lower than that obtained for K_1 after zinc reduction.

Hiroshima et al.[71] have also reported on the fluorometric detection of epoxides of K_1 and MK-4. During these experiments the epoxides were reduced with an acidic mixture of sodium hydrogen sulfite and sodium cyanotrihydridoborate. The limits of detection for epoxides of K_1 and MK-4 achieved by Hiroshima et al.[71] in their open-tubular reactor was about 3 ng. Haroon et al.[45] and Langenberg and Tjaden[72] reported detection limits of about 25 to 60 pg for K_1O in their respective post-column detection systems (Table 1).

2. Assays For Phylloquinone and Phylloquinone 2,3-Epoxide in Plasma

The assay procedures that have been developed for the measurement of K_1O have relied to a great extent on previously developed sample preparation methodologies used for the assay of K_1. These procedures have been extensively reviewed elsewhere.[6-9]

It has been the experience of most investigators[45,72] that K_1O cannot be measured by a single column method. In order to increase the selectivity for the separation of impurities, multistage procedures similar to those used for K_1 assays have been developed for K_1O. A preliminary purification step was required to remove excessive quantities of polar lipids from initial extracts of serum. Both Langenberg and Tjaden[72] and Haroon et al.[45] used conventional low pressure chromatography on columns of silica to obtain bulk separation of nonpolar lipids from polar lipids (phospholipids, steroids, and triglycerides). Because most lipids in plasma samples are more polar than K_1 and K_1O, their early removal greatly reduces the amount of total lipids and preserves column life during subsequent HPLC steps (Figure 9). Hiroshima et al.[71] did not use a preliminary purification step but injected crude lipid extracts directly onto reversed-phase columns.

In addition to the conventional chromatographic step on silica, Haroon et al.[45] found it necessary to further fractionate the sample by semipreparative HPLC on columns of microparticulate silica. These silica columns were found to have sufficient loading capacities for the purification of serum extracts (obtained after conventional silica chromatography) in one injection. In order to avoid interference from fluorescent contaminants in the final reversed-phase stage of the assay, it was necessary to collect the least possible volume of eluent containing K_1, K_1O, and internal standard ($K_1[I-H_2]$) in the semipreparative stage of HPLC. Added to this was the importance of collecting all the internal standard which eluted at a different retention time to K_1 and K_1O (the HPLC system used K_1 and K_1O coeluted). To avoid these problems, a more useful recently developed approach is to replace the semipreparative HPLC step with conventional reversed-phase (C_{18}, type O.D. from Dupont) cartridges.

The highly retentive Zorbax-C_{18} type of packing material in these cartridges was found to be very useful for the resolution of vitamin K_1 compounds from other nonpolar plasma lipids. Another strategy to reduce sample prep-

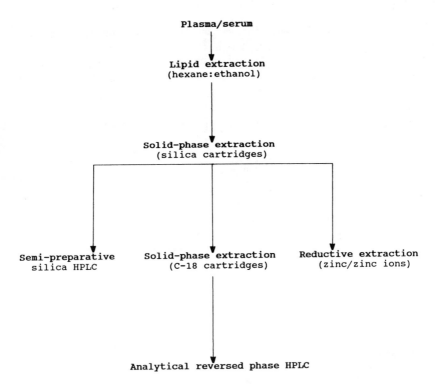

FIGURE 9. Flow diagram for assay procedures for phylloquinone and phylloquinone epoxide.

aration prior to HPLC is to employ a "reductive extraction procedure" (Figure 9). This procedure is only useful for the assays of vitamin K and is not suitable for K-epoxide assays.[45] This extraction method is based on the ability of zinc metal to convert K_1 to K_1 hydroquinone. Vitamin K_1 can be selectively extracted into acetonitrile after conversion to K_1 hydroquinone in acidic mixtures of hexane/acetonitrile containing zinc metal and zinc ions. When this procedure was applied to plasma samples it was found that about 97% of the nonpolar lipids obtained after solid-phase extraction (silica) remained behind in the hexane fraction and 70 to 80% of K_1 was recovered as K_1 hydroquinone in the acetonitrile fraction.

The final resolution of K_1, K_1O and the internal standard was achieved by reversed-phase HPLC. Langenberg and Tjaden[72] used semi-aqueous mobile phases of water and methanol whereas the author resolved K_1 and K_1O with mixtures of dichloromethane in methanol which also contained 10 mM zinc chloride. Figure 10 illustrates the high sensitivity detection of K_1O and K_1 in fasting pooled plasma which was found to contain as little as 50 pg/ml of K_1O and about 500 pg/ml of K_1. Another representative chromatogram of plasma from subjects on anticoagulant therapy is shown in Figure 11. In each case, the peaks of K_1, K_1O, and internal standard were well resolved from contaminating peaks.

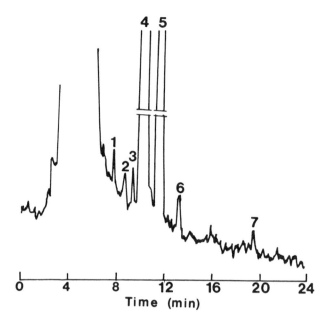

FIGURE 10.   Detection of phylloquinone epoxide (K_1O) and phylloquinone (K_1) in plasma in the absence of anticoagulant therapy. Chromatographic conditions: 17% dichloromethane in methanol containing 10 mM zinc chloride and 0.1 M acetic acid-sodium acetate (pH 4.5). For other chromatographic conditions see Figure 6. (Peaks) 1 = K_1O, 2,3 = unknowns, 4 = K_1, 5 = K_1(I-H_2), 6,7 = unknowns.

To detect endogenous plasma K_1O in the absence of any anticoagulant drugs it was necessary to process 4.0 ml of plasma and inject an equivalent of 3.0 ml on-column; to detect these compounds in plasma samples from anticoagulated subjects, only 0.25 to 0.5 ml of sample needed to be processed. In similar experiments, Langenberg and Tjaden[72] and Hiroshima et al.[71] found that it was not possible to detect plasma K_1O levels in the absence of anticoagulant therapy. Both groups, however, could detect K_1O in plasma from subjects treated with anticoagulant drugs.[71,72]

3. Quantitation and Validation

Because these assays for K_1O are based on multiple chromatographic steps it is essential to correct for any losses during the assay procedure. Both Langenberg and Tjaden[72] and the author used K_1(I-H_2) as internal standards. A theoretical objection of using this particular analogue of K_1 is that K_1(I-H_2) elutes close to the retention volume of MK-6. Recently, MK-6 has been detected in plasma,[44,73] depending on the mobile phase and other chromatographic conditions; it is possible that in some instances coelution and partial resolution of MK-6 and K_1(I-H_2) may occur. This is particularly important when small amounts (100 to 150 pg) of internal standard are added for the

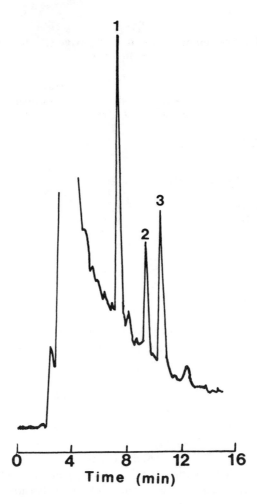

FIGURE 11. Detection of phylloquinone epoxide (K_1O) and phylloquinone (K_1) in the presence of anticoagulant therapy. For conditions see figure 10. peaks: $1 = K_1O$, $2 = K_1$, $3 = K_1(I\text{-}H_2)$.

measurement of fasting levels of K_1O in the absence of anticoagulant drugs. From the preliminary levels of K_1O reported here (Table 2) it is apparent that for the simultaneous measurement of K_1O and K_1 in plasma, it would be more useful to use two different internal standards to quantitate these compounds. The reason for this lies in the finding that K_1O levels in the absence of anticoagulant drugs were about ten times lower than K_1. Thus, for the quantitation of K_1, the amount of internal standard added to obtain similar peak heights for K_1 and internal standard is generally not suitable for the quantitation of the low levels of K_1epoxide (Figure 10).

TABLE 2
Phylloquinone (K₁) and K₁ Epoxide (K₁O) Levels
in Plasma

Plasma type	n	Mean (pg/ml)	Range (pg/ml)	Coefficient of variation (%)	Ratio K₁/K₁O
Fasting pool					
K₁ epoxide	5	50	—	25	
					0.11
K₁	12	460	—	10	
Anticoagulated individuals					
K₁ epoxide	45	1192	170–3520 (150–1200)[a]	—	
					2.30
K₁	45	520	80–3060	—	

[a]   Langenberg and Tjaden.[72]

The reproducibility of the assay for K_1O and K_1, (in plasma from anti-coagulated subjects) employing C_{18} cartridges and metallic zinc reactors was found to be 10 to 13%. For similar plasma samples, Langenberg and Tjaden[72] reported a coefficient of variation of 3.7% for K_1O in their electrofluorometric assay systems. The coefficient of variation for the measurement of K_1O in the absence of anticoagulation and employing zinc as the reductant was found to be 25% (Table 2). This reflects the difficulties in measuring the low picogram levels of K_1O at or about the limits of sensitivity of the method.

More recently, it has been possible to explore the possibility of measuring K_1O and K_1 in both normal (pooled, fasting) plasma and anticoagulated (individual) plasma samples. Preliminary experiments carried out by the author employed C_{18} cartridges for sample purification. The results are summarized in Table 2. Phylloquinone epoxide was quantitated with respect to K_1. Quantitation of K_1 was achieved with internal standardization with $K_1(I-H_2)$. These results are, therefore, considered to be only semiquantitative.

IV. SCOPE OF REACTION DETECTION TECHNIQUES FOR VITAMIN K COMPOUNDS

The last 5 years have seen a considerable increase in both clinical and nutritional knowledge of K vitamins. Perhaps the greatest impact of HPLC assays for vitamin K has been in the area of the pathogenesis of hemorrhagic disease of the newborn (see Chapters 11 and 12).

Chromatographic methods, in conjunction with more sensitive immunological techniques[41] for the detection of undercarboxylated prothrombin molecules is clarifying the pathogenesis of this particular disease and vitamin K prophylaxis. Though symptoms of vitamin K deficiency are often described in neonates the attribution of these symptoms to a nutritional and/or metabolic deficiency of vitamin K and/or enzymes of the vitamin K-epoxide cycle remains in dispute.[74,75] The assay methodologies for K_1 epoxide described here could be an aid for the assessment of vitamin K and K-epoxide metabolism in the neonates. Additionally, the K-epoxide assay may also be useful in pharmacological studies of drugs known to inhibit vitamin K-epoxide reductase. These include several second- and third-generation cephalosporins (containing N-methyl-thiotetrazole [NMTT])[76] and other drugs such as sulfaquinoxaline,[77] lapachol,[78] and salicylates[79] (see Chapter 13).

Information regarding tissue concentrations of menaquinones and their relationship to phylloquinone is also beginning to emerge.[44,73] From the chromatographer's point of view, perhaps the area of greatest challenge is to further improve the detection of K vitamins and their 2,3-epoxy derivatives. The development of new sample preparation methods and their automation for the isolation of K vitamins from complex biological matrices is also an inviting area.

One obvious way to increase sensitivity is to use narrow-bore HPLC columns in conjunction with miniaturized post-column reactors. For this type of system, solid-phase reactors appear to be the most promising. A distinct advantage of the miniaturization of solid-phase reactors would be the saving of expensive reagents; their compactness also makes temperature control and oxygen removal relatively simple.

A second way to improve sensitivity is to optimize the HPLC mobile phase for a particular reaction. For example, the addition of a better HAD than methanol, such as isopropanol may improve the detection of both K_1 and K_1O. Since a carbon-hydrogen bond is broken during the hydrogen abstraction reaction, its strength will influence the efficiency of the reaction. The strong solvent dependencies for the formation of K_1 hydroquinones during photochemical and zinc-dependent reduction reactions suggest that intermolecular hydrogen abstraction play a significant role in these reactions.

Although the detection of phylloquinone by PCCL has been shown to be inferior to UV-detection, the possibility of vitamin K-dependent phosphorescent detection remains largely unexplored. Detection of K vitamins by phosphoresces may be possible in conjunction with photochemical reactors. In these systems excited triplet states of K vitamin are formed. If chromatography is performed in mobile phases containing sodium dodecyl sulfate micelles, than it is possible to protect these triplet states.[28] Triplet states isolated in micelles can be exposed to reagent(s) that induce phosphorescence. Another such system that could be developed may employ triplet-state energy transfer from donor (excited tripletstate vitamin K) to an acceptor that readily phosphoresces. Both these reactions can utilize compounds that can serve as mobile phase additives and post-column reagents. An added advantage of phosphorescence detection is that conventional fluorometers can be used because these detectors do not differentiate between singlet- or triplet-state mediated photons.

As mentioned previously, assays for K vitamins and other fat-soluble vitamins require an immense degree of sample purification prior to HPLC. In this respect, the emerging field of super-critical fluid extraction (SFE) may prove to be a valuable aid.[80] The usefulness of SFE for extracting K_1 from powdered (i.e., dry) infant formula foods has recently been demonstrated.[81] The most important feature of this method would seem to be in the selective extraction of K_1 which enabled direct injection of lipid extracts onto reversed-phase columns, followed by electrochemical detection.[81] Whether this extraction selectivity can be applied to other biological samples with a high water content remains to be established.

ACKNOWLEDGMENTS

The author would like to express his gratitude to Hoffmann-La Roche Inc. for making this possible. Special thanks are owed to Mr. Edward H. Waysek and Dr. Ann G. Goetz also of Hoffmann-La Roche Inc., Nutley, New Jersey, U.S.A., for their lively interest and spiritual support. Finally, I would like to thank Ms. Barbara Pokrywa for the preparation of this manuscript.

REFERENCES

1. **Matschiner, J. T.,** Isolation and identification of vitamin K from animal tissue, in *The Biochemistry, Assay and Nutritional Value of Vitamin K and Related Compounds,* Association of Vitamin Chemists, Chicago, IL, 1971, 21.
2. **Matschiner, J. T., Taggart, W. V., and Amelotti, J. M.,** The vitamin K content of beef liver. Detection of a new form of vitamin K, *Biochemistry,* 6, 1243, 1967.
3. **Matschiner, J. T. and Taggart, W. V.,** Separation of vitamin K and associated lipids by reversed-phase column chromatography, *Anal. Biochem.,* 18, 88, 1967.
4. **Matschiner, J. T. and Amelotti, J. M.,** Characterization of vitamin K from bovine liver, *J. Lipid Res.,* 9, 176, 1968.
5. **Duello, T. J. and Matschiner, J. T.,** Characterization of vitamin K from pig liver and dog liver, *Arch. Biochem. Biophys.,* 144, 330, 1971.
6. **Shearer, M. J.,** High-performance liquid chromatography of K vitamins and their antagonists, *Adv. Chromatogr.,* 21, 243, 1983.
7. **Shearer, M. J.,** Assay of K vitamins in tissues by high-performance liquid chromatography with special reference to ultra-violet detection, in *Methods In Enzymology,* Vol. 123, part H, Chytil, F. and McCormick, D. B., Eds., Academic Press, Orlando, FL, 1986, 235.
8. **Shearer, M. J.,** Vitamins, in *HPLC of Small Molecules — A Practical Approach,* Lim, C. K., Ed., IRL Press, Oxford, 1986, 157.

9. **DeLeeheer, A. P., Nelis, H. J., Lambert, W. E., and Bauwens, R. M.,** Chromatography of fat-soluble vitamin in clinical chemistry, *J. Chromatogr.,* 429, 4, 1988.
10. **Shearer, M. J., Allan, V., Haroon, Y., and Barkhan, P.,** Nutritional aspects of vitamin K in the human, in *Vitamin K Metabolism and Vitamin K-Dependent Proteins,* Suttie, J. W., Ed., University Park Press, Baltimore, 1980, 317.
11. **Haroon, Y., Shearer, M. J., McEnery, G., Allan, V. E., and Barkhan, P.,** Assay of vitamin K_1 (phylloquinone) by high-performance liquid chromatography: values for human milk and cow's milk, *Proc. Nutr. Soc.,* 29, 49A, 1980.
12. **Thompson, J. N., Hatina, G., and Maxwell, W. B.,** Determination of vitamin E and K in food and tissues using high-performance liquid chromatography, in *Trace Organic Analysis: a New Frontier in Analytical Chemistry,* Special Publication 519, National Bureau of Standards, Gaithersburg, 1979, 279.
13. **Lefevere, M. F., DeLeeneer, A. P., and Claeys, A. E.,** High-performance liquid chromatographic assay of vitamin K in human serum, *J. Chromatogr.,* 186, 749, 1979.
14. **Abe, K., Hiroshima, O., Ishibashi, K., Ohmae, M., Kawabe, K., and Katsui, G.,** Fluorometric detection of phylloquinone and menaquinone-4 in biological materials using high-performance liquid chromatography, *Yakugaku Zasshi,* 99, 192, 1979.
15. **Ikenoya, S., Abe, K., Tsuda, T., Yamano, Y., Hiroshima, O., Ohmea, M., and Kawabe, K.,** Electrochemical detector for high-performance liquid chromatography, *Chem. Pharm. Bull.,* 27, 1237, 1979.
16. **Haroon, Y., Shearer, M. J., Rahim, S., Gunn, W. G., McEnery, G., and Barkhan, P.,** The content of phylloquinone (vitamin K_1) in human milk, cow's milk and infant formula foods determined by high-performance liquid chromatography, *J. Nutr.,* 112, 1105, 1982.
17. **Shearer, M. J., Rahim, S., Barkhan, P., and Stimmler, L.,** Plasma vitamin K_1 in mothers and their newborn babies, *Lancet,* ii, 460, 1982.
18. **Lefevere, M. F., DeLeeneer, A. P., Claeys, A. E., Claeys, I. V., and Steyaert, H.,** Multidimensional liquid chromatography: a breakthrough in the assessment of physiological vitamin K levels. *J. Lipid Res.,* 23, 1068, 1982.
19. **Haroon, Y. and Hauschka, P. V.,** Application of high-performance liquid chromatography to assay phylloquinone (vitamin K_1) in rat liver, *J. Lipid Res.,* 24, 481, 1983.
20. **Ueno, T. and Suttie, J. W.,** High-pressure liquid chromatographic-electrochemical detection analysis of serum *trans*-phylloquinone, *Anal. Biochem.,* 133, 62, 1983.
21. **Hart, J. P., Shearer, M. J., McCarthy, P. T., and Rahim, S.,** Voltammetric behavior of phylloquinone (vitamin K_1) at a glassy carbon electrode, and determination of the vitamin in plasma using high-performance liquid chromatography with electrochemical detection, *Analyst,* 109, 477, 1984.
22. **Haroon, Y., Schubert, C. A. W., and Hauschka, P. V.,** Liquid chromatographic dual electrode detection system for vitamin K compounds, *J. Chromatogr., Sci.,* 22, 86, 1984.
23. **Hart, J. P., Shearer, M. J., and McCarthy, P. T.,** Enhanced sensitivity for the determination of endogenous phylloquinone (vitamin K_1) in plasma using high-performance liquid chromatography with dual-electrode electrochemical detection, *Analyst,* 110, 1181, 1984.
24. **Lefevere, M. F., Frei, R. W., Scholton, A. H., and Brinkman, U. A.,** Photochemical reaction detection of phylloquinone and menaquinones. A comparison with chemical post-column reduction for fluorescence detection, *Chromatographia,* 17, 125, 1983.
25. **Langenberg, J. P. and Tjaden, U. R.,** Determination of (endogenous) vitamin K_1 in plasma by reversed-phase liquid chromatography using fluorometric detection after post-column electrochemical reduction. Comparison with ultraviolet, single and dual electrochemical detection, *J. Chromatogr.,* 305, 61, 1984.
26. **Kusube, K., Abe, K., Hiroshima, O., Ishiguro, Y., Ishikawa, S., and Hoshida, H.,** Determination of vitamin K by high performance chromatography with electrochemical derivatization, *Chem. Pharm. Bull.,* 32, 179, 1984.

27. **Von Kries, R., Shearer, M. J., McCarthy, P. T., Haug, G., Harzer, G., and Göbel, U.**, Vitamin K_1 content of maternal milk: Influence of stage of lactation, lipid composition, and vitamin K_1 supplements given to the mother, *Pediatr., Res.,* 22, 513, 1987.

28. **Chambers, J. Q.**, Electrochemistry of quinones, in *Chemistry of Quinonoid Compounds,* Vol. 2, Patai, S. and Rappoport, Z., Eds., John Wiley & Sons, New York, 1988, chap. 12.

29. **Frei, R. W.**, Reaction detection in liquid chromatography, in *Chemical Derivatization in Analytical Chemistry,* Vol. 1, Frei, R. W. and Lawrence, J. F., Eds., Plenum, New York, 1981.

30. **Poulsen, J. R. and Birks, J. W.**, Photoreduction fluorescence detection of quinones in high-performance liquid chromatography, *Anal. Chem.,* 61, 2267, 1989.

31. **Haroon, Y., Bacon, D. S., and Sadowski, J. A.**, Reduction of quinones with zinc metal in the presence of zinc ions: application of post-column reactor for the fluorometric detection of vitamin K compounds, *Biomed. Chromatogr.,* 2, 4, 1987.

32. **Murov, S. L., Ed.,** *Handbook of Photochemistry,* Marcel Dekker, New York, 1973.

33. **Haroon, Y.,** unpublished data, 1987.

34. **Haroon, Y., Bacon, D. S., and Sadowski, J. A.**, Chemical reduction system for the detection of phylloquinone (vitamin K_1) and menaquinones (vitamin K_2), *J. Chromatogr.,* 384, 383, 1987.

35. **Haroon, Y., Shearer, M. J., and Barkhan, P.**, Resolution of phylloquinone (vitamin K_1), phylloquinone 2,3-epoxide, 2-chlorophylloquinone and their geometric isomers by high-performance liquid chromatography, *J. Chromatogr.,* 200, 293, 1980.

36. **Haroon, Y., Shearer, M. J., and Barkhan, P.**, Resolution of menaquinones (vitamins K_2) by high-performance liquid chromatography, *J. Chromatogr.,* 206, 333, 1981.

37. **Mummah-Schendel, L. L. and Suttie, J. W.**, Serum phylloquinone concentrations in a normal adult population, *Am. J. Clin. Nutr.,* 44, 686, 1986.

38. **van Haard, P. M. M., Engel, R., and Pietersma-de Bruyn, A. L. J. M.**, Quantitation of trans-vitamin K_1 in serum samples by off-line multidimensional liquid chromatography, *Clin. Chim. Acta,* 157, 221, 1986.

39. **Hirauchi, K., Sakano, T., and Morimoto, A.**, Measurement of vitamin K in human and animal plasma by high-performance liquid chromatography with fluorometric detection, *Chem. Pharm. Bull.,* 34, 845, 1986.

40. **Guillaumont, M., Leclercq, M., Gosselet, H., Makala, K., and Vignal, B.**, HPLC determination of serum vitamin K_1 by fluorometric detection after post-column electrochemical detection, *J. Micronutr. Anal.,* 4, 285, 1988.

41. **Pietersma-de Bruyn, A. L. J. M., van Haard, P. M. M., Beunis, M. H., Hamulyák, K., and Kuijpers, J. C.**, Vitamin K_1 levels and coagulation factors in healthy newborns till 4 weeks after birth, *Haemostasis,* 20, 8, 1990.

42. **Hudlicky, P.,** *Reductions in Organic Chemistry,* Ellis Horwood, 1894, 1–218.

43. **Rylander, P. N.,** *Hydrogenation Methods,* Academic Press, New York, 1985, 1–157.

44. **Shino, M.**, Determination of endogenous vitamin K (phylloquinone and menaquinone-n) in plasma by high-performance liquid chromatography using platinum oxide catalyst reduction and fluorescence detection, *Analyst,* 113, 393, 1988.

45. **Haroon, Y., Bacon, D. S., and Sadowski, J. A.**, Liquid chromatographic determination of vitamin K_1 in plasma, with fluorometric detection, *Clin. Chem.,* 32, 1925, 1986.

46. **Turro, N. J.,** in *Modern Molecular Photochemistry,* Benjamin, A. W., Ed., New York, 1981, 362–408.

47. **Sakano, T., Nagaoka, T., Moromoto, A., and Hirauchi, K.**, Measurement of K vitamins in human and animal feces by high-performance liquid chromatography with fluorometric detection, *Chem. Pharm. Bull.,* 34, 4322, 1986.

48. **Dunphy, P. J. and Brodie, A. F.**, The structure and function of quinones in respiratory metabolism, in *Methods in Enzymology,* Vol. 18, Part C, McCormick, D. B., and Wright, L. D., Eds., Academic Press, New York, 1971, 407.

49. **Lambert, W. E., DeLeeneer, A. P., and Lefevere, M. F.,** Determination of vitamin K in serum using HPLC with post-column reaction and fluorescence detection, *J. Chromatogr. Sci.,* 24, 78, 1986.

50. **Lambert, W. E., DeLeeneer, A. P., and Baert, E. J.,** Wet-chemical postcolumn reaction and fluorescence detection analysis of the reference interval of endogenous serum vitamin $K_{1(20)}$, *Anal. Biochem.,* 158, 257, 1986.

51. **Lambert, W., De Leeheer, A., Tassaneeyakul, W., and Widdershoven, J.,** Study of vitamin $K_{1(20)}$ in the newborn by HPLC with wet-chemical reduction and fluorescence detection, in *Current Advances in Vitamin K Research,* Suttie, J. W., Ed., Elsevier, New York, 1988, 509.

52. **Poulsen, J. R. and Birks, J. W.,** Photocatalytic chemiluminescence detection of quinones on high-performance liquid chromatography, *Anal. Chem.,* 62, 1242, 1990.

53. **Carlson, S. A. and Hercules, D. M.,** Delayed thermal fluorescence of anthroquinone in solution, *J. Am. Chem. Soc.,* 93, 5611, 1971.

54. **Lamola, A. A. and Hammond, G. S.,** Mechanisms of photochemical reaction in solution. XXXIII. Intersystem crossing efficiencies, *J. Chem. Phys.,* 43, 2129, 1971.

55. **Hamanoue, H., Kajiwara, Y., Miyake, T., Nakayama, T., Hirase, S., and Teranishi, H.,** Solvents effects on the nonradiative relaxation of processes of the lowest excited singlet of meso-substituted bromoanthrancenes, *Chem. Phys. Lett.,* 94, 276, 1983.

56. **Leary, G. and Porter, G.,** The phytochemistry of two phytyl quinones: alpha-tocopherylquinone and vitamin K_1, *J. Chem. Soc. A,* 92, 2273, 1970.

57. **Snyder, C. D. and Rapoport, G.,** Photooxydation of phylloquinone and menaquinones, *J. Am. Chem. Soc.,* 91, 731, 1969.

58. **Wilson, R. M., Walsh, T. F., and Gee, S. K.,** Laser photochemistry: the wavelength dependent oxidative photodegradation of K vitamin analogs, *Tetrahedron Lett.,* 21, 3459, 1980.

59. **Vire, J. C., Patriarche, G. J., and Christian, G. D.,** Electrochemical study of the degradation of vitamin K_3 and vitamin K_3 bisulfite, *Anal. Chem.,* 51, 752, 1979.

60. **van Zoonen, P., Kamminga, D. A., Gooijer, C., Velthorst, N. H., and Frei, P. W.,** Quenched peroxyoxalate chemiluminescence as a new detection principle in flow injection analysis and liquid chromatography, *Anal. Chem.,* 58, 1245, 1986.

61. **Birks, J. W. and Frei, R. W.,** Photochemical reaction detection in HPLC, *Trends in Anal. Chem.,* 1, 361, 1982.

62. **Poulsen, J. R. and Birks, J. W.,** in *Chemilumenescence and Photochemical Reaction Detection in Chromatography,* Birks, J. W., Ed., VCH Publishers, New York, 1989, 149–230.

63. **Underfriend, S. L.,** *Fluorescence Assays in Biology and Medicine,* Academic Press, New York, 1962.

64. **Krull, I. S.,** in *Reaction Detection in Liquid Chromatography,* Krull, I. S., Ed., Marcel Dekker, New York, 1986, 303–352.

65. **MacCrehan, W. A. and May, W. E.,** Oxygen removal in liquid chromatography with zinc oxygen-scrubber column, *Anal. Chem.,* 56, 625, 1984.

66. **Matschiner, J. T., Bell, R. G., Amelotti, J. M., and Knauer, T. E.,** Isolation and characterization of a new metabolite of phylloquinone in the rat. *Biochim. Biophys. Acta,* 201, 309, 1970.

67. **Bell, R. G. and Matschiner, J. T.,** Vitamin K activity of phylloquinone oxide, *Arch. Biochem. Biophys.,* 141, 473, 1970.

68. **Willingham, A. K. and Matschiner, J. T.,** Changes in phylloquinone epoxidase activity related to prothrombin synthesis and microsomal clotting activity in the rat, *Biochem. J.,* 140, 435, 1974.

69. **Suttie, J. W.,** Recent advances in the hepatic vitamin K metabolism and function, *Hepatology,* 7, 367, 1987.

70. **Shearer, M. J., McBurney, A., and Barkhan, P.,** Studies on the absorption and metabolism of phylloquinone (vitamin K$_1$) in man, *Vitam. Horm.,* 32, 513, 1974.

71. **Hiroshima, O., Abe, K., Ikenota, S., Ohmae, M., and Kawabe, K.,** Determination of phylloquinone-2,3-epoxide and menaquinone-4 2,3-epoxide in biological materials by highperformance liquid chromatography and fluorometric reaction detection, *Yakugaku Zasshi,* 99, 1007, 1979.

72. **Langenberg, J. P. and Tjaden, U. R.,** Improved method for the determination of vitamin K$_1$ epoxide in human plasma with electrofluorimetric reaction detection, *J. Chromatogr.,* 289, 377, 1984.

73. **Shearer, M. J., McCarthy, P. T., Compton, O. E., and Mattock, M. B.,** The assessment of human vitamin K status from tissue measurements, in *Current Advances in Vitamin K Research,* Suttie, J. W., Ed., Elsevier, New York, 1988, 437.

74. **Kries, R. V., Shearer, M. J., and Göbel, U.,** Vitamin K in infancy, *Eur. J. Pediatr.,* 147, 106, 1988.

75. **Guillaumont, M., Sann, L., Leclercq, M., Dostalova, L., Vignal, B., and Frederich, A.,** Changes in the hepatic vitamin K$_1$ after prophylactic administration to the new-born, *Am. J. Clin. Nutr.,* 1990.

76. **Shearer, M. J., Bechtold, H., Andrassy, K., Koderisch, J., McCarthy, P. T., Trenk, D., Jähnchen, E., and Ritz, E.,** Mechanism of cephalosporin-induced hypoprothrombinemia: relation to cephalosporin side chain, vitamin K metabolism and vitamin K status, *J. Clin. Pharmacol.,* 28, 88, 1988.

77. **Preusch, P. C., Hazelett, S. E., and Lemasters, K. K.,** Sulphaquinoxaline inhibition of vitamin K quinone reductase, *Arch. Biochem. Biophys.,* 269, 18, 1989.

78. **Preusch, P. C. and Suttie, J. W.,** Lapachol inhibition of vitamin K epoxide reductase and vitamin K quinone reductase, *Arch. Biochem. Biophys.,* 234, 405, 1984.

79. **Creedon, K. A. and Suttie, J. W.,** Effect of N-methyl-thiotetrazole on vitamin K epoxide reductase, *Thrombos. Res.,* 44, 147, 1986.

80. **Hawthorne, S. B.,** Analytical-scale supercritical fluid extraction, *Anal. Chem.,* 62, 633A, 1990.

81. **Schneiderman, M. A., Sharma, A. K., Mahanama, K. R. R. and Locke, D. C.,** Determination of vitamin K$_1$ in powdered infant formulas, using supercritical fluid extraction and liquid chromatography with electrochemical detection, *J. Assoc. Off. Anal. Chem.,* 71, 815, 1988.

Chapter 4

ADVANCES IN THE ASSESSMENT OF ACTIVATION STATES OF FACTOR VII IN HYPERCOAGULABLE STATE: SOME EPIDEMIOLOGICAL ASPECTS AND LABORATORY APPROACHES FOR ASSAYS OF FACTOR VII AND TISSUE FACTOR PATHWAY INHIBITOR

M. J. Seghatchian

TABLE OF CONTENTS

I. INTRODUCTION

There is extensive epidemiological evidence supported by laboratory findings suggesting that elevated factor (F)VII is associated with hypercoagulability related to thrombogenesis. Since native clotting factors are mostly present in considerable excess concentration in circulation to produce thrombin, a high concentration of native FVII *per se* is unlikely to be the cause of thrombogenesis. This is despite the laboratory findings which show that a high concentration of FVII is associated with a higher rate of thrombin generation *in vitro*. Instead the changes in the activation of FVII and/or formation of intermediate complexes (such as ternary and quarternary complexes VIIa-TF-IXa, VIIa-PL-IXa-VIII), which dramatically enhance the rate of thrombin generation, are considered to be more likely candidates for FVII-induced thrombogenesis or ischemic heart predisposition.[1-3]

The underlying mechanisms involved in triggering of a prethrombotic state still remains a major scientific challenge requiring a broad spectrum of assays for a better characterization of its components and the determination of the activation state of each of the components involved. In this respect, there has been a resurgence of interest to characterize the activation states of FVII and to develop assays for the quantative estimation of various forms of FVII as well as assays of the specific inhibitor of extrinsic tissue factor pathway inhibitor (EPI).

In this manuscript, after a brief review of epidemiological aspects of elevated factor VII levels associated with ischemic heart disease (IHD) predisposition, some of the preliminary works on the characterization of activation states of FVII, using new generation assay procedures are described. Two new chromogenic procedures consisting of a modified two-stage chromogenic assay for the assessment of FVII concentrations and one-stage chromogenic assay which differentiates FVIIa from native FVII on the basis of shortening the lag phase of activation (rate of FXa generation) and nonparallelism in biometrical assays are described and the results obtained on the same sets of samples are compared with the results of clotting and tritiated FX assay of FVII. Finally, the characteristic properties of assays for the extrinsic pathway inhibitor are briefly summarized.

II. EPIDEMIOLOGICAL ASPECTS RELATED TO ELEVATED FACTOR VII AND ISCHEMIC HEART DISEASE PREDISPOSITION

In a series of epidemiological studies Meade et al.[1-3] indicated a strong relationship between hypercoagulability as defined by an elevated FVII and the outcome of thrombogenesis in IHD. Thus the higher the FVII activity, in prospective studies, the higher the risk of dying from IHD. Furthermore, the cause and effect relationship, in the same group, revealed that high FVII activity is found with increasing age, with increasing obesity, with increasing use of oral contraceptives, after the menopause and in diabetes.[4] On the other hand, FVII levels is low in black populations (compared with white populations) and in vegetarians. These findings are consistent with the lower incidence of IHD in the black population of the U.K. than in the white population and in vegetarians than nonvegetarians.[5]

More importantly, the results of recent randomized controlled trials (e.g., Dutch Sixty-Plus Reinfarction Study) have provided useful information of the pathogenesis of myocardial infarction and its clinical management. The collective results of these trials, indicated a 20% reduction in mortality. Furthermore, substantial benefit, in terms of the prevention of reinfarction and other thromboembolic episodes was shown in patients in whom proportionate reductions in vitamin K-dependent clotting factors attributable to oral anticoagulant therapy were more than 50%.[5] This striking result on the secondary prevention of IHD strongly supports the view that FVII is involved in its onset.[5]

In the laboratory too, evidence has been obtained that the increase in FVII activity in plasma during cold activation is very closely related to the level of thrombin activity.[6] These results clearly suggest that hypercoagulability should no longer be viewed simply as a concept but is a real phenomenon based on evidence in terms of changes in the activation states FVII activity.[6]

The study was based on the dietary fat hypothesis, particularly that the intake of saturated fat leads to high blood cholesterol levels and in turn the promotion of atherosclerosis can also be interpreted by the elevated or changed activation states of FVII.[7] The dietary influences on coagulation may, nevertheless, be operating through contactase[6,7] (with chylomicrons and very low density as the source of a negatively charged surface) and the elevated intrinsic/extrinsic tenase leading to a burst of thrombin generation.[8]

On the basis of collective evidence Meade[5] suggests that IHD is best defined as an over reactivity of the procoagulatory system, whereas hypercoagulability, leading to various thrombogeneses, is manifested predominantly as an under reactivity of the natural anticoagulant-inhibitory system (i.e., protein C, protein S, AT III).

A. EXPERIMENTAL EVIDENCE FOR CHANGES IN FACTOR VII ACTIVATION STATES

Several properties of FVII strengthen the view that a change in the activation state of FVII is the most likely cause in the induced hypercoagulability. These are briefly summarized here:

1. The importance of FVII in hypercoagulability is evident by virtue of its molecular nature, as (unlike other clotting factors) it circulates in a partially active form.
2. The native molecule is easily activated by tissue factor (TF).
3. FVII interconnects the intrinsic and other pathways at an earlier stage than tenase complexes (XII and IXa can activate VII and vice versa).[8]
4. A rise in other procoagulant factors (II, IX, X) and proteins S, Z, and M increases the coagulant activity of factor VII, due to the conversion of native FVII (single chain) to α-VIIa (double chain form); this results in a 100-fold increase in the procoagulant activity.
5. FVIIa activity is inhibited slowly in plasma making it a useful marker of procoagulant potential.
6. Native VII competes with VIIa for its specific inhibitor allowing VIIa to perform its procoagulant function.

Several other lines of recent experimental evidence have strengthened the view that hypercoagulability due to FVII is more likely to be associated with an activation of the molecule rather than simply an increase in its synthesis. These are briefly summarized below:

1. Phospholipase C-Sensitive Form of Factor VII

Based on a study in a small group of subjects (age 40), Dalakar et al.[9] reported that the increased level of FVII procoagulant activity (approximately 16%), in the risk group, was apparently due to an increase of phospholipase C-sensitive form of FVII in their plasma. We have confirmed their findings and additionally shown that where hypercoagulability is associated with increased levels of both FVII and FVIII clotting activity (VII:C & VIII:C) phospholipase also reduced FVIII:C to normal values (Seghatchian and Stirling unpublished observation).

2. Thrombin-Like and Kallikrein-Like Activities of Plasma

Plasma contains significant amounts of proteases in complexes which are easily determined by chromogenic assay. On the basis of low grade proteolytic enzyme activity of plasma[10,11] and cold activation[6] we have obtained experimental evidence that elevated VIII:C or VII:C might be related to the formation of a ternary or quarternary circulating complexes in which phospholipid or apoprotein may play a major role in protecting the enzyme from plasmatic proteolytic inhibitors. Nevertheless, the true proof for a hypercoagulable state would be if we were able to directly measure thrombin production in the circulation and show that the amount produced was proportional to the degree of hypercoagulability. It is still debatable whether thrombin is produced continuously at below threshold concentrations or only locally in certain conditions. When thrombin is generated, however, it is rapidly mopped up by endothelial cells; there are also more than 25 substrates for thrombin in circulatory blood.[11]

Meade et al[12] showed that despite its very short half-life (3 min) the presence of circulating fibrinopeptide A (FPA) provides unequivocal evidence of myocardial infarction, provided blood samples were taken within a relatively short time of the onset of chest pain. FPA was found to be much higher in post-mortem blood from those who had died suddenly of IHD compared with those who died suddenly from other reasons. This is further corroborated by the observation that elevated FVII correlated with the FPA level in the Northwick Park Heart Study. The cold activation of FVII, following exposure of plasma for 4 h at 4°C is another example of parallel increase in FVII and thrombin as measured by FPA.[6]

In a collaborative study with Northwick Park, the author found that although the elevated patterns of low-grade proteolytic enzymes of plasma thrombin-like activity (TLA) and FPA were found to follow the same trend in paired sample analysis, thrombin-like enzymes did not correlate with FPA despite the good correlation of TLA with FVII and the elevated FVIII activities (unpublished observation). Nevertheless, this simple screening procedure is useful in assessing hypercoagulability in various pathophysiological states.

3. Parallel Decrease/Increase in Vitamin K, Factor VII, Cholesterol in Dietary Study

It has been indicated[7,13] that increased levels of FVII:C correlates with the fat content of diet, by influencing triglyceride and the very low-density lipoprotein (LDL) concentrations of plasma. This hyperactivity could be associated with either FVII activation or increased in total levels of VII:C or both. The interaction of vitamin K-dependent proteins with LDL is associated with complex formation having different charge properties and different functional activity. In collaboration with colleagues at Northwick Park Hospitals, Shearer and Seghatchian have evaluated the vitamin K levels of some individuals who were involved in the dietary fat experiments.[7] Parallel increase and decreases in FVII, and LDL and vitamin K were observed in the same subjects (unpublished observation). These preliminary results suggest the possibility that changes in FVII may, at least, be partially influenced by the different individual, either by affecting the rate of synthesis of FVII or its rate of clearance.

Nevertheless it is not possible to ignore the view that lipids may contribute to FVII activation by inducing a conformational change in the FVII molecule. Alternatively, the triglycerides may affect the clearance rate of FVII (i.e., prolonging its short half-life) which would account for the observed individual variation seen in these types of studies.

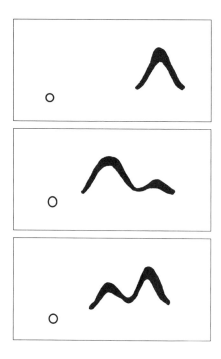

FIGURE 1. Crossed immunoelectrophoresis of purified apoprotein B (low-density lipoprotein), alone (top), and after 30 min incubation with purified factor VII containing factor X (middle), and the same following activation with factor Xa generated by Russell's Viper Venom (bottom) at the same concentration (20 µg/ml). The first dimension electrophoresis (3 h, 30 V/cm) was carried out in 1% agarose (A37) in Veronal buffer at pH 8.6 and I = 0.02. The second dimension was performed using anti-APO B, overnight at 3.5 V/cm. Note the appearance of double peaks of apoprotein, with complete immunologic identity line in mixtures containing factor X and VII or Xa and VIIa, as evidence for complex formation.

B. INFLUENCING FACTORS TO INDUCED HYPOCOAGULABILITY

Various factors such as circulating lipoproteins and activated platelets can influence the development of arterial thrombosis in which vitamin K-dependent proteins can also play a major role.

The role of lipoproteins and in particular, the low-density lipoprotein fraction rich in apoprotein B, has been of interest because LDL is considered to be the most important component of the cholesterol atherogen.

The interaction between apoprotein B and vitamin K-dependent clotting factors can be demonstrated by electrophoresis in agarose using gel cutting,[14] or tracer[15] and/or crossed immunoelectrophoresis.[16,17] Figure 1 shows a representative crossed immunoelectrophoresis pattern of the incubated mixtures of partially purified FVII/VIIa containing FX or FXa and apoprotein B, as evidence for complex formation between LDL and vitamin K-dependent proteins. The binding of LDL to activated vitamin K-dependent proteins may play an important role at the endothelial cell level which by the virtue of its capacity for internalization or localization may contribute to the clearance or contact activation of intermediate components. In this respect, genetic disturbances of LDL uptake could have implication for cardiovascular risk due to reduced clearance.

C. THERAPY WITH VITAMIN K-DEPENDENT PROTEIN, CONCENTRATES OR RECOMBINANT FACTOR VII AND INDUCED HYPERCOAGULABILITY

Essentially four different products have shown to be capable of correcting hemostasis in patients with inhibitors to FVIII and FIX. These are:

1. Prothrombin complexed concentrates (PCC) and activated PCC products (APC).
2. FXa complexed with phosphatidyl-choline-phospatidyl serine vesicles.
3. Bovine apoprotein-TF (AP-TF) deplipidated.
4. FVIIa prepared by recombinant technology.[18]

The thromboembolic complications and the reported booster effect of FVIII antibodies following the administration of vitamin K-dependent concentrates (PCC/APCC) are among major complications of this type of therapy. The former has been attributed to the content of activated factors, in particular to the presence of phospholipids of platelet origin which are thought to protect the active enzymes from inactivation by proteolytic inhibitors.

On a theoretical basis any agents capable of activating the prothrombinase complex, independently of the active FVIII or -IX, may be useful in the treatment of inhibitors. FXa-PL complexes are thought to be a useful candidate as such an agent, though it should be noted that high concentrations of phospholipids may cause a disseminated intravascular coagulation (DIC) syndrome, as the consequence of activation of protein C (initiated by the generated thrombin), and leading in turn to the extensive degradation of FVIII and FV. The infusion of free FXa appears not to be an effective therapy because it is promptly inhibited by antithrombin (AT III) and EPI.

The infusion of TF also induces thrombus, thrombocytopenia and defibrination and the delipidated protein moiety of TF appears to be inactive by itself though *in vivo* it may become relipidated with some beneficial effect.

Recombinant FVIIa can activate FIX and FX directly, especially at the site of injury where TF and activated platelets are exposed.[18] In addition VIIa is not significantly inhibited by plasma levels of AT III.

The clinical experience so far seems to justify the conclusion that recombinant (rVIIa) at 70 to 90 μg/kg is hemostatically active in major surgery and in life-threatening bleeding, particularly when used in combination with antifibrinolytic therapy. No thrombotic complications have been reported with use of rVIIa.[18]

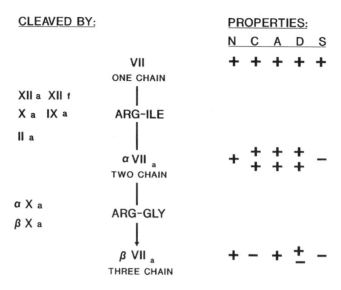

FIGURE 2. The biochemical properties of various forms of native factor VII (VII zymogen). (N) Nucleophilic residue; (C) coagulant activity; (A) amidolytic activity; (D) ability to incorporate DFP; and (S) serine specificity.

The monitoring of rVIIa treatment still remains an unresolved problem though *in vitro* experience has shown a normalization of the APTT (activated partial thromboplastin time) subsequent to the addition of 3.8 μg/ml of rVIIa approximately corresponding to 140 μ/ml. The use of one stage chromogenic assays which provide information both on the lag phase and reaction rate may prove useful in the assessment of rVIIa activity. Current information reveals that a stringent standardization of each component of the assay including diluted TF is essential if the interlaboratory variation in potency estimation is to be improved.[19,20]

III. CHARACTERISTIC PROPERTIES OF VARIOUS FORMS OF FACTOR VII

Since several variables may lead to the elevation of FVII activity *in vivo*, it is often difficult to correctly identify whether an elevated FVII is due to increased synthesis (total circulatory VII) or activation and/or a combination of the two. Accordingly, the accurate estimation of FVII procoagulant activity, as the major indicator of hypercoagulability associated with IHD, requires critical biochemical and methodological considerations. Figure 2 shows the biochemical characteristics of various forms of FVII. Ideally the laboratory monitoring FVII function should be able to differentiate the native from the activated forms. In this respect the clotting assay which is an indirect measurement of coagulation factors at the end of the cascade is not expected to fulfill this requirement. Therefore, efforts have been made to develop methods for measuring the concentration of FVII and to assess FVII activity states on the basis of the ratio of the functional activity to its concentration.

At least 5 methods for the evaluation of FVII are currently available. These include:

1. An ELISA method, which measures immunologically the total concentration of FVII.
2. The two stage amidolytic method, based on the optimal FXa generation.[21] This reflects total FXa generation induced by both FVII/VIIa produced in the first stage and the measurement of Xa by S2222 or S2337, providing measures of FVII concentration.
3. The tritiated FX method of FVII which again measures the activity of fully converted FVIIa (i.e., serum FVII), on the basis of releasing tritiated peptide from tritiated FX.
4. The one-stage clotting assay using both the conventional reagent and reagent from different species to make the assay more sensitive to FVIIa.
5. A newly developed one stage amidolytic assay (VII:Am₁) which like the one-stage FVII assay measures the rate of FXa generation but has a higher sensitivity and specificity by using purified FX in excess. Some characteristic properties of FVII: Am₁ are described below.

A. DEVELOPMENT OF A FUNCTIONAL ASSAY OF FACTOR VII BY AMIDOLYTIC METHOD

The classical two stage assay[21] of FVII consisting of TF/VII/calcium-induced activation of purified FX, in the first step, followed by the measurement of the generated FXa, (after chelating calcium with EDTA), using Synthetic Substrate (S2222 or S2337) is a cumbersome procedure, having too many subsampling steps. This procedure has been modified by eliminating the EDTA quenching step and measuring the generated FXa; subsequent to optimal activation at pH 7.4. The modified procedure like the classical method measures the FVII concentration and is not affected by changes in the activation state of FVII as found in cold-activated or clotted samples.

In contrast to the modified two-stage amidolytic procedure, by incorporating S2337 in the assay system prior to the activation (i.e., before the addition of calcium) a simplified procedure is designed which measures progressive TF-induced FVII activation by an one stage, amidolytic method. This assay, like the coagulation assay, is sensitive to the presence of the activated FVII in the test sample. In addition, on the basis of the reaction rate and the shortening of the lag phase, this procedure will provide some indication for the presence of FVIIa in the test samples.

The one-stage amidolytic procedure (VII:Am₁) in contrast to clotting assays is not affected by the variation in other plasmatic components including the presence of thrombin as corroborated by the addition of one unit of heparin or hirudin in the test samples. The characteristic of various amidolytic assays, for the purpose of a comparative analysis are shown in the flow diagram.

FLOW DIAGRAM
Amidolytic Assays

Two-stage assay (subsampling)	Modified two-stage assay	One-stage assay (No-subsampling)

Common Procedure

50 μl Plasma dilution (diln) in TBS (1/100, 1/200, 1/400)

+

50 μl Thromboplastin (MCR 1/5 diln in TBS)

+

100 μl FX 1.4 μ/ml in TBS, pH = 7.5

Two-stage (nonsubsampling)

Two-stage assay (subsampling)	Modified two-stage assay	One-stage assay (No-subsampling)
25 μl 25-mM CaCl$_2$	25 μl 25mM CaCl$_2$	25 μl 4-mM S2337
↓ 5 min	+	+
250 μl 0.3-M EDTA	25 μl TBS	25 μl 25-mM CaCl$_2$
↓	↓ 3 min	↓ 3 min
Subsampling step (100 μl to 600 μl TBS, pH 7.8)	25 μl 4-mM S2337	25 μl TBS (pH 7.5)
+	↓ 5 min	↓ 5 min
100 μl 2-mM S2337	↓	↓
Stop reaction with 200 μl of glacial acetic acid	Stop reaction with 200 μl of glacial acetic acid	Stop reaction with 200 μl of glacial acidic

Note: TBS = Tris-buffered saline; and MCR = Manchester Comparative Reagent.

Some of the useful characteristics of the one-stage amidolytic assays of FVII are indicated below:

1.   The FVII:Am$_1$ procedure with a coefficient of variation of 6% is extremely sensitive to the different forms of FVII and lends itself to automation.
2.   The components of the assay can be "tuned" and standardized for the assessment of low and high concentration of FVII. This is extremely important as the rate of Xa generation is dependent upon FVII concentration (Figure 3).

THE RATE OF FACTOR X ACTIVATION IS DEPENDENT
UPON VII CONCENTRATION

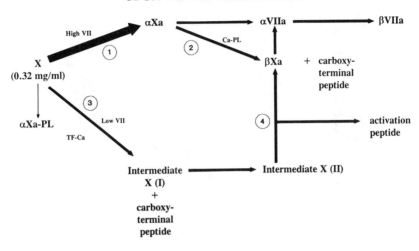

FIGURE 3. The rate of factor X activation is dependent upon factor VII concentration and formation intermediate products. The intermediate products have no coagulant activity and only following release of activation peptide the coagulant molecular forms are formed. α and βXa have similar coagulant activity. The formation of factor Xa is fast in the presence of high concentrations of factor VII (reaction ①). The αXa formed can either undergo autocatalytic degradation or be converted to βXa in the presence of calcium (Ca) and phospholipid (PL) (reaction ②). Both αXa and βXa are able to convert native factor VII to αVIIa and subsequently to βVIIa (see also Figure 2). In contrast to reaction ① with high concentrations of factor VII, the generation of factor Xa in the presence of low concentrations of factor VII (reaction ③) is relatively slow, passing through two intermediate forms of factor X (I and II) before conversion to βXa (reaction ④).

3.　The one-stage $VII:Am_1$ correlates ($r = 0.85$, $p = 0.001$) with the one-stage coagulation assays (Figure 4).

4.　The $VII:Am_1$, like VII:C is also found to be useful to differentiate between native and activated VII (i.e., cold activator and post-coagulation samples showing non-parallelism in the multiple-dose biometrical assay as shown in Figure 5).

5.　The one-stage amidolytic assay is particularly sensitive to FVIIa, which on the basis of the shortening of the lag phase could identify the presence of FVIIa in the assay mixture (not shown).

6.　$VII:Am_1$ is also useful for measuring the electrophoretic distribution of FVII in agarose or polyacrylamide gel (see Figure 6) helping to differentiate various forms of FVII based on their functional and biochemical properties.

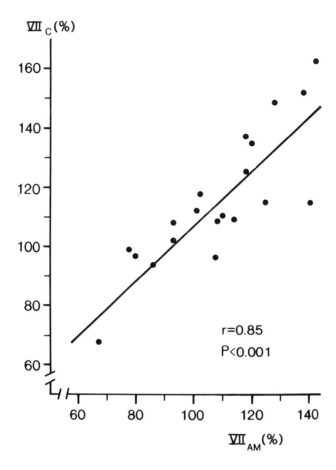

FIGURE 4. The relationship between factor VII activity measured by one-stage clotting (VII:C) and one-stage amidolytic assay (VII:Am$_1$). Significant correlation is found using paired one-stage procedures on the same samples.

B. COMPARATIVE ANALYSES OF FACTOR VII POTENCY EVALUATED BY VII:C, VII:Am$_1$, VII:Am$_2$, AND VII:T

FVII activity has been classically measured by either the correction of the clotting time of FVII deficient plasma (VII:C) which is sensitive to the presence of activated factors including VIIa or the two-stage coupled amidolytic assay (VII:Am$_2$) which is not affected by the activation state of FVII as in the first stage FVII is fully activated. The other popular assays are the two-stage tritiated factor assay which reflects various forms of FVII which may be present in serum, and the one-stage amidolytic assay (VII:Am$_1$), as described here, which measures the progressive FXa generation in a diluted system, using purified FX, hence eliminating the need for FVII deficient plasma which is essential for the clotting assay.

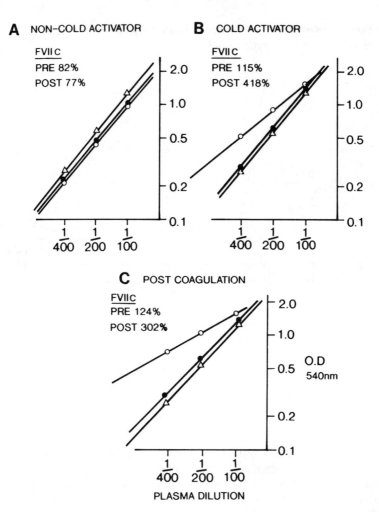

FIGURE 5. Assay of paired "non-cold" and "cold activator" samples by clotting and amidolytic assay showing induction of nonparallelism in the chromogenic assay (VII:Am$_1$). Plasma samples from two persons with "cold activator" and "non-cold activator" properties (A and B) or serum from a "non-cold activator" (C) were analyzed by clotting assay (values shown as inserts to each figure), then assayed by a one-stage amidolytic assay of factor VII using a multiple-dose biometrical assay. *Note*, the divergence in the "cold-activator" and serum samples indicating the formation of factor VIIa in these samples. (●), Reference plasma; (△), before cold activation; and (○), after cold activation.

In collaborative work with the staff of the Northwick Park Hospital the author has examined the mean potency of FVII in 42 normal donors as measured in four methods. The potency was calculated as a percent of a commercial reference plasma. The results are summarized below:

Distribution of VII activity in polyacrylamide gel as determined
by one-stage amidolytic assay

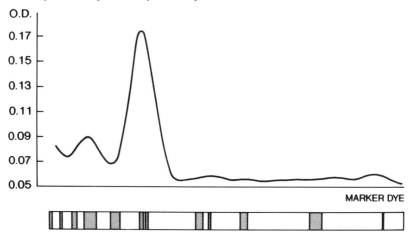

FIGURE 6. Electrophoretic distribution of FVII in standard polyacrylamide gel. Comparison between the protein stain and one-stage amidolytic activity (O.D.) measured by one stage amidolytic assay using the gel-cutting procedure.

The Mean FVII Potency in 42 Normal Donors

$FVII_c$	106.9 ± 21.6
$FVII_{am}$ one stage	122.0 ± 29.7
$FVII_{am}$ modified two stage	126.3 ± 33.1
FVIIT	133.1 ± 21.6

The one-way ANOVA results are very highly significant ($p < 0.0001$; F value = 39.9). The difference between clotting and tritiated assays is the largest. The only difference not exceeding $p = 0.05$ is between the two amidolytic assays with $p = 0.05$.

The difference between one-stage procedures reflects the different sensitivity of the two test systems for various forms of FVII and the possible interference of other plasmatic components, including FVII inhibitors in the clotting assay. This is clearly not the case in the amidolytic assay which uses purified FX and a very high dilution of the test samples (1:100 to 1:400). The differences between one-stage and two-stage procedures resides in the fact that in the latter, FVII is fully activated in the first-stage hence the assay measures only serum or activated VII-induced FXa generation capability. This is substantiated by the comparison between the serum (containing VIIa) and plasma as shown in Table 1.

The ratio of functional activity to concentration measured by one-stage and two-stage procedures, respectively, are often used for the assessment of the activity state of FVII. Although, in general, the parallel increase of FVII activity and concentration may imply that the increase is related either to the

TABLE 1
Comparison Between Potency of Plasmas and Sera from
11 Normal Donors as Assayed by Four
Different Assays

	Plasma (mean ± SD)	Serum (mean ± SD)	Difference	S.E. of difference
$FVII_c$	97.5 ± 21.2	340.8 ± 76.1	243.3	20.1
$FVII_{Am_1}$	112.0 ± 23.0	148.4 ± 34.8*	36.4	4.0
$FVII_{Am_2}$	109.5 ± 24.7	109.8 ± 27.0	0.4	1.6
$FVII_T$	128.5 ± 26.4	136.1 ± 39.5	7.6	6.2

Note: It should be emphasized that the value obtained for the serum cannot be called a "true" potency because the assay is performed against reference plasma and, in a majority of the cases, the dose-response curves, in particular for the VII_{Am_1} assay, were nonparallel.

synthesis or a slower catabolism or clearance the disparity between the results suggests activation has occurred.

This interpretation is complicated by the fact that there are at least five possible activated products of FVII with different properties (Figure 2) and this is even more complicated by the fact that the activation of FX is dependent on FVII concentration (Figure 3) making it difficult to produce a standardized functional assay.

The possible causes of increased FVII potency in hypercoagulable states still remains elusive and might be due to:

1.   Increased synthesis of FVII zymogen
2.   Release of TF
3.   Increase in alpha VII_a concentration
4.   Formation of a ternary intermediate complex, (VII-TF-Xa), the essential catalyst of FIX activation
5.   Other activated factors and their biologically active intermediates

The application of these new procedures such as electrophoretic procedures either based on interacting components or on gel cutting and/or nonparallelism in biometrical assays. (Figures 4 through 6) nevertheless will undoubtedly lead to a better characterization of the molecular forms of FVII involved in thrombogenesis.

IV. EXTRINSIC PATHWAY INHIBITOR OR LIPOPROTEIN ASSOCIATED COAGULATION INHIBITOR (EPI/LACI)

The initiation of coagulation by FVII-thromboplastin is controlled by a newly characterized lipoprotein, the so-called EPI or lipoprotein associated coagulation inhibitor (LACI). The circulating LACI is a 38-kDa molecule with a kinetic constant (Ki) of 130 pmol for recombinant VIIa.[22]

It is well established that a mixture containing a suspension of TF and FVII triggers coagulation, first by activating FX and FIX, and second the TF as surface helps in rapidly recruiting other components required for the formation of tenase(s).

A. CHARACTERISTIC PROPERTIES OF EPI/LACI

EPI/LACI has been recently identified as a natural constituent of cells, which inhibits binding of FVII to TF.[23,24] The inhibitory effect was found to be FXa-dependent[23,24] suggesting that this mechanism could be important in turning off TF-induced coagulation (i.e., at a wound site). It is known that EPI has 5 characteristic structural features which contribute to its inhibitory effect at the endothelial cell level.

These include positively charged (NH_2) and negatively charged (COOH) domains, and 3 Kunitz type inhibitory domains. Inhibition is a two-step reaction: first, FXa binds to an arginine residue in the second kunitz domain to form a FXa-EPI complex; second, the FXa-EPI complex forms a complex (stoichiometrically) with VIIa/TF leading to the formation of a quarternary Xa/EPI/VIIa/TF complex which is essential for inhibition of the catalytic activity of VIIa. The presence of lysine residue in the kunitz domain is essential for the second step and for endothelial binding.

Three pools of EPI activity have been identified

1. A plasma pool in which EPI circulates in association with plasma lipoproteins
2. A platelet pool from which EPI may be released when platelets are activated at a wound site
3. A pool of EPI bound to glycosaminoglycans on the luminal surface of vascular endothelial cells, which is releasible into plasma by the administration of heparin; the latter might be responsible for anti-Xa, activity of heparin.

The plasma concentration of EPI varies but is approximately 100 ng/ml. The plasma levels remain unchanged in patients with decompensated hepatocellular disease.[24]

B. COMPARISON BETWEEN ASSAY PROCEDURES
1. End Point Chromogenic Assay

This is a three-step assay in which various components of the assay are preincubated for 10 min at 37°C to achieve optimal inhibitory development. In Step 1, 50 μl of VIIa (0.0125 mg/ml) is mixed with 50 μl TF (1/50 dilution), 50 μl Ca^{++} (75 mM) 50 ml factor X (0.025 μl/ml) to generate optimal levels of extrinsic Xa. In Step 2, 50 μl of plasma is added to the incubation mixture for 10 min to form an EPIXa complex. In Step 3, 50 μl of factor X (0.4 μl/ml) is added to assess the residual ternary complexes of VIIa/TF/Xa remaining active. The 50-μl synthetic substrate, S2222 (2.7 m M), is used to monitor Xa-like activity in this test system. The greater the ability of the EPI/Xa complex to inhibit the generation of FXa the lower will be the amount of S2222 cleaved.

2. Dynamic PT Method

This method is based on measurements of the prolongation of the prothrombin time (PT) by EPI. The EPI is titrated against dilutions of TF and PT measured in a modified assay consisting of incubation (2 min, 37°C) of 100 μl Ca^{++} (25 mM), 100 μl TF (15 μg/ml) and 100 μl of plasma, recording the clotting time. The time required to reach a set at optical density using a chromogenic substrate (as is used in end point assays) is also applicable.[19]

The dynamic assay needs to be strictly standardized for TF to give a clotting time of about 200 s. At high levels of TF the inhibitory effect of EPI is dramatically swamped.

3. Immunological Assay and Disparity Between Assays

This is a sandwich type ELISA using an antibody raised against the NH_2 terminus of EPI. The assay consists of the following steps:

1. Plasma is incubated in PVC multiwell plates at 4°C, allowing the plasma components to stick to the plate.
2. Rabbit anti-EPI is added and the unbound antibody is washed.
3. Peroxidase gold antirabbit immunoglobulin is added followed by color development.

The preliminary results suggest that the functional heterogeneity of EPI leads to methodological disparity in the results given by the three assays. The levels of EPI by chromogenic assay were found to be much higher in patients with thromboembolic disease (133 $\pm$ 38%) than in normals whereas the results of diluted PT(s) were much lower in patients (92.5 $\pm$ 22 s) than in normal population (134.4 $\pm$ 24 s).[25] Less antigenic components were observed in a patient population of 65 $\pm$ 15 as compared to a normal population of 82 $\pm$ 21. It is possible that the complexed forms of EPI remain active in synthetic substrate assays, contributing to some of the disparity between results.

V. FUTURE TRENDS

The key event initiating blood coagulation after tissue injury is exposure of FVII to TF rather than contact activation leading to FXIa formation as attested by the frequent occurrence of life-threatening bleeding in severe deficiency of FVII as compared to patients lacking FXI who rarely have a bleeding problem. For effective hemostasis, enzyme/cofactor complexes must form on a cell surface (TF/VII can initiate FX and FIX activation leading to both ternary and quarternary complex). Natural anticoagulants act by regulating the activity of these enzyme complexes. The inhibitor effect requires the presence of FXa which is both a direct and indirect product of the action of FVIIa/TF upon its substrates.

Many advances in the characterization of the activity state of FVII have been made and more remains to be done in both quantitative determination of various forms of FVII and EPI which was recently called TF inhibitor. The role of the endothelial cell in modulating and/or influencing the time course of hypercoagulability in the ''normal'' population compared to patients in various pathophysiological states will remain as an area of active search in the 1990s.

For more detailed information on TF pathway inhibitors the reader should take note of excellent recent reviews.[26-28]

ACKNOWLEGMENTS

The author wishes to express his special thanks to all his colleagues at Northwick Park Hospital for their efforts in setting up these new techniques. My sincere thanks go to M. Vickers, for her help with the various chromogenic factor VII assays, D. Howarth for tritiated FVII assays, and Y. Stirling for the overall laboratory aspects. Special thanks are also due to J. F. Stivala for the computerized slides and M. Shearer for joint editorial review. Part of the data reported here were presented in BSHT, 1984.

REFERENCES

1. **Meade, T. W., Mellow, S., Brozovic, M., Miller, G. J., Chakrabsarti, R., North, W. R. S., Haines, A. P., Stirling, Y., Imeson, J. D., and Thomson, S. G.,** Haemostatic function and ischaemic heart disease: principal results of the Northwick Park Heart Study, Lancet, ii, 533, 1986.
2. **Meade, T. W., Brozovic, M., Chakrabarti, R., Haines, A. P., North, W. R. S., and Stirling, Y.** Ethnic group comparisons of variables associated with ischaemic heart disease, *Br. Heart J.,* 40, 789, 1978.
3. **Meade, T. W., Stirling, Y., Thomson, S. G., Vickers, M. V., Woolf, L., Ajdukiewicz, A. B., Stewart, G., Davidson, J. F., Walker, I. D., Douglas, A. S., Richardson, I. M., Weir, R. D., Aromaa, A., Impivaara, O. M., Maatela, J., and HJladovec, C.,** An international and interregional comparison of haemostatic variables in the study of ischaemic heart disease, *Int. J. Epidemiol.,* 15, 331, 1986.
4. **Meade, T. W., Ed.,** Clotting factors and ischaemic heart disease: the epidemiological evidence, in *Anticoagulants and Myocardial Infarction,* John Wiley & Sons, London, 1984, 91.
5. **Meade, T. W.,** Hypercoagulability and ischaemic heart disease, *Blood Rev.,* 1, 2, 1987.
6. **Miller, G., J., Seghatchian, M. J., Walter, S. J., Howorth, D., Thomson, S. G., Esnouf, P., and Meade, T. W.,** An association between the factor VII coagulant activity and thrombin activity induced by surface/cold exposure of normal human plasma, *Br. J. Haematol.,* 62, 379, 1986.

7. **Miller, G. J., Martin, J. C., Webster, J., Wilkes, H., Miller, N. E., Wilkinson, W. H., and Meade, T. W.,** Association between dietary fat intake and plasma factor VII coagulant activity — a predictor of cardiovascular mortality, *Atherosclerosis,* 60, 269, 1986.
8. **Rao, L. M., Rapaport, S. I., and Bajaj, S. P.,** Activation of human factor VII in the initiation of tissue factor dependent coagulation, *Blood,* 68, 685, 1986.
9. **Dalaker, K., Hjermann, I., and Prydz, H.,** A novel form of factor VII in plasma from men at risk for cardiovascular disease, *Br. J. Haematol.,* 61, 315, 1985.
10. **Seghatchian, M. J.,** Prothrombinase in factor IX concentrates as the potential thrombogenic components, in *Thrombosis and Hemorrhagic Diseases,* Urutin, O. N., and Vinazzer, H., Eds., Gozlem, Turkey, 1986, 132.
11. **Seghatchian, M. J.,** Low grade activated factors in plasma; a new approach for screening prethrombotic states, in *Thrombosis and Hemorrhagic Disease,* Ulutin, O. N. and Vinazzer, H., Eds., Gozlem, Turkey, 1986, 165.
12. **Meade, T. W., Howarth, D. J., and Stirling, Y.,** Fibrinopeptide A and sudden coronary death, Lancet, ii, 607, 1984.
13. **Constantino, M., Merskey, C., Kudzma, D. J., and Zucker, M. B.,** Increased activity of vitamin K-dependent clotting factors in human hyperlipoproteinemia — association with cholesterol and triglyceride levels, *Thromb. Haemostas.,* 38, 465, 1977.
14. **Seghatchian, M. J.,** Assessment of thrombin heterogenicity with quantitative electrophoresis, *Thromb. Res.,* 19, 757, 1980.
15. **Seghatchian, M. J. and Mackie, I. J.,** Factor VIII coagulant antigen in clinical factor IX concentrates: characterisation of the molecular forms with the use of radiolabelled factor VIII:C antibodies, *Thromb. Res.,* 24, 473, 1981.
16. **Seghatchian, M. J.,** An agarose gel method for evaluating FVIII procoagulant electrophoretic distribution, *Ann. NY Acad. Sci.,* 370, 236, 1981.
17. **Lombardi, R., Mannucci, P. M., Seghatchian, M. J., Vicente Garcia, V., and Coppola, R.,** Alterations of factor VIII von Willebrand factor in clinical conditions associated with an increase in its plasma concentration, *Br. J. Haematol.,* 49, 61, 1981.
18. **Hedner, U.,** Factor VIIa in the treatment of haemophilia, *Blood Coag. Fibrinol.,* 1, 307, 1990.
19. **Seghatchian, M. J.,** Advances in amidolytic assays of FVIII: Variables affecting the rate of Xa generation, In Factor VIII — Von Willebrand Factor, Seghatchian, M. J. and Savidge, G. F., Eds., CRC Press, FL, 1989, 97.
20. **Osterud, B.,** How to measure factor VII and factor VII activation, *Haemostasis,* 13, 161, 1983.
21. **Seligsohn, U., Osterud, B., Griffin, J. H., and Rapaport, S. I.,** Evidence for the participation of both activated FXII and activated FIX in cold promoted activation of factor VII, *Thromb. Res.,* 13, 1049, 1978.
22. **Rao, L. W. M. and Rapaport, S. I.,** Studies of a mechanism inhibition of the initiation of the extrinsic pathway of coagulation, *Blood,* 69, 645, 1987.
23. **Hubbard, A. R. and Jennings, C. A.,** Inhibition of tissue thromboplatin — mediated blood coagulation, *Thromb. Res.,* 42, 489, 1986.
24. **Carson, S. D.,** Tissue factor (coagulation factor III) inhibition by apolipoprotein II, *J. Biol. Chem.,* 262, 718, 1987.
25. **Goodwin, C. E., Melissari, E., Kakkar, V. V., and Scully, M. F.,** Lipoprotein-associated coagulation inhibitor levels in normal and thrombophylic individuals, *Br. J. Haematol.,* 77 (Suppl. 1), 61, 1991.
26. **Broze, G. J., Jr., Gerard, T. J., and Novotny, W. F.,** Regulation of coagulation by a multivalent kunitze-lype inhibitor, *Biochemistry,* 29, 7539, 1990.
27. **Broze, G. J., Jr, Gerard, T. J., and Novotny, W. F.,** The lipoprotein associated coagulation inhibitor, in *Progress in Haemostasis and Thrombosis,* Vol. 10, Collen, B. S., Ed., W. B. Saunders, Philadelphia, 1990, 243.
28. **Rapaport, S. I.,** The extrinsic pathway inhibitor. A regulator of tissue factor-dependent blood coagulation, *Thrombos. Haemostas.,* 66, 6, 1991.

Chapter 5

AN ACTIVATED FORM OF FACTOR VII IN PLASMA, A NEW LINK BETWEEN LIPIDS AND CLOTTING*

Hans Prydz

TABLE OF CONTENTS

* Data in this chapter represents a submission date of 1989.

I. INTRODUCTION

The importance of the thrombo-hemorrhagic balance for the tendency to develop atherosclerosis is again the focus of much interest. It is, of course, a revival of the Duguid-Rokitansky theory[1] although in a partially different form. More emphasis is placed on the acute effects of the clotting process, especially the multiple effects of thrombin as a mitogen, a chemotactic substance and a releasing factor for various platelet and endothelial cell products. This has, in turn, led to an increased interest in factors or processes which alter the thrombo-hemorrhagic balance in the direction of clotting, i.e., formation of thrombin and fibrin. Factor VII (FVII) is a prime candidate for such studies, being the first factor to interact with thromboplastin in the powerful extrinsic clotting system (Figure 1).

Even greater interest in this factor has arisen from the observation reported by Meade et al.[2,3] that the level of FVII activity in a prospective study emerged as a highly significant predictive factor for the development of cardiovascular disease.

FVII is a member of the family of vitamin K-dependent plasma glycoproteins. It is mainly produced in the liver[4] and has a short half-life in plasma (4 to 6 h).[5-7] Due to its very low plasma level, about 0.5 μg/ml,[8] our knowledge of its primary structure lagged behind for many years. All we knew was its approximate M_r from gels, estimated to be about 50 kDa for the bovine[9,10] and about 45 to 48 kDa for the human factor.[11] This situation improved greatly when Hagen et al.[12] reported the cloning of the complete cDNA for FVII. The nucleotide sequence translated into a protein of 466 amino acids with a propeptide of 60 residues.

The structure has a number of interesting features. As expected, the N-terminal end of the mature protein consists of a glutamic acid-rich sequence of 34 amino acids, of which 10 are glutamic acid residues modified in the vitamin K-dependent carboxylation reaction. Following, are two epidermal growth factor-like domains each of about 40 residues. In the first of these domains, a rather novel posttranslational modification was detected in bovine FVII; one aspartic acid residue was hydroxylated on the β-carbon. In human FVII, aspartic acid was not hydroxylated.[13] FVII displayed the classical serine protease mechanism and its active site structure with a histidine (253), an asparagine (302), and a serine (404).

II. ACTIVATION OF FACTOR VII

Like other clotting factors in plasma, FVII is a proenzyme (zymogen) and needs some sort of activation to be able to play its role in coagulation. With other clotting factors the activated state renders the factor able to participate as an active enzyme or cofactor in the subsequent reaction of the coagulation pathway. This is not always true for FVII. There are presently

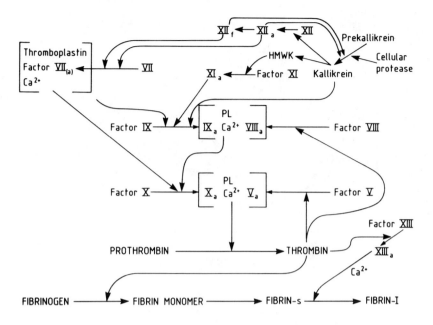

FIGURE 1. A simplified version of the clotting system.

three established ways for its activation. Only one of these clearly leads to the formation of an active factor in the above sense. These three ways are

1. Factor VII from human and bovine sources can undergo a proteolytic nick cleaving an Arg-Ile bond, giving rise to a two-chain disulfide linked molecule.[8,14,15] The product consists of a light chain of 152 amino acids derived from the N-terminal part of the native factor, and a heavy chain of 254 amino acids, which contains the enzymatically active part.[11] FIXa,[16,17] FXa,[9,18,19] and FXIIa[20,21] activate FVII in this way. Two chain FVII has a much higher specific activity (30- to 100-fold) than the single-chain form in a thromboplastin-triggered test system[8,14,15] and it has been suggested by Østerud[22] that purified two-chain FVII in the presence of Ca^{2+} and phospholipid can activate FX.

2. The classical activation of FVII by formation of a complex with Ca^{2+} and thromboplastin. This complex can activate FIX and X, i.e., FVII is "properly" activated. It is still unclear whether this activation is irreversible, i.e., involves a proteolytic nick as discussed above. Certain observations from our laboratory[23] suggested that subsequent to the activation, inactivation of thromboplastin by phospholipase C (PLC) and removal by ultrafiltration might allow FVII to retain at least some of its factor X-activating (Xa) capacity. Traces of FXa were present during the activation part of these experiments, and probably, activated FVII by limited proteolysis. Other data[24] suggest that the activation is

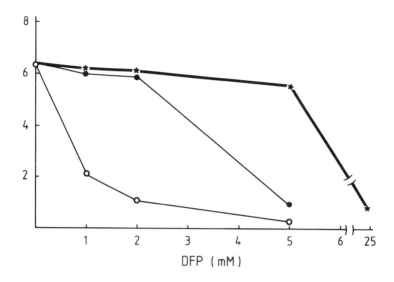

FIGURE 2.   Effect of DFP on activity of FVII. (— o —) FVII + thromboplastin + Ca^2; (— ● —) FVII + thromboplastin; (— * —) FVII alone. (From Prydz, H. and Lyberg, T., in *Protides the Biological Fluids,* Peeters, H., Ed., Pergamon Press, 1980, 241. With permission.)

due to a conformational change in the FVII molecule upon binding. Human FVII in its native state is fairly resistant to inactivation by the serine protease inhibitor diisopropyl fluorophosphate (DFP). In the presence of thromboplastin and Ca^{2+} its sensitivity is markedly increased, suggesting that the active site is more easily accessible to the inhibitor (Figure 2). The binding of FVII to thromboplastin has been utilized in affinity purification of the protein component of thromboplastin.[25]

3.   The third way of activation constitutes the subject of this contribution and will be described in more detail.

It is an old observation that FVII activity is high in pregnancy.[26,27] Departing from our studies on thromboplastin and its interaction with FVII,[23,28,29] we looked for such complexes in plasma from pregnant women. To our surprise, we detected a circulating form of activated FVII which was extremely sensitive to PLC but which neither sedimented in the ultracentrifuge, nor reacted with a neutralizing antibody to thromboplastin and thus clearly was not a thromboplastin FVII complex. This form of activated FVII was not present in plasma from healthy, nonpregnant women of comparable age.[30] The level of complexity increased towards the end of pregnancy (Figure 3) to reach a two- to three-fold activation. The activation of FVII appeared to be fully reversible when the complex was treated with PLC and was therefore not due to a conversion of single chain to two-chain form. After PLC the FVII activity returned to a normal level as defined by the activity in pooled plasma from age-matched nonpregnant women.[29]

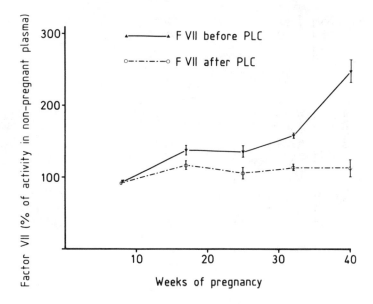

FIGURE 3. The effect of phospholipase C on FVII activity during pregnancy. Each value is the mean ± SEM of samples from 10 to 18 women at each time point. (From Dalaker, K., *Br. J. Obstet. Gynaecol.*, 93, 17, 1986. With permission.)

III. CHARACTERIZATION OF THE FVII COMPLEX

The FVII activity in plasma samples containing the activated complex form was as sensitive to neutralization by an antiserum to FVII as was the FVII activity in normal nonpregnant plasma[31] (Figure 4). By gel filtration we could show that the PLC-sensitive FVII activity eluted from the column ahead of the "normal" FVII corresponding to an estimated M_r of about 66 to 72 kDa, and that after PLC treatment it returned to a normal elution pattern (Figure 5).

From these data it seemed most likely that the activation was due to the formation of a complex between FVII and (an)other compound(s) and not to any covalent or irreversible modification of FVII. The sensitivity to PLC, so far, constitutes the only established evidence concerning the nature of the other component(s). This highly purified enzyme from *Bacillus cereus*[32,33] is active towards phosphatidylcholine (PC), phosphatidylethanolamine (PE) and phosphatidylserine (PS) and has no activity towards phosphatidylinositol (PI).[34,35] It has no proteolytic activity and especially no effect on "normal" FVII even under prolonged incubations. The quality of the enzyme is crucial for proper estimation of the level of the PLC-sensitive form.

Our best guess at this stage, therefore, is that the activated FVII is present as a complex with phospholipids. Assuming this, and in addition that the FVII-phospholipid complex shows normal hydrodynamic behavior, it is

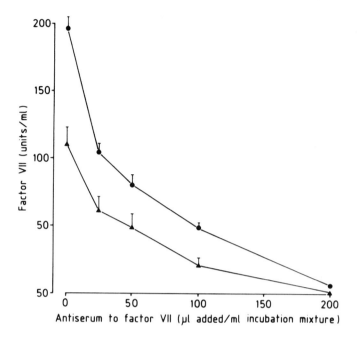

FIGURE 4. The effect of antiserum to FVII on its activity in plasma before (— ● —) and after (— ▲ —) treatment with phospholipase C. Plasma and various dilutions of antiserum were incubated for 30 min at room temperature, centrifuged for 10 min at 1500 x*g* and tested for remaining FVII activity. (From Dalaker, K., Skartlien, A.-H., and Prydz, H., *Scand. J. Haematol.*, 36, 430, 1986. With permission.)

possible to estimate the stoichiometry of the complex to be one molecule of FVII complexed to about 20 to 25 molecules of phospholipids.

The FVII molecule contains some rather hydrophobic sequences, but it is a matter of speculation whether the assumed binding to phospholipids is hydrophobic, mediated via Ca^{2+} or mixed. There is other direct evidence for the binding of FVII to phospholipid membranes in the presence of Ca^{2+}.[36,37]

It is interesting to note that FVII when present in this complex acquires a DFP sensitivity very similar to that seen when FVII is bound to thromboplastin in the presence of Ca^{2+} (Figure 6). The suggestion then is that this binding of FVII to the phospholipids results in a similar conformational change, making the serine residue 404 accessible.[31] This DFP sensitivity is reversible after PLC treatment and explains the increased specific activity of FVII in the complex.

The complex is very stable (for weeks) when kept at $-80°C$ but decays over 2 to 3 d at room temperature. The complex did not survive $BaSO_4$ adsorption nor did it survive the high ionic strength necessary for lipoprotein flotation. After trying several methods we found that precipitation with phosphotungstate and $MgCl_2$ gave a clear separation of PLC-sensitive FVII from normal FVII.[38] The non-PLCsensitive FVII remained in the supernatant.

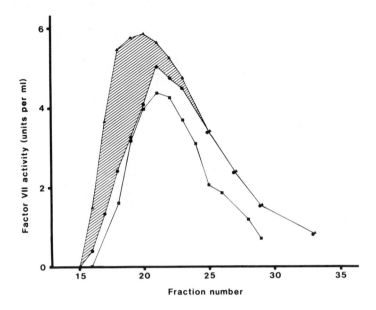

FIGURE 5. Gel filtration of plasma from normal (— ● —) and pregnant (— ▲ —) women on Sephadex G-100. The column was equilibrated and eluted with barbital-buffered saline; (— ■ —) remaining FVII activity after phospholipase C treatment of pregnant plasma. (From Dalaker, K. and Prydz, H., *Br. J. Haematol.*, 56, 233, 1984. With permission.)

Further studies towards elucidation of the nature of these complexes are under way in several laboratories.

IV. ASSAY OF PLC-SENSITIVE FVII COMPLEX

At present we use two different assay systems for this activated state of FVII. In both, the test sample (usually plasma) is incubated for 10 min at 37°C with highly purified PLC from *B. cereus* (final concentration 5 μg/ml). The control sample is incubated under identical conditions with an equivalent volume of the buffer without PLC (The buffer is barbital-buffered saline).

In one test then, these pretreated plasma samples are tested for FVII activity in a one-stage clotting system using congenitally FVII deficient plasma as the substrate and thromboplastin as the trigger. The plasma sample, thromboplastin, and Ca^{2+} are incubated separately for 3 min and clotting started by mixing them. An alternative assay system we have used[39] is Normotest® (Nycomed, Oslo, Norway) which functions as well for the purpose.

V. PLC-SENSITIVE FVII ACTIVITY IN PLASMA FROM PREGNANT WOMEN

The activity of FVII in plasma drawn at 35 to 40 weeks of gestation was two- to threefold higher than in nonpregnant women. This increase was

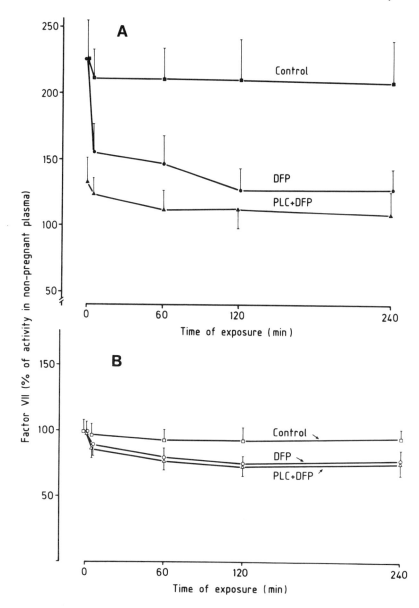

FIGURE 6. The effect of DFP on FVII activity in plasma from pregnant (A) and nonpregnant (B) women. (Modified from Dalaker, K., *Br. J. Obstet. Gynaecol.*, 93, 17, 1986. With permission.)

abolished completely by treating the plasma with PLC purified from *Bacillus cereus*. The enzyme had no effect at all on factors II and X, neither in plasma from normal nor from pregnant women, although the activities of these factors also increase moderately during pregnancy.

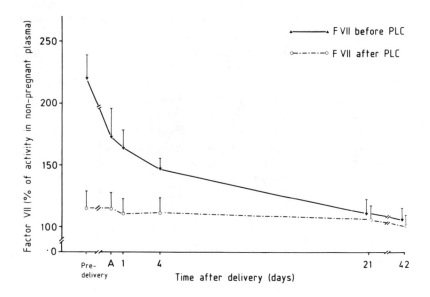

FIGURE 7.   PLC-sensitive FVII activity in pregnant women.

A low level of PLC-sensitive FVII activity was observed as early as 17 weeks and increased significantly from 32 weeks to term (Figure 3). After delivery a marked drop (about two-thirds) in FVII activity took place within 30 min, the remaining PLC-sensitive activity decayed slowly over a period of about 3 weeks (Figure 7).

Using bivariate regression analyses the level of the PLC sensitive complex in plasma, from pregnant women at term, showed a highly significant positive correlation with serum triglycerides and with the blood platelet count.[40]

VI. PLC-SENSITIVE FVII ACTIVITY IN PLASMA FROM MEN AT RISK FOR CARDIOVASCULAR DISEASE

Meade et al.[2] reported that the level of FVII activity at recruitment to the prospective Northwick Park Heart Study appeared to be an independent risk factor for cardiovascular death. Their data suggested an increase in FVII activity and not in mass. We initially investigated 36 men of age 42 years drawn from the Oslo Heart Study. Of the 36, 25 men belonged to a high-risk group as defined by a risk factor score comprising cholesterol, cigarette smoking, and blood pressure;[41] and 11 men belonged to a low-risk group by the same criteria. The high-risk group had significantly higher PLC-sensitive FVII activity than did the low-risk group (31 vs. 2%).[42] The correlation of PLC-sensitive FVII and plasma triglycerides was highly significant ($r = 0.79$, $p < 0.0001$) whereas its correlation with cholesterol only reached borderline values.

We have also carried out two prospective studies to see if the level of FVII complex has predictive value. In one study, we studied 100 patients from a group of 475 male infarct survivors. The subjects were grouped in four categories according to age and risk factor score,[41] and represented the high and low quintiles of the original patient population. Although all of these patients had survived a well-documented myocardial infarct, and thus by one definition are at risk, the low-risk groups had average conventional risk scores of three and four. All groups had average levels of PLC-sensitive FVII activity of 20 to 36%, i.e., clearly increased[43] and there was again a highly significant positive correlation with serum triglycerides (r = 0.88, p <0.0001). We are now following up on these 100 men to see if any correlation between the level of complex and cardiovascular events can be detected.

In another study, also currently in the follow-up stage, we have determined the level of PLC-sensitive FVII in plasma samples from about 271 healthy men of age 42 drawn from the Oslo Heart Study. Finally, we have shown[44] that the level of this complex is amenable to dietary intervention, in that the alteration (decline or increase) in PLC-sensitive FVII correlated very closely with the change in triglyceride levels in the same person over a 3 month intervention period. Similarly, a decrease in complex levels was seen after increased ω-3 fatty acid intake (Levorsen, Ose, Grøn, and Prydz, unpublished data, 1987).

VII. RELATED OBSERVATIONS BY OTHER LABORATORIES

As stated above, the interest in FVII levels in relation to cardiovascular disease is based on the observations by Meade et al.,[2,3] later confirmed by Balleisen et al.,[45] Hoffman et al.,[46,47] Carvalho de Sousa,[48] and Sandset et al.,[49] in addition to our own results described above.*

The presence of a PLC-sensitive FVII complex in such patients has been confirmed by Sandset et al.[49] and by Hoffman et al.[47] although the latter authors reached another conclusion based upon an apparent misinterpretation of their assays which actually show the opposite of what they stated. The relationship between triglycerides and FVII activity has been confirmed by Miller et al.[50,51]

VIII. PRESENCE IN OTHER DISEASE STATES

We have looked at various other disease states and groups of women (such as women taking oral contraceptives). In the first sample of 19 diabetics (type I), the PLC-sensitive FVII activity was markedly increased in 6 adult

---

* Heinrich et al.,[50] however, reported in 1991 that further analysis of their Procam-study revealed no significant predictive value of FVII.

TABLE 1
Plasma FVII Activity Before and After
Treatment with PLC

Factor VII activity (U/ml) PLC treatment		Cholesterol	Triglycerides
Before	After	(mmol/l)	(mmol/l)
107	19	6.5	5.1
108	44	6.1	4.0
90	46	5.0	0.9
171	51	11.3	4.3
230	9	n.t.	n.t.

patients with $HbA_1 > 10\%$, but not in 5 apparently better-controlled patients ($HbA_1 < 10\%$) nor in 8 adolescent patients with poorly controlled disease.[38] In a large group of diabetics, however, these data were not confirmed. There was no correlation between HbA_1 and PLC-sensitive FVII levels.

During these studies we made some astonishing observations in the controls. Of 40 healthy men, 5 had extremely high levels of complex (Table 1). Three of these men had an apparently normal level of FVII activity (90 to 108%) prior to PLC-treatment. In all five, the level of FVII activity after treatment was surprisingly low (9 to 51%) as if a congenital deficiency was compensated for by formation of complex. This was in marked contrast to the pregnant women and the men at risk for cardiovascular disease, in whom the level of FVII activity after PLC always approached normal levels. We are now starting a follow-up study on these men to see if their FVII complex levels have changed.

IX. FURTHER RESEARCH

It would be preferable for further studies on the mechanism of formation of these PLC-sensitive complexes to be able to establish an animal model. By taking advantage of the existence of a colony of deeply FVII deficient dogs as a source of substrate plasma for a canine test system and using dog brain thromboplastin, we have demonstrated that PLC-sensitive complexes are found and can be induced by feeding special diets (Spurling and Prydz, unpublished data). After further characterization this animal model may be useful for metabolic studies to elucidate the formation of the complexes. An obvious hypothesis is that PLC-sensitive FVII is formed postprandially, by some interaction of FVII and chylomicrons or VLDL.

In pregnant women the kinetics of disappearance of the complex after the birth of the placenta suggest that this organ, itself extremely rich in thromboplastin, may be involved in the formation of the PLC-sensitive FVII activity.

Although the complexes in men appear to be physically similar to those in women, they may have a different pathogenesis. Alternatively, the rapid decay in complex levels postpartum might be due to rapid and preferential consumption of the complex.

So far, there are no really good data to allow more than speculation about the origin of the PLC-sensitive FVII complexes. The answer(s) may be interesting and important.

ACKNOWLEDGMENTS

Work in the author's laboratory was supported by the Norwegian Council on Cardiovascular Diseases and the Norwegian Medical Research Council/NAVF.

REFERENCES

1. **Duguid, J. B.,** Thrombosis as a factor in the pathogenesis of coronary atherosclerosis, *J. Pathol. Bacteriol.,* 58, 207, 1946.
2. **Meade, T. W., North, W. R. S., Chakrabarti, R., Stirling, Y., Haines, A. P., Thompson, S. G., and Brozovic, M.,** Haemostatic function and cardiovascular death: early results of a prospective study, *Lancet,* i, 1050, 1980.
3. **Meade, T. W., Brozovic, M., Chakrabarti, R. R., Haines, A. P., Imeson, J. D., Mellows, S., Miller, G. J., North, W. R. S., Stirling, Y., and Thompson, S. G.,** Haemostatic function and ischaemic heart disease: principal results of the Northwick Park Heart Study, *Lancet,* ii, 533, 1986.
4. **Prydz, H.,** Studies on proconvertin (factor VII). V. Biosynthesis in suspension cultures of rat liver cells, *Scand. J. Clin. Lab. Invest.,* 16, 540, 1964.
5. **Hasselback, R. and Hjort, P. F.,** Effect of heparin on in vivo turnover of clotting factors, *J. Appl. Physiol.,* 15, 945, 1980.
6. **Hellemans, J., Vorlat, M., and Verstraete, M.,** Survival time of prothrombin and factors VII, IX and X after completely synthesis blocking doses of coumarin derivatives, *Br. J. Haematol.,* 9, 506, 1983.
7. **Josso, F., ProuWartelle, O., and Ménaché, D.,** Durée de vie de la proconvertine (facteur VII), *Nouvelle Rev. Franc. d'Hématol.,* 4, 572, 1964.
8. **Fair, D. S.,** Quantitation of factor VII in plasma of normal and warfarin-treated individuals by radioimmunoassay, *Blood,* 62, 784, 1983.
9. **Broze, G. J. and Majerus, P. W.,** Purification and properties of human coagulation factor VII, *J. Biol. Chem.,* 225, 1242, 1980.
10. **Radcliffe, R. and Nemerson, Y.,** The activation and control factor VII by activated factor X and thrombin. Isolation and characterization of a single chain form of factor VII, *J. Biol. Chem.,* 250, 388, 1975.
11. **Gladhaug, A. and Prydz, H.,** Purification of the coagulation factors VII and X from human serum. Some properties of factor VII, *Biochim. Biophys. Acta,* 215, 105, 1970.
12. **Hagen, F. S., Gray, C. L., O'Hara, P., Grant, F. J., Saari, G. C., Woodbury, R. G., Hart, C. E., Insley, M., Kisiel, W., Kurachi, K., and Davie E. W.,** Characterization of a cDNA coding for human factor VII, *Proc. Nat. Acad. Sci. U.S.A.,* 83, 2412, 1986.

13. **Thim, L., Bjoern, S., Christensen, M., Nicolaisen, E. M., Lund-Hansen, T., Pedersen, A. H., and Hedner, U.,** Amino acid sequence and posttranslational modifications of human factor VII$_a$ from plasma and transfected baby hamster kidney cells, *Biochemistry,* 27, 7785, 1988.
14. **Goodnight, S. H., Jr., Feinstein, D. I., Østerud, B., and Rapaport, S. I.,** Factor VII antibody-neutralizing material in hereditary and acquired factor VII deficiency, *Blood,* 38, 1, 1971.
15. **Gjønnaess, H.,** Cold promoted activation of factor VII. III. Relation to the kallikrein system, *Thromb. Diath. Haemor.,* 28, 182, 1972.
16. **Laake, K. and Østerud, B.,** Activation of purified plasma factor VII by human plasmin, plasma kallikrein, and activated components of the human intrinsic blood coagulation system, *Thromb. Res.,* 5, 759, 1974.
17. **Seligsohn, U., Østerud, B., Brown, S. F., Griffin, J. H., and Rapaport, S. I.,** Activation of human factor VII in plasma and in purified system. Roles of activated factor IX, kallikrein and activated factor XII, *J. Clin. Invest.,* 64, 1056, 1979.
18. **Jesty, J. and Silverberg, S. A.,** Kinetics of the tissue factordependent activation of coagulation factors IX and X in a bovine plasma system, *J. Biol. Chem.,* 254, 12,337, 1979.
19. **Østerud, B.,** The intrinsic and extrinsic activation of factor IX, in *Protides of Biological Fluids,* Peeters, H., Ed., Pergamon, Oxford, 1988, 233.
20. **Kisiel, W., Fujikawa, K., and Davie, E. W.,** Activation of bovine factor VII (proconvertin) by factor XII$_a$ (activated Hageman factor), *Biochemistry,* 16, 4189, 1977.
21. **Radcliffe, R. A., Bagdasarian, R., Colman, R., and Nemerson Y.,** Activation of bovine factor VII by Hageman factor fragments, *Blood,* 50, 611, 1977.
22. **Østerud, B.,** How to measure factor VII and factor VII activation, *Haemostasis,* 13, 161, 1983.
23. **Østerud, B., Berre, A., Otnaess, A.-B., Bjørklid, E., and Prydz H.,** Activation of coagulation factor VII by tissue thromboplastin and calcium, *Biochemistry,* 11, 2853, 1972.
24. **Prydz, H. and Lyberg, T.,** Tissue thromboplastin — molecular and cellular biology, in *Protides of the Biological Fluids,* Peeters, H., Ed., Pergamon Press, Oxford, 1980, 241.
25. **Guha, A., Bach, R., Konigsberg, W., and Nemerson, Y.,** Affinity purification of human tissue factor: interaction of factor VII and tissue factor in detergent micelles, *Proc. Natl. Acad. Sci. U.S.A.,* 83, 299, 1986.
26. **Alexander, B., Meyer, L., Kenny, J., Goldstein, R., Gurewich, V., and Grinspoon, L.,** Blood coagulation in pregnancy: proconvertin and prothrombin, and the hypercoagulable state, *New Engl. J. Med.,* 254, 358, 1956.
27. **Loeliger, A. and Koller, F.,** Behavior of factor VII and prothrombin in late pregnancy and in the newborn, *Acta Haematol.,* 7, 157, 1952.
28. **Bjørklid, E., Storm, E., and Prydz, H.,** The protein component of human brain thromboplastin. *Biochem. Biophys. Res. Commun.,* 55, 969, 1973.
29. **Bjørklid, E. and Storm, E.,** Purification and some properties of the protein component of tissue thromboplastin from human brain, *Biochem. J.,* 165, 89, 1977.
30. **Dalaker, K. and Prydz, H.,** The coagulation factor VII in pregnancy, *Br. J. Haematol.,* 56, 233, 1984.
31. **Dalaker, K.,** Clotting factor VII during pregnancy, delivery and puerperium, *Br. J. Obstet. Gynaecol.,* 93, 17, 1986.
32. **Otnaess, A.-B., Prydz, H., Bjørklid, E., and Berre, A.,** Phospholipase C from *Bacillus cereus* and its use in studies of tissue thromboplastin, *Eur. J. Biochem.,* 27, 238, 1972.
33. **Little, C., Aurebekk, B., and Otnaess, A.-B.,** Purification by affinity chromatography of phospholipase from *Bacillus cereus, FEBS Lett.,* 2, 175, 1975.

34. **Otnaess, A.-B., Little, C., Sletten, K., Wallin, R., Johnsen, S., Flengsrud, R., and Prydz, H.,** Some characteristics of phospholipase C from *Bacillus cereus, Eur. J. Biochem.,* 79, 459, 1977.

35. **Roberts, M. F., Otnaess, A.-B., Kensil, C. A., and Dennis, E. A.,** The specificity of phospholipase A2 and phospholipase C in a mixed micellar, *J. Biol. Chem.,* 253, 1252, 1978.

36. **Bjørklid, E., Storm, E., Østerud, B., and Prydz, H.,** The interaction of the protein and phospholipid components of tissue thromboplastin (factor III) with the factors VII and X, *Scand. J. Haematol.,* 14, 65, 1975.

37. **Ruf, W., Rehemtulla, A., Morrissey, J. H., and Edgington, T. S.,** "The isolated extracellular domain of tissue factor is functional on phospholipid surfaces," XIIth Congr. Int. Soc. Thrombosis and Haemostasis, 1989, Abstract.

38. **Dalaker, K., Skartlien, A.-H., and Prydz, H.,** A new form of coagulation factor VII in plasma, *Scand. J. Haematol.,* 36, 430, 1986.

39. **Dalaker, K., Janson, T. L., Johnsen, B., Skartlien, A.-H., and Prydz, H.,** A simple method for determination of the factor VII-phospholipid complex using Normotest, *Thromb. Res.,* 47, 287, 1987.

40. **Dalaker, K., Ingebretsen, O. C., Rasmussen, S., Nordbø Berge, L., and Prydz, H.,** Phospholipase C-sensitive factor VII activity in normal pregnancy, *Acta Obstet. Gynecol. Scand.,* 69, 111, 1990.

41. **Leren, P., Askevold, E. M., Foss, O. P., Frøili, A., Grymyr, D., Helgeland, A., Hjermann, I., Holme, I., Lund-Larsen, P. G., and Norum, K. R.,** The Oslo Study. Cardiovascular disease in middle-aged and young Oslo men, *Acta Med. Scand.,* 199, Suppl. 588, 1975.

42. **Dalaker, K., Hjermann, I., and Prydz, H.,** A novel form of factor VII in plasma from men at risk for cardiovascular disease, *Br. J. Haematol.,* 61, 315, 1985.

43. **Dalaker, K., Smith, P., Arnesen, H., and Prydz, H.,** Factor VII-phospholipid complex in male survivors of acute myocardial infarction, *Acta Med. Scand.,* 222, 111, 1987.

44. **Skartlien, A.-H., Lyberg Beckmann, S., Holme, I., Hjermann, I., and Prydz, H.,** Effect of alteration in triglyceride levels on factor VII-phospholipid complexes in plasma, *Arteriosclerosis,* 9, 798, 1989.

45. **Balleisen, L., Schulte, H., and Assmann, G.,** Coagulation factors and the progress of coronary heart disease, *Lancet,* ii, 461, 1987.

46. **Hoffman, C., Shah, A., Sodums, M., and Hultin, M. B.,** Factor VII activity state in coronary artery disease, *Blood,* 68, Suppl. 1, 1988.

47. **Hoffman, C., Shah, A., Sodums, M., and Hultin, M. B.,** Factor VII activity state in coronary artery disease, *J. Lab. Clin. Med.,* 4, 475, 1988.

48. **Carvalho de Sousa, J., Azevedo, J., Soria, C., Barros, F., Ribeiro, C., Parreira, F., Caen, J. P.,** Factor VII hyperactivity in acute myocardial thrombosis. A relation to the coagulation activation, *Thrombosis Res.,* 51, 165, 1988.

49. **Sandset, P. M., Sirnes, P. A., and Abildgaard, U.,** Factor VII and extrinsic pathway inhibitor in acute coronary disease, *Br. J. Haematol.,* 72, 391, 1989.

50. **Heinrich, J., Schulte, H., Balleisen, L., Assman, G., and van de Loo, J.,** Predictive value of haemostatic variables in the Procam-Study, *Thromb. Haemostas.* 65(6) Abstract 466, 1990.

51. **Miller, G. J., Walter, S. J., Stirling, Y., Thompson, S. G., and Esnouf, M. P.,** Assay of factor VII activity by two techniques — evidence for increased conversion of VII to αVII$_a$ in hyperlipidemia, with possible implications for ischaemic heart disease, *Br. J. Haematol.,* 59, 249, 1985.

52. **Miller, G. J., Martin, J. C., Webster, J., Wilkes, H., Miller, N. E., Wilkinson, W. H., and Meade, T. W.,** Association between dietary fat intake and plasma factor VII coagulant activity — a predictor of cardiovascular mortality, *Atherosclerosis,* 60, 269, 1986.

53. **Prydz, H., Spurling, N. W., Boyce. A. J., and Mifsud, C. V. J.,** Phospholipase C-sensitive factor VII complexes in dog plasma, *Thromb. Res.,* 64, 387–394, 1991.

Chapter 6

CHANGES IN THE ACTIVITY STATE OF THE PROTEIN C AND PROTEIN S SYSTEMS AND HYPERCOAGULABILITY: SOME LABORATORY CONSIDERATIONS

M. J. Seghatchian

TABLE OF CONTENTS

0-8493-6423-X/93/$0.00 + $.50

I. INTRODUCTION

Considerable interest has developed over the last 2 decades in the characterization of the natural anticoagulant activities of vitamin K-dependent anticoagulant proteins.[1-8] A schematic representation of the subcomponents of the protein C (PC) and protein S (PS) anticoagulant pathway, including the inhibitor of activated PC (APC) is shown in Chapter 1, Figure 3. In considering assessment of the activity state of PC and PS anticoagulant, the analyst needs to rely not only on the development of reliable functional and immunological assays, but also on biochemical procedures, to differentiate various forms of PC and PS and to reduce the influence of the interfering components. This article addresses some of the related issues and provides a new approach for identification of APC and APC-inhibitor complexes.

II. VARIABLES INFLUENCING PROTEIN C AND S ASSAYS

Variables influencing the activation states of PC and PS are numerous. Some of these, together with the currently used assays, are described below. Two types of functional assays are commonly used for PC:

1. Assays in which the plasma is first absorbed with barium citrate or aluminum hydroxide to separate PC from des-γ-carboxy PC and the inhibitor of APC. The eluted PC is then activated with thrombin/thrombomodulin. The APC formed is measured either by a chromogenic substrate or a clotting method.
2. Assays in which the PC is directly activated with "Protac", (a PC activator isolated from the venom of the Copperhead snake, *Agkistrodom contorix*) and the APC formed is measured with a chromogenic substrate or with a clotting method.[8]

The different types of reported assays[10-15] generally give comparable results for plasma samples obtained from normal subjects and from patients, except when the patients are being treated with oral anticoagulants. A possible explanation for this abnormality may reside in the relative sensitivity of various assays to the concentration of APC-PC inhibitor complexes. Abnormality in the clearance of the altered molecular forms of PC, can also contribute to above disparity, as certain assays are sensitive to partially carboxylated forms of PC.

The situation seems to be even more complicated with respect to PS assays, due to the fact that PS in plasma is present as a free form (having APC cofactor activity) and as a complex with C4b binding protein (having no APC cofactor activity). Several functional assays of PS have been described.[16-22] This includes a new procedure using factor Va (FVa) as a substrate for APC and diluted plasma.[22] In immunological assays apart from the measurement of total PS one is more often interested in the measurement of free PS. This can be accomplished by treating the plasma with polyethylene glycol (PEG) prior to the analysis to selectively precipitate the complexed C4b-bound PS leaving the free PS to be assayed in the supernatant.[20] Crossed immunoelectrophoresis is often used for further characterization of the electrophoretic heterogeneity of PC and PS. This is described here in some detail.

Although several kindreds of PC and PS deficiency associated with recurrent thrombosis have been described,[4,5,17] a simple causative association has been called into question by the work on blood donors by Miletich et al.[16] who suggest that coinheritance of other factors may be necessary for the expression of a thrombotic tendency.

Another important variable is the level of various proteolytic inhibitors, including PC inhibitor (PCI), which circulates in plasma at concentrations of about 5 μg/ml; this specifically blocks the activity of APC by forming a 1:1 molecular complex and yielding a carboxy-terminal peptide that remains bound to APC.[9] Like antithrombin III (AT III) and heparin cofactor II (HPC II), the activity of PCI is accelerated several-fold by sulfated polysaccharides, such as heparin and dextran sulfate. Both free PCI and its complexes with proteases bind to solid matrix heparin. In normal plasma 10 to 15% of PCI appears in complexes with proteases such as kallikrein (kk), APC, and urokinase.[23] In outdated blood, almost all of the PCI is inactivated or complexed with kk. The inactivated form of the inhibitor is also identified when the contact system has been activated with dextran sulfate. Soya bean trypsin inhibitor (SBTI) an effective inhibitor of plasma kk leaves the PCI in its native form. Although C_1 esterase and α-2 macroglobulin are also considered to be the dominating plasma kk inhibitors, the second-order rate constant of kk for PCI is, nevertheless, two times higher than the inactivation of kk by C_1-esterase inhibitor.

A. METHODOLOGICAL UNCERTAINTIES IN PROTEINS C AND S ASSAYS

A major problem associated with functional assays of the protein C system lies in the difficulty in activating PC to APC without interfering with the activity of clotting factors. This is true even for the most commonly used procedure which uses snake venom (''Protac'') for the activation of PC. This is because Protac inactivates factor (F)V and FVIII both directly and indirectly through APC. Variability between assays also exists in immunological assays, possibly due to the molecular heterogenicity of PC (i.e., abnormal molecules, partially carboxylated and PC in complex with other plasma proteins including PS and PCI) which are depicted to a variable degree by different methods.

Similar problems are encountered with the assay of PS which circulates in plasma in bound and unbound forms of which only the free form is functional as the cofactor for APC. Inadequacy in the concentration of any of the subcomponents of PC and PS assays can also dramatically alter the outcome.

A functional assay of PS is based on *activated partial thromboplastin time* (APTT)-like activity using a low concentration of contact activator and using FVa as the substrate.[14,24] In this assay 100 μl of test plasma (1:10 dilution) in veronal acetate buffer (pH 7.4), 100 μl PS-deficient plasma containing cephalin as the source of phospholipids, 100 μl of APC (1U/ml), are mixed followed by 100 μl of FVa (0.16 U/ml) containing 12.5×10^{-3} g/ml kaolin. The coagulation is triggered after 2 min incubation at 37°C by the addition of 100 mM calcium. The method is reportedly unaffected by heparin (up to 11 μl/ml) and insensitive to all other procoagulant factors and inhibitors of the coagulation system.

Recently Vigano et al.[24] have evaluated commercial APTT reagents for their sensitivity to the cofactor effects of PS by comparing APC-dependent clotting time prolongation for normal plasma and for PS depleted plasma. For some reagents, abnormalities in dose-response curves were found in normal and in PS-depleted plasma, which is attributed to the difference in the phospholipid content and composition of some APTT reagents.[24] It should be noted that the APTT test reflects only the time taken to reach a threshold concentration of thrombin and not differences in amounts of thrombin produced.

Similarly the accuracy of the immunological assay is dependent on the characteristic properties of reagents; such as specificity, the titer of antibody, complete immunological identity, the avidity of the antibody and their detection limits for accurate diagnosis and decision on the therapeutic modality. Nevertheless, with the improved precision in the purification and characterization of coagulant proteins and quality control of reagents used by laboratories (including the choice of control plasma and anticoagulant), we are able to choose specific molecular markers to provide accurate information for specific pathophysiological states.[25,26] The development of monoclonal antibodies for vitamin K-dependent proteins and the use of ELISA tests for improving the sensitivity down to picogram amounts has improved the accuracy of the current methodology considerably, hence reducing uncertainty.

B. METHODOLOGICAL UNCERTAINTIES IN PROTEIN C INHIBITOR ASSAYS

New advances are also being made in the characterization of PCI and its complex formation with APC and other proteases. PCI is a member of the serpin family. It is a single-chain glycoprotein with a MW of 57,000 which inhibits APC with a K_d of 5.0×10^{-8} M by formation of a 1:1 complex. PCI also inhibits other serine proteases *in vitro* (e.g., thrombin, FXa, FXIa, kk, urokinase, and tissue plasminogen activator). The inhibition (except for kk) is accelerated by heparin and sodium dextran sulfate and glycosaminoglycans. Prolongation of the modified prothrombin time (M-PT) or the kaolin-cephalin clotting time (KCCT) are used to assess the inhibition of APC as shown below:

Modified prothrombin time (M-PT)	Kaolin Cephalin Clotting Time (KCCT)
	[100 μl plasma]
	[100 μl in 5 mg kaolin/ml cephalin]
	[80 μl of patient plasma]
100 μl Plasma	↓ 4.45 min at 37°C
+	
20 μl APC (0.2 μg/ml)	+20 μl (APC 0.2 μg/ml)
↓ 5 min	↓ 15 s at 37°C
100 μl thromboplastin	100 μl Ca^{++} (25 mM)
	Clotting time
+	
100 μl$^+$ Ca^{++} (25 mM)	
Normal 18 s	Normal KCCT 95
	which is prolonged in patients

PCI does not appear to circulate as an irreversible complex with APC, since the PC could readily be separated by aluminium hydroxide absorption.

The heparin dependent inhibition of APC by PCI is completely neutralized by histidine-rich glycoprotein (HRG). At physiological concentrations of Zn^{++} (20 μM) significant enhancement of the neutralization by HRG of the heparin-dependent activity of PCI occurs which is attributable to the increased affinity of HRG for heparin in the presence of Zn^{++}.

Despite the methodological advances in the assessment of the subcomponents of the PC pathway, the full potential of such measurements will not be fully realized until various assays are validated against each other and applied to specific clinical cases in attempts to define how minor modifications in reagents can accurately depict the changes in the activation states of these vitamin K anticoagulant proteins.

III. EXPERIMENTAL FINDINGS ON CHANGES IN PROTEIN C ACTIVATION STATES IN WOMEN ON ORAL CONTRACEPTIVES

The recognition of the potent anticoagulant properties of PC has led to a resurgence of interest in monitoring the plasma levels and activity states of this protein in relation to hypercoagulability and to establish whether there is a relationship between the elevated level of PC and induced states of hyper-coagulability.

The initial large scale studies on the blood donor population by Miletich et al.[16] and by Dolan et al.[27] have revealed male donors have a higher functional PC (1.07 μ/ml) than female donors (1.01 μ/ml) The differences between the two groups decreases with age possibly due to an increased concentration in older women. Furthermore there is a significant difference in PC levels between ABO blood-type groups (in order AB being highest followed by O, A, and then B).

In a collaborative study with Meade et al.[28] the author compared factor VII:C, thrombin-like activity (TLA), and PC levels in 24 women taking oral contraceptives (OC), with 24 matched controls. PC antigen levels were found to be higher in women of the same age and of the same degree of obesity who were using OC (see Table below). In the pooled data for 48 women investigated there was an increase in PC of about 1% (of standard) for each 1.00 mm increase in skinfold thickness.

Furthermore, the mean FVII level in the OC users was also higher than in nonusers as was the low-grade proteolytic enzyme measured by thrombin substrate S2238, (see Table below).

It is possible that the increase in PC in OC users counteracts the increase in procoagulatory factors such as the activated FVII and TLA, thus helping to ensure that the thrombogenic potential as a whole is not altered.

The good correlation between PC, FVII, and TLA levels (measured by chromogenic assay at 540 nm reported here in arbitrary units (A.U.) of plasma suggests that higher levels of thrombin are produced in OC users leading to the activation of PC and its complexes with a host of plasmatic inhibitors, including PCI; the latter possibly remains active on synthetic substrate assay.

MEAN VALUES (S.D.) OF FOUR VARIABLES IN OC USERS AND NONUSERS

	OC Users	Nonusers	Difference	P-value
FVII:C, %	97.4(24.5)	82.2(31.2)	15.2(41.3)	0.003
PC, %	153.0(41.4)	124.0(34.4)	29.0(35.4)	0.0003
TLA, (A.U.)	538.6(246)	407.6(182)	89.0(238)	0.001
FPA, ng/ml	15.7(30.6)	13.7(29.3)	2.2(31.8)	0.14

IV. CHANGES IN THE ACTIVITY STATES OF PROTEIN C SUBSEQUENT TO ORAL ANTICOAGULANT INTAKE

PC is a recently recognized vitamin K-dependent protein involved in the modulation of hemostasis. A decrease in both PC antigen and PC functional activity is observed during anticoagulant therapy.

In anticoagulated (warfarinized) plasma, it is suggested that crossed immunoelectrophoresis in a calcium medium is the method of choice for differentiation of the normal from the abnormal (PIVKA — *p*roteins *i*nduced by *v*itamin *K* *a*ntagonists) molecule. Since the immunological technique, using polyclonal antibodies does not provide information on the activity state of the protein, a comparative study has been carried out on normal and warfarinized plasmas in both calcium and EDTA to determine whether PC activity is associated with the PC antigen and whether electrophoresis in EDTA can help in differentiating various forms of PC in oral anticoagulant condition.

A. COMPARATIVE ANALYSIS OF PROTEIN C IN NORMAL AND WARFARINIZED PLASMA

A comparative study of the PC functional activity (PC: *Act*) and the electrophoretic distribution patterns of protein C antigen (PC: *Ag*) has been carried out on normal and warfarinized plasmas in both calcium and EDTA containing systems. Two-dimensional (crossed) electrophoresis was carried out according to the method of Vigano,[14] but with the following modifications.

COMPARISON OF TWO CROSSED-IMMUNOELECTROPHORETIC METHODS FOR PROTEIN C

	Original Method (Vigano et al.[14])	Modified Method (Seghatchian and Stirling)
Sample Load	70 μl	300 μl Reptilase-treated plasma
Well size	9 × 5.5 mm	20 × 5.5 mm
Agarose	1%	1%
Depth of agarose	1.5 mm	3 mm
Electrophoresis in first dimension	Barb. buffer pH 8.6 EDTA or Ca lactate 0.002 *M*	Barb. buffer pH 8.6 EDTA or Ca lactate 0.002 *M* 5 V/cm, 6 h Two transverses of the plate as 6 V/cm 4 h by bromo-phenol blue marker
Electrophoresis in second dimension	No EDTA in 2 V/cm 20 h	As for first dimension: 3 V/cm 20 h
Conc. of antiserum	0.25%	0.375%
Wicks	3 *M* Chromatography paper	12 sheet thickness Whatman No. 1 filter paper

Note: Each plasma was set up in duplicate.

After first dimension electrophoresis, one gel was run in the second dimension into PC antibody containing agarose and its duplicate was cut in the direction of migration into 2.0 × 0.5 cm segments and each assayed directly for PC functional activity by a modification of Bertina's method.[5,10] This assay measures the level of alumina-adsorbed PC using commercially available thrombin and standardized Al(OH)$_3$ for APC. (Adsorption of normal plasma for 30 s with a one-tenth volume of Al(OH)$_3$ giving a prothrombin time of around 100 s). Of the PC 90% is adsorbed as measured by Laurell

TABLE 1
Protein C Functional Activity and Antigen Levels in Normal Plasmas

Protein C activity %	Protein C antigen %[a]	Ratio activity/antigen
119	100	1.19
85	97	0.88
120	115	1.04
132	142	0.92
88	64	1.37
111	77	1.44
86	73	1.118
102	106	0.96
Mean = 105.4	96.9	1.09

(Ratio range 0.88–1.44) mean 1.09.
(Ratio range 0.64–1.37) mean 0.97 (Bertina et al.[5]).

[a] of standard

rocket. In contrast to Bertina's method, the $Al(OH)_3$ is present during the activation stage, (2 h at 37°C) to provide an activation surface. After neutralization of the thrombin by incubation for 20 min at 37°C with a fivefold excess molar concentration of AT III/heparin, APC was measured by addition of chromogenic substrate S2366 at a concentration of 2 K_m. The reaction was stopped after 10 min with glacial acetic acid. A diazotization reaction is used to convert and enhance the color of the trace amounts of p-nitroaniline released which is read at 540 nm.

The assay appears to be specific (PC depleted plasma OD 0.05) and compares well with the results in plasma obtained by Bertina as indicated in Tables 1 and 2.

Comparative analyses of PC:Act and PC:Ag indicate that in normal and mildly anticoagulated plasmas with values of the prothrombin ratio (PTR) up to 1.9, PC:Act and PC:Ag correlate fairly well. The presence of elevated circulating APC and/or its complexes (not inhibited by AT III/heparin) and remaining active on the chromogenic substrate might contribute to the higher PC:Act/PC:Ag ratio in some samples. Between a PTR of 2.0 to 2.9, PC:Act and PC:Ag are both decreased giving a ratio which is still in the normal range. Above PTR values of 3.0, PC:Act is decreased to a greater degree than PC:Ag (an approximately twofold increase of antigen over activity) resulting in a low PC:Act/PC:Ag ratio. The lower activity level would confirm Bertina's[5] suggestion that only carboxylated PC is adsorbed onto $Al(OH)_3$. The low antigen level is possibly due to either a decrease in synthesis due to the presence of acarboxylated (des-α-carboxy) forms or the failure of the antibody

TABLE 2
Protein C Functional Activity and Antigen Levels in Warfarinized Plasmas

Prothrombin ratio	Protein C activity %	Protein C antigen %[a]	Ratio activity/antigen
Range 1.0–1.9			
1.31	61	73	0.84
1.69	85	60	1.42
1.77	100	81	1.23
	80.5 Mean	68 Mean	1.2 Mean
Range 2.0–2.9			
2.3	39	43	0.91
2.38	41	44	0.93
2.77	38	49	0.77
	39.3 Mean	45.3 Mean	0.87 Mean
Range 3.0–4.0			
3.00	37	45	0.82
3.46	35	64	0.55
3.69	23	55	0.42
	32 Mean	55	0.58 Mean
Range) 4.0–4.16			
4.6	15	35	0.43
5.38	18	51	0.35
8.54	17	39	0.44
10.46	18	36	0.5
	11.5	21	0.55
	16 Mean	36 Mean	0.44 Mean

Bertina et al.[5]

2.7	0.39	0.47	0.83
3.1	0.37	0.43	0.86
3.7	0.28	0.41	0.68
4.5	0.27	0.40	0.67

[a] of standard

to recognize the acarboxylated form to the same extent as the fully and/or partially carboxylated form.

Comparative two-dimensional electrophoresis of normal and warfarinized plasma (shown in Figure 1) revealed the following results. First, in buffers containing either calcium or EDTA a heterogenous pattern of PC:*Ag* was apparent in normal and anticoagulated plasmas with a lower level of antigen seen in the anticoagulated samples. In EDTA, there is a suggestion that this decrease may be in the higher mobility component. In calcium (but not in EDTA), the acarboxylated form could be clearly differentiated from the fully carboxylated form by its faster migration. In calcium, the distribution of

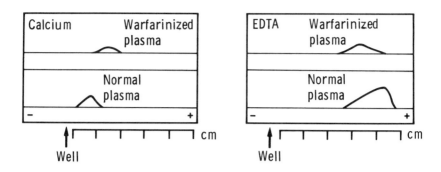

FIGURE 1. Electrophoretic distribution of protein C in normal and warfarinized plasma in calcium and EDTA containing buffers (See text for details).

antigen and activity were coincident in both normal and warfarinized plasma, whereas in the EDTA the functional activity peak appeared in the same area as in calcium, but the antigen peak was shifted more towards the anodic region. This would suggest that in EDTA the immunological and functional assays are measuring two different properties of the same molecule. The role of calcium in maintaining the structural and functional integrity of PC remains to be explored, but it is possible that native and/or APC in this system may bind to a differing extent to other plasma proteins (including PCI).

In a second set of results from a further experiment run under the same conditions, one gel was cut after the first dimension and tested (in addition to PC:*Act*) for the presence of free plasma proteases or their chromogenically active complexes. The gel sections were eluted in 0.313% tridodium citrate containing 1% bovine albumin, pH 7.5, and incubated (without AT III and heparin) with chromogenic substrate S2238 for 1 h at 37°C. The reaction was stopped with glacial acetic acid, color converted and read at 540 nm (for details see Chapter 1, reference 18 and Chapter 4, references 10 and 11). The main peak of free proteases occurred nearer the well region than did PC act, but with some overlap into this latter region. The lack of inhibition by AT III/heparin, the longer incubation time, and the use of chromogenic substrate S2238 with greater specificity for thrombin and APC would account for the very high peak of plasma proteases in comparison with that of PC:*Act*.

Simultaneous assessment by functional and immunological assay after electrophoretic separation is a new approach to the characterization of plasma proteins. The modification of the two-dimensional electrophoresis gives greater resolution while the direct assay of gel segments for functional activity aid our understanding of the nature of PC. The method could be usefully applied in the characterization and classification of inherited and acquired abnormalities of not only PC, but other plasma proteins as well (see Chapter 4, references 14 to 16).

TABLE 3
Data from One Individual Volunteer
Following a Single Dose of Warfarin

Time	Factor VII activity %[a]	Protein C activity %[a]	Protein C antigen %[a]
0	130	96	100
2	124	94	100
4	124	92	96
8	112	66	64
12	60	54	54
24	30	50	44
48	22	40	34
72	60	70	60

Note: Sequential studies in one individual volunteer following a single dose of warfarin. The fall in protein C level was accompanied by an approximately 30% increase in factors V and VIII which remained high during the period of study, suggesting thrombin-induced activation.

[a] Of standard.

B. EXPERIMENTAL FINDINGS ON CHANGES IN PROTEIN C ACTIVITY STATES IN RELATION TO ORAL ANTICOAGULANT THERAPY

The regulatory function of the PC-thrombomodulin system (PC-TM) following a single dose (15 mg) of the oral anticoagulant warfarin was investigated by Stirling and Seghatchian.[29] Levels of the anticoagulant PC and other known procoagulant factors VII, −X, −IX and −II decrease according to their half-life.

Table 3 shows the sequential changes in FVII end PC antigen and activity during 72 h following a single dose of warfarin.

Thrombin generation in the early phase of oral anticoagulation was indicated by the elevated levels of FVIII and FV. The drop in the level of PC in the early phase was associated with the formation of a transient slow migrating form of PC (possibly a complex of APC with PCI or PS with APC and PCI) (Figure 2). This decrease in the early phase ended 72 h later with concomitant fall in FVIII and FV lower levels than seen in the early phase (Figure 3). These findings indicated that the PC-TM system is activated during the early phase of anticoagulation, possibly in response to thrombin generation. Accordingly, PC-TM has two independent regulatory functions in the thrombin generation system:

1. Feedback inhibition of FVa and FVIIIa and
2. Regulation of PCI attributable to complex formation

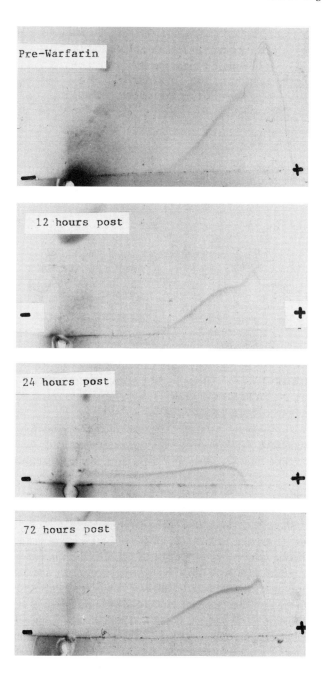

FIGURE 2. Comparative analysis of PC electrophoretic pattern, in plasma obtained following intake of 15 mg warfarin in one individual. The formation of a transient slow migrating forms are possibly indicative of complex formation between APC and its inhibitor (PCI) or between PS, APC, and PCI (for proposed mechanism see Chapter 1, Figure 3).

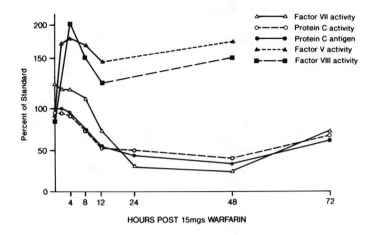

FIGURE 3. Comparative analysis between the levels of some procoagulant and anticoagulant proteins following intake of 15 mg warfarin in one individual. Elevated factors VIII and V in the early phase is either due to the release reaction or thrombin generation due to rapid disbalance between procoagulant and some anticoagulant proteins.

Despite considerable interest in the role of both inherited and acquired deficiencies of the PC system in thrombovascular diseases there is still a lack of clear definition of the cause of deficiency states. Preliminary investigations[29,30] on congenital PC deficiency states have revealed the presence of a large population of PC species having a slower electrophoretic migration as identified by using gel cutting followed by ELISA PC assays on gel slices. A new approach for evaluating the changes in activity state of PC is therefore established, based on the PC electrophoretic migration, using EDTA as buffer. This is described with some details in this chapter.

V. FUTURE TRENDS IN LABORATORY AND/OR CLINICAL ASPECTS OF HYPERCOAGULABILITY

In the past 2 decades we have witnessed a dramatic expansion in the fields of coagulation and hemostatic regulatory mechanisms. New areas such as the inhibitory effect of tissue FVIIa complexes (TFPI/EPI/LACI), thrombin induced release of TPA from endothelial cells, and activation of fibrinolysis by kk, and PC/PS inhibitory system to control formation of intravascular fibrin are now firmly established. Nevertheless it has been much more difficult to establish methods which accurately detect a discrete change in activation of the hemostatic system as observed in hypercoagulable states.

The accurate identification or characterization of any individual vitamin K-dependent protein involved in the generation of hypercoagulable states requires a clear understanding of the components of the membrane associated enzyme complexes (MAEC) procoagulant/anticoagulant systems on the surface of activated platelets. The binding to a surface component is essential to all these regulatory systems, as it confers the dramatic increase in the catalytic efficiency of the reaction processes which can be detected experimentally by the changes of their respective K_m and K_{Cat} values.

One future approach will be to directly measure the released activation peptides together with the enzymatic intermediate complexes, which occur during the conversion of a zymogen to a serine protease, by employing a direct test reflecting the *in vivo* activation using synthetic peptide analogues. An improvement to the current *in vitro* test systems, would be to carry them out in the presence of endothelial cells, a component missing in our past test procedures. Because of the involvement of the activated platelet membrane in both bioactivation and bioattenuation process, efforts should be directed to assess (at least immunologically) the presence of activated vitamin K-dependent proteins on the platelet membrane. This can be carried out either before or after stimulation to differentiate between active and activatable platelets in various pathophysiological states. Efforts in this direction, using flow cytometry principles, are currently in progress.

The true incidence of thromboembolic events in patients with lupus anticoagulant problems are another area of thrombotic complication which has expectedly received a lot of attention in recent years. The incidence is approximately 30% requiring further prospective studies. The question of cause, consequence or coincidence in thrombotic events remains a difficult problem to be resolved. One of the potential pathophysiological mechanisms, includes a decreased generation of APC on the surface of the endothelial cell, a phospholipid-dependent step requiring the presence of thrombin complexed with the endothelial membrane glycoprotein, thrombomodulin. It is becoming clear that in lupus patients the generation of APC on the surface of endothelial cells and/or platelets inhibits effective APC and PS complex formation. The role of β_2-glycoprotein (apolipoprotein II), another physiological inhibitor of the intrinsic pathway of coagulation, also remains to be elucidated as it is not clear whether this protein is also involved in the expression of lupus activity. The clinical management of lupus and associated thromboembolic events is controversial requiring prospective trials. Despite this, it is safe to say that the use of molecular markers to detect in induced hypercoagulability (due to vitamin K-dependent proteins) is no longer a concept but a reality, carried out effectively by many nonexpert laboratories.

Sickle cell (HbSS) patients have also had a predisposition to generate more thrombin end plasmin *in vivo* than normal subjects. This is probably due to the fact that hemostasis in sickle cell patients is less tightly regulated as compared to HbAA controls, contributing to the initiation of vaso-occlusive processes associated with the painful crisis of sickle cell disease.

According to Herenberg[31] prothrombotic state reflects an imbalance between the coagulant and natural anticoagulant mechanism that could eventually develop into overt thrombotic phenomena in response to a thrombogenic stimulus. This is substantiated experimentally with an increased thrombin antithrombin complex concentration as an indication of hypercoagulability.[32]

The elevated circulatory thrombin/antithrombin (TAT) is apparently associated with increased FVII consumption *in vivo*.[33] Since the proteolyzed FVII is less reactive with monoclonal than with polyclonal antibodies, comparative analyses using these two types of antibodies will provide a new and accurate marker for FVII consumption.[33,34]

Increased levels of fibrin D-dimer are also observed in sickle cell disease, indicating increased production of fibrin and its lysis by plasmin as a compensatory physiological response to the increased endogenous coagulation.[3] Nevertheless in contrast to previously established hemostatic abnormality associated with hypercoagulability (i.e., DIC [disseminated intravascular coagulation], DVT [deep venous thrombosis], acute leukemia, and liver disease) there is no significant correlation between FVII and other markers of hypercoagulability in sickle cell disease. Hence, the biochemical mechanism underlying the hypercoagulable tendencies in sickle cell disease, that may contribute to the vaso-occlusive process, remains to be fully elucidated. Both leukocytosis (with enhanced leukocyte adhesion to the endothelium) and inflammatory events have been linked to thrombotic processes involving different cellular interactions and could contribute to the disruption of the multicellular metabolic processes in such a disorderly microcirculatory phenomena.[34]

The epidemiological approach will undoubtedly receive further attention. Already studies in thousands of probands have revealed that plasma levels of fibrinogen and FVII:C may be useful predictors of an increased coronary risk. The results of the Northwick Park Heart Study has been critically reviewed and preventative measures using low dose warfarin is now on the way with apparent success. Another line of development is to elucidate the role of the vitamin K-dependent proteins in progressive stenosis, in which, both the increase and the narrowing of the vessel may influence the activation states of bioamplification and bioattenuation systems.

Finally with respect to methodological aspects, new biochemical and immunological tests have become available which allow the detection of picogram levels of activated peptides and intravascular thrombin generation (as well as platelet specific proteins such as platelet factor 4 and beta thromboglobulin). These assays need to be further validated to assess their usefulness. The recent development of ELISA methods for assessing modified AT III, EPI, or TFPI quaternary complexes and APC-PCI complexes provide new markers of hypercoagulability with reasonable *in vivo* half-lives, which closely reflect ongoing prothrombotic states as well as helping to assess the changes in the activation states of pro- and anticoagulant vitamin K-dependent proteins. More recently, attention has been focused on the involvement and role of cellular components (endothelium, platelets, monocytes, and macrophases) in hypercoagulability.

Electrophoretic distribution of protein C
as compared to fx

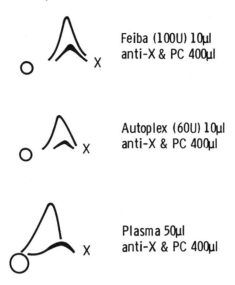

FIGURE 4. Crossed electrophoretic distribution pattern of PC as compared to factor X in human plasma and two types of commercial vitamin K-dependant concentrates ("Feiba" or "Autoplex"), using mixed anti-X and anti-PC antibodies — changes in the relative electrophoretic migration are indicative of processing-induced alteration in the activity states of these proteins or selective enrichment of some molecular forms of PC and/or factor X present in plasma.

Endothelial dependent mechanisms of the procoagulant and anticoagulant pathways clearly will be in focus in coming years. For example it is becoming established that blocking the activity of FIXa or FXa results in inhibition of intravenous coagulation. However in contrast to blocking FXa activity FIXa activity does not interfere with extravenous hemostasis. This opens a new area of development work for searching of potential agents which block FIXa-cell surface interaction selectively.

We might also expect to see a lot of new developments with respect to the supply of human plasma-derived proteins. For example, the supply of plasma-derived PC and PS might be insufficient to meet the modest estimate of clinical demand of these naturally occurring vitamin K anticoagulants. Recently, large transgenic animals (e.g., sheep) have been developed which contain the human PC gene and which produce a milligram-per-milliliter quantity of PC in their milk. This product is now among many other new-generation products awaiting clinical trials and a comparison with plasma derived products. The latter, as indicated in Figure 4 may be partially proteolyzed as indicated by changes in electrophoretic migration.

Combination therapy with APC and urokinase has also provided improved efficiency in their antithrombotic effects without impairing hemostatic function. Further clinical trails in this direction are already on the way.

Various genetic engineering strategies based on single amino acid or more extensive sequence changes have resulted in analogs with significantly improved pharmacodynamics, clinical safety and efficiency. This strategic area requires much further in-depth investigation. Standardization in methodology is another developing area in the future.

ACKNOWLEDGMENTS

The author wishes to express his sincere thanks to Yvonne Stirling for her expert technical contribution in these collaborative studies. Her dedication and vigilance in pursuing various laboratory aspects of this work has contributed to some of the new findings described in this chapter. Special thanks are also due to M. J. Shearer for joint editorial review of this manuscript. The data reported here were presented in part at the ICTH Congress (1985) and to the British Society of Hematology.

REFERENCES

1. **Stenflo, J.,** A new vitamin K dependent protein, *J. Biol. Chem.,* 251, 355, 1976.
2. **Comp, P. C. and Esmon, C. T.,** Activated protein C inhibits platelet prothrombin converting activity, *Blood,* 54, 1272, 1979.
3. **Kisiel, W.,** Human plasma protein C, *J. Clin. Invest.,* 64, 761, 1979.
4. **Walker, F. J.,** Regulation of activated protein C by a new protein, *J. Biol. Chem.,* 255, 1260, 1980.
5. **Bertina, R. M., Broekmans, A. W., Van Der Linde, I. D., and Meriens, K.,** Protein C deficiency in a Dutch family with thrombotic disease, *Thromb. Haemostas.,* 48, 1, 1981.
6. **Griffin, J. H., Evatt, B., Zimmermann, T. S., Kleiss, A. J., and Wideman, V.,** Deficiency of protein C in congenital thrombotic disease, *J. Clin. Invest.,* 40, 1370, 1981.
7. **Owen, W. G. and Esmon, C. T.,** Functional properties of an endothelial cell cofactor of thrombin catalyzed activation of protein C, *J. Biol. Chem.,* 256, 5532, 1981.
8. **Francis, R. B. and Patch, M. J.,** A functional assay for protein C in human plasma, *Thromb. Res.,* 32, 605, 1983.
9. **Suzuki, K., Nishioka, J., and Hasimato, S.,** Protein C inhibitor-purification from human plasma and characterization, *J. Biol. Chem.,* 258, 163, 1983.
10. **Bertina, R. M., Broekmans, A. W., Frommenhock-Ran, E. C., and Van Wijngaarden, A.,** The use of a functional and immunologic assay for plasma protein C in the study of heterogeneity of congenital protein C deficiency, *Thromb. Haemostas.,* 51, 1984.
11. **Boyer, C., Rotschild, C., Wolf, M., Amiral, J., Meyer, D., and Larrieu, M. J.,** A new method for the estimation of protein C by ELISA, *Thromb. Res.,* 36, 579, 1984.
12. **Comp, P. C., Nixon, R. R., and Esmon, C. T.,** Determination of functional levels of protein C, an antithrombotic protein, using thrombin, thrombomodulin complex, *Blood,* 63, 15, 1984.
13. **Salam, N.,** A functional assay of protein C in human plasma, *Blood,* 63, 671, 1984.

14. **Vigano, S., Mannucci, P. M., Solinas, S., Botasso, B., and Mariani, G.,** Decrease in protein C antigen and formation of an abnormal protein soon after starting oral anticoagulant therapy, *Br. J. Haematol.,* 57, 213, 1984.

15. **Amiral, J., Boyer, C., Rotschild, C., and Wolf, M.,** Determination of protein C by an immunoenzymatic assay, in *Protein C — Biochemical and Medical Aspects,* I. Witt, Ed., Walter de Grluyter, Berlin, 1985, 67.

16. **Miletich, J., Sherman, L., and Broze, G.,** Absence of thrombosis in subjects with heterozygous protein C deficiency, *N. Engl. J. Med.,* 317, 991, 1987.

17. **Comp, P. C., Nixon, R. R., Cooper, M. R., and Esmon, C. T.,** Familial protein S deficiency is associated with recurrent thrombosis, *J. Clin. Invest.,* 74, 2082, 1984.

18. **Walker, F. J.,** Protein S and the regulation of activated protein C, *Thromb. Haemostas.,* 100, 131, 1984.

19. **Kamiya, T., Sugihara, T., Ogata, K., Saito, H., Suziki, K., Nishioka, J., Hashimoto, S., and Yamagata, K.,** Inherited deficiency of protein S in a Japanese family with recurrent venous thrombosis. A study of three generations, *Blood,* 67, 406, 1986.

20. **D'Angelo, A., Vigano-D'Angelo, S., Esmon, C. T., and Comp, P. C.,** Acquired deficiencies of protein S, *J. Clin. Invest.,* 81, 1445, 1988.

21. **Suzuki, K. and Nishioka, J.,** Plasma protein S activity measured using Protac a snake venom derived activator of protein C, *Thromb. Res.,* 49, 241 1988.

22. **Wolf, M., Boyer-Neumann, C., Martinoli, J. L., Leroy-Matheron, C., Amiral, J., Meyer, D., Larrieu, M. J.,** A new functional assay for human protein S activity using activated factor V as substrate, *Thromb. Haemostas.,* 62, 1144, 1989.

23. **Laurell, M. and Stenflo, J.,** Protein C inhibitor from human plasma: characterisation of native and cleaved inhibitor and demonstration of inhibitor complexes with plasma kallikrein, *Thromb. Haemostas.,* 62, 885, 1989.

24. **Vigano, D., Angelo, S., Gilardoni, F. D., and Angelo, A.,** Evaluation of coagulometric assays in the assessment of protein C anticoagulant activity variable sensitivity of commercial APTT reagents to the cofactor effect of protein S, *Thromb. Haemostas.,* 62, 861, 1989.

25. **Kitchens, C. S.,** Concept of hypercoagulability a review of its development clinical application and recent progress, *Semin. Thromb. Hemostas.,* 11, 293, 1985.

26. **Rosenberg, R. D.,** The biochemistry and pathophysiology of the prethrombotic state, *Ann. Dev. Med.,* 38, 493, 1987.

27. **Dolan, G., Cooper, P., Jackson, P., Brown, P., Sampson, B., Forman, K., and Preston, F. E.,** Variation in plasma protein C concentration in well healthy volunteers and the significance of low values, *Br. J. Haematol.,* 77 (Suppl. 1), 61, 1991.

28. **Meade, T. M., Stirling, Y., Howarth, D. Y., and Seghatchian, M. J.,** Effect of oral contraceptives on protein C and thrombin production (unpublished observation, 1991).

29. **Stirling, Y. and Seghatchian, M. J.,** Sequential studies on vitamin K dependent protein in one individual following a single dose (15 mg) of Warfarin (unpublished observation, 1991).

30. **Seghatchian, M. J., Conard, J., and Samama, M.,** Heterogeneity in protein C electrophotetic migration evaluated by gel cutting and protein C functional assay by ELISA assay. (unpublished observation, 1991).

31. **Herenberg, J., Hass, R., and Zimmerman, R.,** Plasma hypercoagulability after termination of oral anticoagulants, *Thromb. Res.,* 29, 627, 1982.

32. **Boisclair, M. D., Lane, D. A., Wilde, J. T., Ireland, H., Preston, F. E., and Ofosu, F. A.** A comparative evaluation of assays for markers of activated coagulation and/or fibrinolysis: thrombin-antithrombin complex, D-dimer and fibrinogen, fibrin fragment E antigen, *Br. J. Haematol.,* 74, 421, 1990.

33. **Offosu, F. A., Leclerc, J., Delrone, F., Craven, S., Shafi, S., Pewin, I., and Blachman, M. A.,** The low molecular weight heparin (ex-oxaparine) inhibits in vivo factor VII consumption and prothrombin activation associated with elective knee replacement surgery, *Thrombos. Haemostas.,* 65, 1298, 1991.

34. **Lipowsky, H. H. and Chein, S.,** Role of leucocyte endothelium adhesion in affecting recovery from ischemic episodes, *Ann. NY Acad. Sci.,* 565, 308, 1989.

Chapter 7

PROTEIN C AND PROTEIN S: METHODOLOGICAL AND CLINICAL ASPECTS

Catherine Boyer-Neumann, Martine Wolf, and Mary-Jo Larrieu

TABLE OF CONTENTS

0-8493-6423-X/93/$0.00 + $.50
© 1993 by CRC Press, Inc.

Enhancement of the coagulation pathway may favor the development of thrombosis and is prevented by defense mechanisms, in which inhibitors play an important role. Protein C and protein S are vitamin K-dependent glycoproteins; protein C, activated by the thrombin-thrombomodulin complex on the endothelial surface, is responsible for the inactivation of factors Va and VIIIa.[1] Protein S serves as a cofactor for activated protein C (APC), by enhancing the rate of inactivation of both factors Va and VIIIa by APC (Figure 1).[2] The clinical importance of protein C and protein S is supported by the association between recurrent thromboembolic diseases and inherited deficiencies of one of these two proteins.[3] This chapter will summarize current physiological and methodological aspects of both inhibitors and clinical evidence that protein C and S are important regulators of thrombosis.

I. PROTEIN C

A. PHYSIOLOGICAL ASPECTS

Protein C is a vitamin K-dependent glycoprotein with a molecular mass of 62,000 Da[4] present in plasma at a concentration of approximately 4 μg/ ml.[5] Its site of synthesis appears to be unique to the hepatocyte.[6] The complete primary structure of protein C has now been determined[7] and its gene is found to be located on chromosome 2.[8] Protein C consists of a heavy chain (41,000 Da) and a light chain (21,000 Da) linked by a single disulfide bridge.[9] The active site, serine, is located on the heavy chain, and the γ-carboxyglutamic acid (Gla) residues on the light chain; the Gla residues facilitate binding to calcium cell membranes.[10,11] Protein C circulates in plasma as a zymogen which is converted to its active form, APC, by the thrombin-thrombomodulin complex.[12] This process involves a single cleavage (Arg12 Leu13) in the heavy chain, with the release of an activation peptide with a molecular mass of 1400 Da.[4] APC exerts its anticoagulant function by inactivating factors Va and VIIIa, two non-enzymic cofactors of coagulation,[13,14] and is itself slowly neutralized by a specific plasma protease inhibitor which has a molecular mass of 57,000 Da.[15,16] The rate of inactivation of factors Va and VIIIa by APC is greatly enhanced by protein S,[2] which increases the affinity of APC for the phospholipid membrane surface. In addition, human APC potentiates fibrinolysis *in vitro*[17] and *in vivo*,[18] by decreasing plasminogen activator inhibitor (PAI) activity. This anticoagulant system is controlled by two distinct types of inhibitors: a heparin-dependent plasma inhibitor named protein C inhibitor[19] and a heparin-independent one, which has been shown to be α-1-antitrypsin.[20]

B. METHODOLOGICAL ASPECTS
1. Functional Assays of Protein C

Functional assays should be used for laboratory screening tests because qualitative defects will remain undetected if only immunological methods are performed.

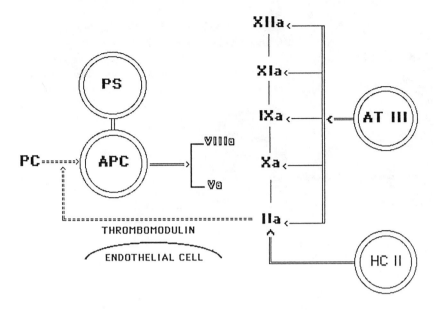

FIGURE 1. Schematic representation of the target sites of the physiological inhibitors of the coagulation pathway. This figure illustrates mainly the protein C pathway: thrombin (IIa) forms a complex with the endothelial cells surface protein, thrombomodulin, which activates protein C (PC). Activated protein C (APC) linked to its cofactor protein S (PS) inhibits both factors Va and VIIIa by limited proteolysis.

A number of functional assays have been described and recently reviewed.[21] Usually, these methods involve three steps: separation of protein C from its plasma inhibitor by adsorption with aluminium hydroxide,[22] barium citrate,[23,24] or a monoclonal antibody;[25] activation of the zymogen by thrombin alone[22,24] or thrombin-thrombomodulin complex;[23,25] and, finally, measurement of protein C activity. This estimation may be performed either by clotting methods (prolongation of activated partial thromboplastin time (APTT) or of factor Xa clotting time) or by amidolytic assays using different synthetic substrates. The main characteristics of these three step techniques are summarized in Table 1. These methods, however, are time consuming and their complexity results in a potential source of errors.

The recent identification of a venom of the Southern Copperhead (*Agkistrodon contortrix contortrix,* named Protac®), which specifically activates protein C, has allowed the development of simple and rapid assays for protein C activity.[26,27] Activation by Protac is sufficiently fast to enable the measurement of protein C directly in plasma, thereby bypassing the adsorption step. Kinetic analysis of these venom enzymes indicate that they activate protein C as efficiently as the thrombin-thrombomodulin complex.[28] Measurements of APC may then be performed either by clotting,[26] or amidolytic[27] methods (Table 1).

TABLE 1

Functional Assays of Protein C

Assay (Ref.)	Protein C separation	Protein C activation	Measurement of APC[a]
Bertina et al.[22]	Aluminium hydroxide	Human thrombin without Ca^{2+}	Amidolytic (S-2366)
Sala et al.[23]	Barium citrate	Human thrombin rabbit thrombomodulin + Ca^{2+}	Amidolytic (S-2366)
Francis et al.[24]	Barium citrate	Human thrombin without Ca^{2+}	Clotting (APTT)
Vigano D'Angelo et al.[25]	Monoclonal antibody	bovine thrombin rabbit thrombomodulin + Ca^{2+}	Amidolytic or clotting
Martinoli et al.[26]	None	Protac	Clotting
Kobayashi et al.[27]	None	Protac	Amidolytic (S-2366)

[a] APC: activated protein C.

The assays described above are able to detect congenital protein C deficiency, either quantitative (type I) or qualitative (type II). However, in clinical practice, a rapid and accurate assay is needed for screening purposes and methods using Protac as an activator appear the most appropriate. As a vitamin K-dependent protein the levels of protein C are invariably decreased in patients undergoing oral anticoagulant treatment; the extent of this decrease varies with the type of assay. Since des-γ-carboxylated protein C retains its capacity to split chromogenic substrates, only clotting assays can evaluate all the dysfunctional defects of protein C in vitamin K-deficient states.

2. Immunological Assays of Protein C

Since the introduction of the first immunological assay for plasma protein C,[29] several methods have now been described: electroimmunodiffusion (EID) with polyclonal antibodies in the presence of EDTA,[29] enzyme-linked immunoabsorbent assay (ELISA) or radioimmunoassay using polyclonal[30,31] or monoclonal[32] antibodies.

Studies evaluating the sensitivity and specificity of immunological assays have been reported.[21,33-35] Although all the methods are specific for protein C antigens, EID is less sensitive, and cannot detect levels under 10% of the normal range. Nevertheless, protein C levels are quite similar in normal subjects whatever the assay used. Similarly in most clinical conditions or situations such as myocardial infarction, chronic liver disease or during the post-operative period, protein C antigen is detected with equal efficiency by all assays. Significant methodological discrepancies, however, have been observed in two groups; namely in patients on anticoagulant therapy and in patients with disseminated intravascular coagulation (DIC). Thus, in patients taking oral anticoagulant drugs, measurements of protein C antigen by ELISA methods seem to be consistently lower than those measured by EID in the presence of EDTA. This could be related to the presence in anticoagulated patients of undercarboxylated (des-γ-carboxy) species of protein C and to differences in their electrophoretic mobility from the fully carboxylated form. Even more pronounced discrepancies are found for protein C measurements made in patients with DIC and this may be due to the presence in this condition of complexes of APC with its specific inhibitor (PCI). The formation of such complexes results in a loss of antigenicity and levels of protein C measured by ELISA are about half those measured by EID.

Finally, functional assays are more advisable when screening for congenital protein C deficiency. When a defect is found, immunological methods will allow further characterization.

3. Physiological Variations

Plasma protein C levels in healthy adults range from 67 to 125% of a normal pool.[36] In newborns, protein C is decreased and progressively increases from the second week, reaching the adult values after the sixth month.[37,38] In women taking oral contraceptives, protein C is 20% higher than in controls. Similarly, protein C levels increase during pregnancy, averaging about 130% of normal: peak concentrations of protein C are reached during the second trimester, then its level progressively decreases until delivery and returns to normal in the post-partum period.[39]

C. CLINICAL ASPECTS
1. Congenital Protein C Deficiency

Since the first description in 1981 by Griffin et al.[40] of a kindred in whom a decreased protein C concentration was associated with recurrent thrombotic events, several other families with hereditary protein C deficiency have now been reported.[41,42] This disorder is inherited as an autosomal codominant mode. The majority of the patients are heterozygotes with levels of the zymogen averaging 50% of normal. In a few cases, extremely low or undetectable levels of protein C are found in newborns and the family analysis reveals that the disorder is consistent with homozygosity (or double heterozygosity) in such infants.[43,44] Recently, DNA analysis has allowed the identification of the genetic abnormality in some kindreds: total or partial gene deletion, nonsense or missense mutations.[45]

In a relatively large study from the Netherlands the prevalence of protein C deficiency in the Dutch population has been estimated to be about 1 per 16,000.[46] However, Miletich et al.[47] found a much higher frequency of heterozygous protein C deficiency in a healthy population of blood donors, i.e., 1 per 200 to 300, and all the affected subjects are asymptomatic.[47] These data however need to be confirmed by further prospective studies. The prevalence of the defect in a young population with thrombotic manifestations has been estimated to be 7% which is similar to protein S deficiency but higher than antithrombin III (AT III) deficiency (Table 2).[46]

TABLE 2
Incidence of Protein C
and Protein S
Deficiencies in Young
Patients with
Thrombotic Disease

Protein	Incidence (%)
Protein C	7
Protein S	5–10
Antithrombin III	2–3
Plasminogen	1–2
Fibrinogen	1

The clinical manifestations of heterozygous protein C deficiency are essentially those associated with recurrent deep or superficial venous thrombosis, which in about 40% of cases is complicated by pulmonary embolism. In fact, the clinical profile is quite similar to that seen in AT III deficiency, except that arterial thrombosis may also be observed. A characteristic feature of protein C deficiency is the development of cerebral thrombophlebitis which may be due to the absence of thrombomodulin in the microcirculation of brain tissue. Another typical complication of this defect is the skin necrosis observed during the early phase of oral anticoagulant treatment: the rapid decrease in the already low protein C level, due to its short half-life (6 to 7 h), leads to thrombosis in the microvasculature.[48,49]

The first thrombotic event may appear spontaneously or in conjunction with known risk factors, such as major trauma, surgery, pregnancy, and the post-partum period. The age of onset of thrombotic episodes ranges from 15 to 35 years of age with a mean of 24 years. Although affected patients rarely show any symptoms before the age of 15, approximately 65% have suffered from recurrent thrombotic episodes before the age of 50. In contrast, homozygous protein C deficiency is always associated with severe clinical symptoms, beginning in early infancy, and presenting as fulminans purpura or massive thrombosis with fatal issue.[43,44,50,51] The severity of thrombosis in infants with homozygous protein C deficiency, with dramatic symptoms occurring soon after birth, justifies a prenatal diagnosis when possible, or an early diagnosis after birth and immediate substitutive therapy (see below).

Although major thrombotic complications are observed in most of the heterozygous patients, some affected subjects remain asymptomatic. In fact, individuals with protein C deficiency do not appear equally predisposed to thrombosis. Some studies have shown that in families with homozygous deficiency, the heterozygous parents with a partial deficiency have no history of thrombosis.[43] Bauer et al.[52] studying heterozygous protein C deficient patients, with similar plasma protein C levels, demonstrated that some of

TABLE 3
Variants (Type II) of Protein C Deficiency: Characteristics of Five Cases

Protein C variant (Ref.)	Functional defect	Mutation
Protein C Cadiz[53]	Normal activation; abnormal serine-protease activity	—
Faioni et al.[54]	Normal activation; normal binding to phospholipids and protein S; abnormal serine-protease activity	Near the active site
Protein C Rouen[55]	Normal activation; normal serine-protease activity; abnormal anticoagulant activity	—
Protein C Tochigi[56]	Abnormal activation	Arg169 Trp
Protein C London I[57]	Abnormal activation	Agr169 Trp

them have a significant decrease in the protein C activation peptide (PCP) and a significant increase in the prothrombin fragment F.1 + 2 (F1 + 2). These authors were unable, however, to establish any significant correlation between the variations of these markers and the occurrence of thrombosis. This implies that other factors, such as thrombomodulin levels, PCI activity or protein S interaction may play a role in the onset of thrombosis *in vivo*.

The majority of patients with congenital protein C deficiency are heterozygotes with a quantitative (type I) deficiency characterized by a similar decrease, close to 50%, of both immunological and functional levels of protein C. In a few cases, a qualitative (type II) defect has been reported, with reduced levels of protein C activity but normal levels of protein C antigen.[22,53-57] The functional abnormality of these molecular variants can affect either the catalytic domain, the activation site or the N-terminal part of the molecule involved in the binding to phospholipids (Table 3).

Recently, the isolation of cDNA for protein C gene has allowed the characterization of the mutations of type I or type II defects. In type I, distinct mutations have been described, including splice site, non-sense and missense mutations.[58] In type II, the mutation has been characterized at the activation site (Arg 169 → Trp) in two cases: protein C Tochigi[56] and protein C London I[57] (Table 3). In protein C Tochigi, this mutation is associated with a type I deficiency due to a complete deletion of one protein C gene.

2. Acquired Protein C Deficiency

Acquired deficiency of protein C often reflects pathological states or is induced by drugs (Table 4). In 1982, Mannucci et al.[59] reported an extensive study of protein C deficiency in various disease conditions, commonly associated with combined defects in the other coagulation proteins. Chronic or acute liver disease and DIC remain the two major causes of these acquired deficiencies. Protein C levels are low in chronic liver disease, by degrees roughly proportional to the severity of the disease and to the impairment of

TABLE 4
Acquired Deficiencies of Protein C

Pathological states
Liver disease
Disseminated intravascular coagulation
Respiratory distress syndrome
Acute leukemias
Post-operative period
Lupus-like anticoagulants

Drug-induced
Vitamin K-antagonists
L-Asparaginase

protein synthesis, thus confirming that the liver is the site of synthesis of this inhibitor. However, one cannot rule out the possibility that low plasma levels of protein C are due to an increased turnover, as previously demonstrated for other hemostatic components in chronic liver disease. In our experience, protein C appears to be a very sensitive marker of liver function.

In clinical conditions associated with DIC, protein C levels are usually very low and sometimes unmeasurable.[5,60] The most likely explanation for this is that protein C, when activated by thrombin during DIC, forms complexes with PCI leading to a more rapid clearance from the circulation. It is possible that during DIC, anoxia, and/or endotoxin, damage to endothelial cells may occur so that thrombomodulin becomes more available at the endothelial surface; hence, APC would be much enhanced and its clearance from plasma accelerated. This hypothesis is supported by the finding of very low or undetectable levels of protein C in adult respiratory distress syndrome, a condition characterized by extensive pulmonary endothelial damage. Protein C is also decreased in patients with acute leukemia and hyperleucocytosis. It seems that liver dysfunction, more pronounced in patients with hyperleucocytosis, is the major determinant of low protein C levels in acute leukemia.[60]

The period immediately following minor or major surgery is associated with an acquired defect of protein C. A possible explanation is that during surgery, and immediately after, tissue damage induces an *in vivo* activation of blood clotting, resulting in increased thrombin formation. In conjunction with thrombomodulin, thrombin might in turn activate protein C, leading to its faster removal from the circulation.[59]

Patients with lupus-like anticoagulant may develop thrombotic complications associated with protein C deficiency.[61] The lupus anticoagulant is an abnormal immunoglobulin directed against phospholipids of the endothelial cells. Activation of protein C may be impaired at the endothelial surface, thus enhancing the possibility of thrombosis.

The rates of decrease from the circulation of protein C and the other vitamin K-dependent clotting factors during the early phase of oral anticoagulant therapy have also been studied.[62] The findings indicate that protein

C, like factor VII, has a very short plasma half-life and decreases rapidly; whereas the other vitamin K-dependent clotting factors, with correspondingly much longer plasma half-lives, remain relatively unchanged in the short term. These data might explain the poor antithrombotic effect of early anticoagulant therapy and also the occurrence of skin necrosis in protein C deficient states.[48]

Protein C deficiency found in patients treated with the cytotoxic agent L-asparaginase may be due to the inhibition of protein synthesis in liver.[63]

II. PROTEIN S

A. PHYSIOLOGICAL ASPECTS

Protein S is a vitamin K-dependent glycoprotein with a molecular mass of 70,000 Da[64] present in plasma at a concentration of 25 μg/ml.[65] It acts as a cofactor of APC in the proteolytic inactivation of factors Va and VIIIa. Protein S enhances the binding of APC to the phospholipids of platelets and endothelial cells.[66]

Protein S has the unusual property of circulating in plasma in two forms which are in a dynamic equilibrium: free protein S (40%), the only active form, and inactive protein S (60%) reversibly complexed to the C4b-binding protein (C4bBP). Recently, Dahlbäck et al.[67] have suggested the existence of another plasma component which regulates the interaction between C4bBP and protein S. The complete primary structure of protein S has now been determined,[64] the cDNA has been sequenced[68] and the gene was found to be localized on chromosome 3.[69,70] Protein S consists of a single chain with a N-terminal region homologous to that of other vitamin K-dependent proteins, containing 10 Gla residues and some β-hydroxyaspartic and β-hydroxyas-paragine residues.[71-73] Adjacent to this Gla region is a thrombin sensitive region followed by four epidermal growth factor (EGF) domains.[74] Unlike other vitamin K-dependent proteins, protein S does not contain a serine-protease catalytic domain but has a unique large carboxyterminal structure that bears homology with the androgen binding protein. Protein S exerts its anticoagulant function as a cofactor for APC. It enhances the binding of protein C to a phospholipid and thereby increases the rate of inactivation of factors Va and VIIIa.[2]

B. METHODOLOGICAL ASPECTS

The measurement of protein S levels is complicated by the fact that two forms exist in plasma, one free and the other reversibly complexed with C4bBP. Only the free form is functionally active as a cofactor for the anti-coagulant effect of APC, whereas the complexed one does not contribute to the regulation of coagulation.[75] The presence of these two forms also makes the diagnosis of protein S deficiency more difficult since conventional im-munological assays do not distinguish between them.

1. Immunological Assays of Protein S

Protein S was first determined in native plasma by the Laurell EID method, by ELISA or by radioimmunoassay using polyclonal antibodies against the total protein.[76-79] The relative distribution of both forms may be assessed by two-dimensional immunoelectrophoresis (DDIE).[80] In normal plasma, protein S migrates as two distinct peaks, one remaining near the origin and representing the complexed form, and the other, with a more anodal mobility, corresponding to the free form. However, this method allows only a semi-quantitative estimation of protein S and is not suitable for the diagnosis of protein S deficiency.

For this reason, alternative ways of separating the free and bound forms have been sought. One method is based on the selective precipitation of free and bound protein S with polyethyleneglycol (PEG): thus the addition of 3.75% PEG 8000 to plasma selectively precipitates the complex leaving the free protein in the supernatant.[80] The free form may be then measured by either EID or ELISA. The ELISA method is more sensitive (detection limit: 0.01%) and thus appears to be more suitable. Normal levels of free protein S measured by the PEG precipitation method range from 60 to 120% as compared to a pool of normal donors.[80] A disadvantage of such multistage methods involving separation of free and bound protein S is that they require a high degree of technical expertise. Therefore functional assays appear more convenient.

2. Functional Assays of Protein S

The methods presently available are all based on the ability of protein S to act as a cofactor for APC. The anticoagulant effect of protein S is measured using either the prolongation of the prothrombin time[66,81] or the activated partial thromboplastin time.[82-88] However, these assays are still difficult and may be influenced by other clotting factors. The use of diluted plasma may overcome these problems particularly with regard to the influence of factor II and VIII levels. At the present time, several laboratories use their own in-house assays, so that it is difficult to compare different methods and their correlation with free protein S antigen levels.

3. Physiological Variations

In normal subjects, total protein S ranges from 70 to 130% while free protein S, estimated by either PEG precipitation or functional methods, ranges from 60 to 120%.[80]

Low levels of protein S have been described during pregnancy, in the post-partum period and in women taking oral contraceptives.[89,90] During pregnancy, the plasma concentration of total protein S falls progressively reaching the lowest levels (about 55% of normal) during the second trimester.[89,90] Moreover, free protein S is also reduced and does not return to normal until 12 weeks after delivery. In healthy pregnant women, this low protein S level is compensated by an increased protein C concentration, and thus normal pregnancy may not necessarily predispose women to thrombosis. On the other hand, pregnancy constitutes an obvious added risk factor to women who already have a congenital protein S deficiency, and this may warrant prophylactic anticoagulant treatment.

In healthy newborns, total protein S is about one third of normal adult values.[91] Free protein S represents the predominant form, and this is due to the fact that C4bBP levels at birth are only about 18% of normal. This results in relatively normal levels of free protein S, and it is possible that this may compensate physiologically for the very low protein C levels in the neonatal period.[92]

C. CLINICAL ASPECTS
1. Congenital Protein S Deficiency

In 1984, shortly after the development of immunological assays for protein S, the first families with protein S deficiency were described.[76,77] Subsequently, other reports confirmed the major role of protein S as a physiological antithrombotic protein.[82,83,93] Many heterozygous protein S-deficient patients with thrombotic disease have now been identified. The prevalence of the defect in the global population (1 per 15,000) and its incidence in young patients with thrombosis (about 8%) appears to be similar to that seen for protein C deficiency (Table 2). The disease is inherited as an autosomal dominant trait.[76] The clinical manifestations in the heterozygous state are very similar to those of protein C deficiency, including the occurrence of superficial thrombophlebitis and arterial thrombosis. However, unlike protein C deficiency, the appearance of skin necrosis at the onset of oral anticoagulant treatment is less frequent in protein S deficiency; this is probably due to the longer half-life of protein S compared to protein C. Diagnosis of protein S deficiency is based on low levels of protein S activity and free protein S antigen with total protein S antigen being normal or slightly reduced. Any classification of congenital protein S deficiency is difficult due to the association of the protein with C4bBP. A decrease in free protein S may be caused not only by a quantitative protein S deficiency but also by an abnormal interaction between protein S and C4bBP. Interestingly, the existence of an abnormal C4bBP has recently been demonstrated in a family with complete lack of free protein S.[94] Until now, the only available classification appears to be type I for quantitative deficiency and type II for a qualitative defect.[95] This is complicated, however, by the fact that a phenotypic protein S defect may involve a genetic abnormality of at least three different proteins (protein S, C4bBP, or other regulating component). The gene for protein S is localized on chromosome 3.[69,70] Detailed analysis have revealed the presence of two genes, PSα and a pseudogene PSβ.[96] Presently, only four genetic abnormalities have been reported: two mutations, one in the pseudogene[97] and the other one in the α gene[98] (Heerlen polymorphism: Ser 460 Pro) and two deletions.[99,100]

In the near future it is likely that the development of both functional assays and genomic analysis will allow the identification of numerous mutations and a better understanding of the relationship between structure and function.

2. Acquired Protein S Deficiency

Acquired protein S deficiency occurs in several clinical situations and may constitute an increased risk for thrombosis. The understanding of the pathophysiology is more difficult for protein S than that for the other vitamin K-dependent proteins, since an equilibrium exists in plasma between the functionally active free protein S and its inactive form complexed with C4bBP. As a result of this equilibrium either a decreased level of total protein S antigen or an increase of C4bBP may lead to reduced protein S activity.

In liver disease, plasma levels of protein S are decreased but the degree of reduction of both antigenic and functional levels is much less than for protein C. The most likely explanation for this discrepancy is the demonstration that protein S is synthesized by endothelial cells[101] in addition to hepatocytes whereas protein C is only synthesized by the hepatocyte.[102] On the other hand, C4bBP is also decreased in liver disease by more than protein S itself; because of this, levels of free protein S are only moderately reduced.[86,103]

In patients with DIC, free protein S levels may be normal or slightly decreased. The values are apparently dependent on the C4bBP levels, which may be either increased[86] or normal.[104]

In the nephrotic syndrome, the levels of total protein S, like the other vitamin K-dependent proteins, tend to be high. However, an important increase of C4bBP results in decreased levels of free protein S.[105,106]

As with protein C, protein S activity is markedly decreased during long-term therapy with vitamin K-antagonists such as warfarin: since total protein S antigen is also reduced there is an increase in the ratio between the complexed form and the free one. More importantly, the appearance of des-γcarboxylated forms of protein S in the circulation results in a decrease in the specific activity (ratio of protein S activity: protein S free antigen) to about 0.5.[86,103] Because the half-life of protein S (about 42 h) is much longer than that of protein C (6 to 7 h), the risk of warfarin-induced necrosis at the onset of oral anticoagulant therapy seems to be negligible. One apparent case of warfarin-induced skin necrosis in a patient with protein S deficiency[107] may have been due to other factors predisposing to this condition.

Although a variety of clinical conditions lead to an acquired protein S deficiency it is not known to what extent this may predispose to thrombosis except in patients who already have a congenital protein S deficiency. Further clinical studies are needed to understand the influence of acquired protein S deficiency on thrombotic manifestations.

III. TREATMENT OF PROTEIN C AND PROTEIN S DEFICIENCIES

A. PROPHYLAXIS

Prophylactic anticoagulant treatment is not indicated nor advisable in asymptomatic patients with heterozygous deficiencies. Many affected patients remain quite asymptomatic, with no history of thrombotic complications, and it is therefore unjustified to treat them prophylactically solely on the basis of having the defect. In contrast, longterm oral anticoagulant prophylaxis is imperative when at least one thrombotic episode has occurred. Clinical evidence indicates that vitamin K-antagonists are the most effective therapy to prevent recurrence of thrombosis.[108] Since some patients with protein C deficiency may develop skin necrosis at the onset of oral anticoagulant therapy, low doses may be used at first and the dose progressively increased; heparin should be administered concomitantly for at least 7 to 10 d. When anticoagulants have to be discontinued for surgery, replacement therapy with specific protein C and/or protein S concentrates should be used.

B. CURATIVE

Thrombotic manifestations in patients with congenital deficiency of either protein C or protein S should be treated according to the usual clinical recommendations. Heparin remains the best treatment of the acute phase for all patients whatever the defect. Vitamin-K antagonists should overlap with heparin for at least 5 to 10 d.

The therapeutic approach to purpura fulminans is more complicated since newborns with homozygous protein C deficiency need to receive continuous treatment. Recommendations have recently been given by the ICTH Subcommittee on protein C and protein S:[109] such newborns should receive fresh frozen plasma (10 ml/kg, twice a day) for at least 4 to 10 weeks until all the necrotic lesions disappear. Vitamin K-antagonists should then be used for longterm treatment, with the prothrombin time maintained at an international normalized ratio (INR) of 2.5 to 4.0. In order to prevent the appearance of skin necrosis, infusion of fresh frozen plasma should be maintained until satisfactory prolongation of the prothrombin time is achieved. However, in some cases infusion of fresh frozen plasma appears ineffective or can lead to fluid overload. For this reason, replacement therapy with a concentrate of human protein C and S has been successfully used (100 U/kg protein C given every 48 h over a period of 9 months) allowing the complete resolution of the thrombotic condition.[110] In the future, gene therapy may become available and would seem to offer the best prospects for successful longterm treatment.

REFERENCES

1. **Clause, H. L. and Comp, P. C.,** The regulation of haemostasis: the protein C system, *N. Engl. J. Med.,* 314, 1298, 1986.
2. **Walker, F. J.,** Regulation of activated protein C by a new protein. A possible function for bovine protein S, *J. Biol. Chem.,* 255, 5521, 1980.
3. **Griffin, J. H., Evatt, B., Zimmerman, T. S., Kleiss, A. J., and Wideman, C.,** Deficiency of protein C in congenital thrombotic disease, *J. Clin. Invest.,* 68, 1370, 1981.

4. **Kisiel, W.,** Human plasma protein C. Isolation, characterization, and mechanism of activation by α-thrombin, *J. Clin. Invest.,* 64, 761, 1979.

5. **Griffin, J. H., Mosher, D. F., Zimmerman, T. S., and Kleiss, A. J.,** Protein C, an anhthrombotic protein, is reduced in hospitalized patients with intravascular coagulation, *Blood,* 60, 261, 1982.

6. **Stenflo, J.,** A new vitamin K-dependent protein. Purification from bovine plasma and preliminary characterization, *J. Biol. Chem.,* 251, 355, 1976.

7. **Beckmann, R. J., Schmidth, R. J., Santerre, R. F., Plutzky, T., Crabtree, G. R., and Long, G. L.,** The structure and evolution of a 461 amino acid human protein C precursor and its messenger RNA, based upon the DNA sequence of cloned human liver cDNA, *Nucl. Acids Res.,* 13, 5233, 1985.

8. **Plutzky, J., Hojkins, J. A., Long, G. L., and Crabtree, G. R.,** Evolution and organization of the human protein C gene, *Proc. Nat. Acad. Sci.,* (U.S.A.), 83, 546, 1986.

9. **Kisiel, W.,** Human plasma protein C. Isolation, characterization and mechanism of activation by alpha-thrombin, *J. Clin. Invest.,* 761, 64, 1979.

10. **Fernlund, P. and Stenflo, J.,** Amino acid sequence of the light chain of bovine protein C, *J. Biol. Chem.,* 257, 12,170, 1982.

11. **Stenflo, J. and Fernlund, P.,** Amino acid sequence of the heavy chain of bovine protein C, *J. Biol. Chem.,* 257, 12,180, 1982.

12. **Esmon, C. T. and Owen, W. G.,** Identification of an endothelial cell cofactor for thrombin-catalyzed activation of protein C, *Proc. Nat. Acad. Sci.,* (U.S.A.), 78, 2249, 1981.

13. **Fulcher, C. A., Garoliner, J. E., Griffin, J. H., and Zimmerman, T. S.,** Proteolytic inactivation of human factor VIII procoagulant protein by activated human protein C and its analogy with factor V, *Blood,* 63, 486, 1984.

14. **Kisiel, W., Canfield, W. M., and Ericsson, L. H.,** Anticoagulant properties of bovine plasma protein C following activation by thrombin, *Biochemistry,* 16, 5824, 1977.

15. **Marlar, R. A. and Griffin, J. H.,** Deficiency of protein C inhibitor in combined factor V/VIII deficiency disease, *J. Clin. Invest.,* 66, 1186, 1980.

16. **Suzuki, K., Nishioka, J., and Hashimoto, S.,** Protein C inhibitor, *J. Biol. Chem.,* 258, 1623, 1983.

17. **Sakata, Y., Curriden, S., Lawrence, D., Griffin, J. H., and Loskutoff, D. J.,** Activated protein C stimulates the fibrinolytic activity of cultured endothelial cells and decreases anti-activator activity, *Proc. Nat. Acad. Sci.,* (U.S.A.), 82, 1121, 1985.

18. **Burdick, M. D. and Schaub, R. G.,** Human protein C induces anticoagulation and increased fibrinolytic activity in the cat, *Thromb. Haemost.,* 45, 413, 1987.

19. **Suzuki, K., Deyashiki, Y., Nishioka, J., Kurachi, K., Akiras, M., Yamamoto, S., and Hashimoto, S.,** Characterization of a cDNA for human protein C inhibitor, *J. Biol. Chem.,* 262, 611, 1987.

20. **Heeb, M. J. and Griffin, J. H.,** Physiologic inhibition of human activated protein C by alpha-1antitrypsin, *J. Biol. Chem.,* 263, 11,613, 1988.

21. **Mannucci, P. M., Boyer, C., Tripodi, A., Vigano-D'Angelo, S., Wolf, M., Valsecchi, C., D'Angelo, A., Meyer, D., and Larrieu, M. J.,** Multicenter comparison of five functional and two immunological assays for protein C, *Thromb. Haemost.,* 57, 44, 1987.

22. **Bertina, R. M., Broekmans, A. W., van Es Krommenhoek, C., and van Wijngaarden, A.,** The use of a functional and immunologic assay for plasma protein C in the study of the heterogeneity of congenital protein C deficiency, *Thromb. Haemost.,* 51, 1, 1984.

23. **Sala, N., Owen, W. G., and Collen, D.,** A functional assay of protein C in plasma, *Blood,* 63, 671, 1984.

24. **Francis, R. B. and Patch, M. J.,** A functional assay for protein C in human plasma, *Thromb. Res.,* 32, 605, 1983.

25. **Vigano-D'Angelo, S., Comp, P. C., Esmon, C. T., and D'Angelo, A.,** Relationship between protein C antigen and anticoagulant activity during oral anticoagulant and in selected disease states, *J. Clin. Invest.,* 77, 416, 1986.

26. **Martinoli, J. L. and Stocker, K.**, Fast functional protein C assay using Protac, a novel protein C activator, *Thromb. Res.*, 43, 253, 1986.
27. **Kobayashi, I., Amemiya, N., Endo, T., Motegi, J., Kurlhara, A., Hamaoka, S., Tamura, K., and Kume, S.**, Amidolytic kinetic assay of protein C by selective spectrophotometry in a centrifugal analyser, *Clin. Chem.*, 34, 2260, 1988.
28. **Klein, J. and Walker, F. J.**, Purification of a protein C activator from the venom of the southern Copperhead Snake (Agkistrodon contortrix contortrix), *Biochemistry*, 25, 4175, 1986.
29. **Bertina, R. M., Broekmans, A. W., van der Linden, I. K., and Mertens, K.**, Protein C deficiency in a Dutch family with thrombotic disease, *Thromb. Haemost.*, 48, 1, 1982.
30. **Boyer, C., Rothschild, C., Wolf, M., Amiral, J., Meyer, D., and Larrieu, M. J.**, A new method for the estimation of protein C by ELISA, *Thromb. Res.*, 36, 579, 1984.
31. **Ikeda, K. and Stenflo, J.**, A radioimmuno-assay for protein C, *Thromb. Res.*, 39, 297, 1985.
32. **Suzuki, K., Moriguchi, A., Nagayoshi, A., Mutoh, S., Katsuki, S., and Hashimoto, S.**, Enzyme immunoassay of human protein C by using monoclonal antibodies, *Thromb. Res.*, 38, 611, 1985.
33. **Bertina, R. M.**, An international collaborative study on the performance of protein C antigen assays. Report of the ICTH subcommittee on protein C, *Thromb. Haemost.*, 57, 112, 1987.
34. **Mikami, S. and Tuddenham, E. G.**, Studies on immunological assay of vitamin K dependent factors, *Br. J. Haematol.*, 62, 183, 1986.
35. **Sturk, A., Morrien-Salomon, W. M., Huisman, M. V., Borm, J. J. J., Buller, H. R., and Ten Cate, J. W.**, Analytical and clinical evaluation of commercial protein C assays, *Clin. Chim. Acta*, 165, 263, 1987.
36. **Kluft, C., Bertina, R. M., Preston, F. E., Malia, R. G., Blamey, S. L., Lowe, G. D. O., and Forbes, C. D.**, Protein C, an anticoagulant protein, is increased in healthy volunteers and surgical patients after treatment with stanazolol, *Thromb. Res.*, 33, 297, 1984.
37. **Schettini, F., De Mattia, D., Altomare, M., Montagna, O., Ciavarella, G., and Manzionna, M. M.**, Post-natal development of protein C in full-term newborns, *Acta Paediatr. Scand.*, 74, 226, 1985.
38. **Karpatkin, M., Mannucci, P. M., Bhogal, M., Vigano, S., and Nardi, M.**, Low protein C in the neonatal period, *Br. J. Haematol.*, 62, 137, 1986.
39. **Malm, J., Laurell, M., and Dahlback, B.**, Changes in the plasma levels of vitamin K-dependent proteins C and S and of C4b-binding protein during pregnancy and oral contraception, *Br. J. Haematol.* 68, 437, 1988.
40. **Griffin, J. H., Evatt, B., Zimmerman, T. S., Kleiss, A. J., and Wideman, C.**, Deficiency of protein C in congenital thrombotic disease, *J. Clin. Invest.*, 68, 1370, 1981.
41. **Broekmans, A. W., Veltkamp, J. J., and Bertina, R. M.**, Congenital protein C deficiency and venous thromboembolism: a study of three Dutch families, *N. Engl. J. Med.*, 309, 340, 1983.
42. **Horellou, M. H., Conard, J., Bertina, R. M., and Samama, M.**, Congenital protein C deficiency and thrombotic disease in nine French families, *Br. Med. J.*, 289, 1285, 1984.
43. **Seligsohn, U., Berger, A., Abend, M., Rublin, L., Attias, D., Zivelin, A., and Rapaport, S. I.**, Homozygous protein C deficiency manifested by massive thrombosis in the newborn, *N. Engl. J. Med.*, 310, 559, 1984.
44. **Marciniak, E., Wilson, H. D., and Marlar, R. A.**, Neonatal purpura fulminans: a genetic disorder related to the absence of protein C in blood, *Blood*, 65, 15, 1985.
45. **Romeo, G., Hassan, H. J., Staempeli, S., Roncuzzi, L., Cianetti, L., Leonardi, A., Vicente, V., Mannucci, P. M., Bertina, R. M., Peschle, C., and Cortese, R.**, Hereditary thrombophilia: Identification of non sense and missense mutations in the protein C gene, *Proc. Nat. Acad. Sci.*, (U.S.A.), 84, 2829, 1987.

46. **Broekmans, A. W., van der Linden, I. K., Jansen-Koster, Y., and Bertina, R. M.,** Prevalence of protein C (PC) and protein S (PS) deficiency in patients with thrombotic disease, *Thromb. Res.,* Suppl. VI, 135, 1986.
47. **Miletich, J., Sherman, L., and Broze, G., Jr.,** Absence of thrombosis in subjects with heterozygous protein C deficiency, *N. Engl. J. Med.,* 317, 991, 1987.
48. **Broekmans, A. W., Bertina, R. M., Loeliger, E. A., Hofmann, V., and Klingemann, H. G.,** Protein C and the development of skin necrosis during anticoagulant therapy, *Thromb. Haemost.,* 49, 251, 1983.
49. **Samama, M., Horellou, M. H., Soria, J., Conard, J., and Nicolas, G.,** Successful progressive anticoagulation in a severe protein C deficiency and previous skin necrosis at the initiation of oral anticoagulant treatment, *Thromb. Haemost.,* 51, 132, 1984.
50. **Branson, H. E., Katz, J., Marble, R., Griffin, J. M.,** Inherited protein C deficiency and coumarin responsive chronic relapsing purpura fulminans in a newborn infant, *Lancet,* ii, 1165, 1983.
51. **Estelles, A., Garcia-Plaza, I., Dasi, A., Aznar, J., Duart, M., Sanz, G., Perez-Requejo, J. L., Espana, F., Jimenez, C., and Abeledo, G.,** Severe inherited "homozygous" protein C deficiency in a newborn infant, *Thromb. Haemost.,* 52, 53, 1984.
52. **Bauer, K. A., Broekmans, A. W., Bertina, R. M., Conard, J., Horellou, M. H., Samama, M. M., and Rosenberg, R. D.,** Hemostatic enzyme generation in the blood of patients with hereditary protein C deficiency, *Blood,* 71, 1418, 1988.
53. **Sala, N., Borrell, M., Bauer, K. A., Vigano-D'Angelo, S., Fontcuberta, J., Felez, J., and Rutllant, M. L.,** Dysfunctional activated protein C (PC Cadiz) in a patient with thrombotic disease, *Thromb. Haemost.,* 57, 183, 1987.
54. **Faioni, E. M., Esmon, C. T., Esmon, N. L., and Mannucci, P. M.,** Isolation of an abnormal protein C molecule from the plasma of a patient with thrombotic diathesis, *Blood,* 71, 940, 1988.
55. **Vasse, M., Borg, J. Y., and Monconduit, M.,** Protein C Rouen, a new hereditary protein C abnormality with low anticoagulant but normal amidolytic activities, *Thromb. Res.,* 56, 387, 1989.
56. **Matsuda, M., Teruko, S., Sakata, Y., Murayama, H., Mimuro, J., Tanabe, S., and Yoshitake, S.,** A thrombotic state due to an abnormal protein C, *N. Engl. J. Med.,* 319, 1265, 1988.
57. **Grundy, C., Chitolic, A., Talbot, S., Bevan, N., Kakkar, V., and Cooper, D. N.,** Protein C London I: recurrent mutation at Arg 169 (CGG → TGG) in the protein C gene causing thrombosis, *Nucl. Acids Res.,* 17, 10,513, 1989.
58. **Reitsma, P. H., Poort, S. R., Allaart, C. F., Briet, E., and Bertina, R. M.,** The spectrum of genetic defects in a panel of 40 Dutch families with symptomatic protein C deficiency type I: heterogeneity and founder effects, *Blood,* 78, 890, 1991.
59. **Mannucci, P. M. and Vigano, S.,** Deficiencies of protein C, an inhibitor of blood coagulation, *Lancet,* ii, 463, 1982.
60. **Rodeghiero, R., Vigano, S., Dini, E., and Mannucci, P. M.,** Protein C in acute leukemia with and without disseminated intravascular coagulation, *Thromb. Haemost.,* 51, 349, 1983.
61. **Cariou, R., Tobelem, G., Soria, C., and Caen, J.,** Inhibition of protein C activation by endothelial cells in the presence of lupus anticoagulants, *N. Engl. J. Med.,* 314, 1193, 1986.
62. **Mimuro, J., Sakata, Y., Wakabayashi, K., and Matsuda, M.,** Level of protein C determined by combined assays during disseminated intravascular coagulation and oral anticoagulation, *Blood,* 69, 1704, 1987.
63. **Barbui, T., Finazzi, G., Vigano, S., Mannucci, P. M.,** L-asparaginase lowers protein C antigen, *Thromb. Haemost.,* 52, 216, 1984.
64. **Dahlback, B., Lundwall, A., and Stenflo, J.,** Primary structure of bovine vitamin K-dependent protein S, *Proc. Nat. Acad. Sci. U.S.A.,* 83, 4199, 1986.

65. **Schwarz, H. P., Heeb, M. J., Berretini, M., and Griffin, J. H.,** Quantitative immunoblotting of plasma and platelet protein S, *Thromb. Haemost.,* 56, 382, 1986.
66. **Walker, F. J.,** Protein S and the regulation of activated protein C, Semin. *Thromb. Haemost.,* 10, 131, 1984.
67. **Dahlback, B., Frohm, B., and Nelsestuen, G.,** High affinity interaction between C4b-binding protein and vitamin K-dependent protein S in the presence of calcium. Suggestion of a third component in blood regulating the interaction, *J. Biol. Chem.,* 265, 16,082, 1990.
68. **Lundwall, A., Dackowski, W., Cohen, E., Shaffer, M., Mahr, A., Dahlback, B., Stenflo, J., and Wydro, R.,** Isolation and sequence of the cDNA for human protein S, a regulator of blood coagulation, *Proc. Nat. Acad. Sci. U.S.A.,* 83, 6716, 1986.
69. **Watkins, P. C., Eddy, R., Fukushima, Y., Byers, M. G., Cohen, E. H., Dackowski, W. R., Wydro, R. M., and Shows, T. B.,** The gene for protein S maps near the centromere of human chromosome 3, *Blood,* 71, 238, 1988.
70. **Long, G. L., Marshall, A., Gardner, J. C., and Naylor, S. L.,** Genes for human vitamin K-dependent plasma proteins C and S are located on chromosomes 2 and 3, respectively, *Somatic Cell Mol. Genet.,* 14, 93, 1988.
71. **Discipio, R. G. and Davie, E. W.,** Characterization of protein S, a gamma-carboxy-glutamic acid containing protein from bovine and human plasma, *Biochemistry,* 18, 899, 1979.
72. **Stenflo, J. and Fernlund, P.,** Beta-hydroxyaspartic acid in vitamin K-dependent protein S, *J. Biol. Chem.,* 258, 12,509, 1983.
73. **Dahlback, B., Hildebrand, B., and Linse, S.,** Novel type of very high affinity calcium-binding sites in beta-hydroxy-asparagine containing epidermal growth factor-like domains in vitamin K-dependent protein S, *J. Biol. Chem.,* 265, 18,481, 1990.
74. **Dahlback, B.,** Purification of human vitamin K-dependent protein S and its limited proteolysis by thrombin *Biochem. J.,* 209, 827, 1983.
75. **Dahlback, B. and Stenflo, J.,** High molecular weight complex in human plasma between vitamin K-dependent protein S and complement component C4b-binding protein, *Proc. Nat. Acad. Sci. U.S.A.,* 78, 2512, 1981.
76. **Comp, P. C., Nixon, R. R., Cooper, M. R., and Esmon, C. T.,** Familial protein S deficiency is associated with recurrent thrombosis, *J. Clin. Invest.,* 74, 2082, 1984.
77. **Schwartz, H. P., Fischer, M., Hopmeier, P., Batard, M. A., and Griffin, J. H.,** Plasma protein S deficiency in familial thrombotic disease, *Blood,* 64, 1297, 1984.
78. **Deutz-Terlouw, P. P., Ballering, L., van Wijngaarden, A., and Bertina, R. M.,** Two ELISA's for the measurement of protein S, and their use in the laboratory diagnosis of protein S deficiency, *Clin. Chim. Acta,* 186, 321, 1989.
79. **Bauer, K. A., Kass, B. L., Beeler, D. L., and Rosenberg, R. T. D.,** Detection of protein S activation in humans, *J. Clin. Invest.,* 74, 2033, 1984.
80. **Comp, P. C., Doray, D., Patton, D., Esmon, C. T.,** An abnormal plasma distribution of protein S occurs in functional protein S deficiency, *Blood,* 67, 504, 1986.
81. **Preda, L., Tripodi, A., Valsecchi, C., Lombard, A., Finotto, E., and Mannucci, P. M.,** A prothrombin time-based functional assay of protein S, *Thromb. Res.,* 60, 19, 1990.
82. **Comp, P. C. and Esmon, C. T.,** Recurrent venous thromboembolism in patients with a partial deficiency of protein S, *N. Engl. J. Med.,* 311, 1522, 1984.
83. **Kamiya, T., Sugihara, T., Ogata, K., Saito, H., Suzuki, K., Nishioka, J., Hashimoto, S., and Yamagata, K.,** Inherited deficiency of protein S in a Japanese family with recurrent venous thrombosis: a study of three generations, *Blood,* 67, 406, 1986.
84. **Van de Waart, P., Preissner, K. T., Bechtold, J. R., and Muller-Berghaus, G.,** A functional test for protein S activity in plasma, *Thromb. Res.,* 48, 427, 1987.
85. **Suzuki, K. and Nishioka, J.,** Plasma protein S activity measured using Protac, a snake venom derived activator of protein C, *Thromb. Res.,* 49, 241, 1988.

86. **D'Angelo, A., Vigano-D'Angelo, S., Esmon, C. T., and Comp, P. C.,** Acquired deficiencies of protein S, *J. Clin. Invest.,* 81, 1445, 1988.
87. **Wolf, M., Boyer-Neumann, C., Martinoli, J. L., Leroy-Matheron C., Amiral, J., Meyer, D., and Larrieu, M. J.,** A new functional assay for human protein S activity using activated factor V as substrate, *Thromb. Haemost.,* 62, 1144, 1989.
88. **Wiesel, M. L., Charmantier, J. L., Freyssinet, J. M., Grunebaum, L., Schuhler, S., and Cazenave, J. P.,** Screening of protein S deficiency using a functional assay in patients with venous and arterial thrombosis, *Thromb. Res.,* 58, 461, 1990.
89. **Comp, P. C., Thurnau, G. R., Welsh, J., and Esmon, C. T.,** Functional and immunologic protein S levels are decreased during pregnancy, *Blood,* 68, 881, 1986.
90. **Malm, J., Laurell, M., and Dahlback, B.,** Changes in the plasma levels of vitamin K-dependent proteins C and S and of C4b-binding protein during pregnancy and oral contraception, *Br. J. Haematol.,* 68, 437, 1988.
91. **Malm, J., Bennhagen, R., Holmber, L., and Dahlback, B.,** Plasma concentrations of C4b-binding protein and vitamin K-dependent protein S in term and preterm infants: low levels of protein S-C4b-binding protein complexes, *Br. J. Haematol.,* 68, 445, 1988.
92. **Melissari, E., Nicolaides, K. H., Scully, M. F., and Kakkar, V. V.,** Protein S and C4b-binding protein in fetal and neonatal blood, *Br. J. Haematol.,* 70, 199, 1988.
93. **Sas, G., Blasko, G., Petro I., and Griffin, J. M.,** A protein S deficient family with portal vein thrombosis, *Thromb. Haemost.,* 54, 724, 1985.
94. **Bona, R. D., Weinstein, R. E., and Walker, F. J.,** Pseudo protein S deficiency due to a defect in C4bBP, *Blood,* 76, 500a (abstract), 1990.
95. **Mannucci, P. M., Valsecchi, C., Krachmalnicoff, A., Faioni, E. M., and Tripodi, A.,** Familial dysfunction of protein S, *Thromb. Haemost.,* 62, 763, 1989.
96. **Ploos van Amstel, H., van de Zanden, A. L., Bakker, E., Reitsma, P., and Bertina, R. M.,** Two genes homologous with human protein S cDNA are located on chromosome 3, *Thromb. Haemost.,* 58, 982, 1987.
97. **Ploos van Amstel, H., Reitsma, P., Hamulyak, K., De Die-Smulders, C., Mannucci, P. M., and Bertina, R.,** A mutation in the protein S pseudogene is linked to protein S deficiency in a thrombophilic family, *Thromb. Haemost.,* 62, 897, 1989.
98. **Bertina, R., Ploos van Amstel, H., van Wijngaarden, A., Coenen, J., Leemhuis, M., Deutz-Terlouw, P., van der Linden, I., and Reitsma, P.,** Heerlen polymorphism of protein S, an immunologic polymorphism due to dimorphism of residue 460, *Blood,* 76, 538, 1990.
99. **Ploos van Amstel, H., Huisman, M., Reitsma P., Ten Cate, J. W., and Bertina R.,** Partial protein S gene deletion in a family with hereditary thrombophilia, *Blood,* 73, 479, 1989.
100. **Schmidel, D., Nelson, R., Broxon, E., Comp, P., Marlar, R., Log, G.,** A 5,3-kb deletion including exon XIII of protein S α gene occurs in two protein S-deficient families, *Blood,* 77, 551, 1991.
101. **Fair, D. S., Marlar, R. A., and Levin, E. G.,** Human endothelial cells synthesize protein S, *Blood,* 67, 1168, 1986.
102. **Fair, D. S. and Marlar, R. A.,** Biosynthesis and secretion of factor VII, protein C, protein S and the protein C inhibitor from a human hepatoma cell line, *Blood,* 67, 64, 1986.
103. **Wolf, M., Boyer-Neumann, C., Leroy-Matheron, C., Martinoli, J. L., Contant, G., Amiral, J., Meyer, D., and Larrieu, M. J.,** Functional assay of protein S in 70 patients with congenital and acquired disorders, *Blood Coagulation Fibrinolysis,* 2, 705, 1991.
104. **Bertina, R. M., van Wijngaarden, A., Reinalda-Poot, J., and Bom, V. J. J.,** Determination of plasma protein S: the protein cofactor of activated protein C, *Thromb. Haemost.,* 53, 268, 1985.
105. **Casio, F. G., Harker, C., Batard, M. A., Brandt, J. T., and Griffin, J. H.,** Plasma concentrations of the natural anticoagulants protein C and protein S in patients with proteinuria, *J. Lab. Clin. Med.,* 106, 218, 1985.

106. **Vigano-D'Angelo, S., D'Angelo, A., Kaufman, C. E., Sholer, C., Esmon, C. T., and Comp, P. C.,** Protein S deficiency occurs in the nephrotic syndrome, *Ann. Inter. Med.,* 107, 42, 1987.

107. **Friedman, K. D., Marlar, R. A., Houston, J. G., and Montgomery, R. R.,** Warfarin-induced skin necrosis in a patient with protein S deficiency, *Blood,* 68, 333a (Abstr.), 1986.

108. **Broekmans, A. W., Bertina, R. M., Reinalda-Poot, J., Engesser, L., Muller, H. P., Leeuw, J. A., Michiels, J. J., Brommer, E. J. P., and Briet, E.,** Hereditary protein S deficiency and venous thromboembolism. A study in three Dutch families, *Thromb. Haemost.,* 53, 273, 1985.

109. **Marlar, R. A., Montgomery, R. R., Broekmans, A. W.,** and the Working Party, Diagnosis and treatment of homozygous protein C deficiency, *J. Pediatr.,* 114, 528, 1989.

110. **Vukovich, T., Auberger, K., Weil, J., Engelmann, H., Knöbl, P., and Hadorn, H. B.,** Replacement therapy for a homozygous protein C deficiency-state using a concentrate of human protein C and S, *Br. J. Haematol.,* 70, 435, 1988.

Chapter 8

CONGENITAL DEFICIENCIES OF THE VITAMIN K-DEPENDENT CLOTTING FACTORS

Guglielmo Mariani, A. Ghirardini, and G. Iacopino

TABLE OF CONTENTS

0-8493-6423-X/93/$0.00 + $.50

I. INTRODUCTION

Congenital deficiencies of vitamin K-dependent clotting factors represent a heterogeneous group of hemorrhagic disorders with different patterns of inheritance as well as fairly different clinical pictures. In spite of this heterogeneity, factors IX, VII, II, and X (FIX, FVII, FII, and FX, respectively) have close biochemical homologies, the most striking of which is due to the presence, in their molecules, of a number of γ-carboxyglutamic acid (Gla) residues, which are an essential trigger for their serine protease activity; another homology lies with their site of production, (i.e., the hepatocyte), and with the biochemical events of post-translational processing leading to the addition of the Gla residues. These are common to all of the above-mentioned clotting factors as well as to protein C and protein S. Each of the FII, FVII, FIX, and FX act at different stages of blood coagulation but their severe deficiency is invariably characterized, clinically, by moderate to severe hemorrhagic disorders.

II. HISTORICAL BACKGROUND

Hemophilia has been recognized, for centuries, as a global bleeding disorder, but it was not until 1947 that Pavlovsky[1] demonstrated the existence of two main and distinct types of hemophilia and Aggeler et al.[2] and Biggs et al.[3] characterized the nature of the disease.

A congenital deficiency of FVII was first described in 1952 by Alexander et al.[4] Subsequently, cases previously diagnosed as FVII deficiency were reevaluated and found to be deficient in a "new" factor first denoted "Stuart factor"[5] and then FX. By this time the existence of prothrombin as a vitamin K-dependent coagulation protein had been known for more than 20 years; in fact, in 1939, Seegers et al.,[6] had purified the protein almost to homogeneity. The discovery of prothrombin, however, did not result from any inherited coagulation defect.

III. EPIDEMIOLOGY

Hemophilia B is the most common among the vitamin K-dependent clotting factor deficiencies; its prevalence can be indirectly calculated on the basis of its incidence in the whole hemophilia population, since the ratio of hemophilia A to hemophilia B (from 4:1 to 5:1) is fairly constant.[7] By using this indirect method of calculation, and assuming an average hemophilia frequency of 5 per 100,000, the number of cases of FIX deficiency should be approximately 1 per 100,000 individuals.[7] This figure differs, but not substantially, from the estimated prevalence in the U.K. of 1 per 30,000 males, as reported by McKee.[8]

To date, the frequency of congenital deficiencies of the other vitamin K dependent-clotting factors in the population has not been established with any certainty. It would seem that FVII deficiency is the most common among these "rare" hemorrhagic disorders with an estimated frequency of 1 per 500,000 persons,[9] and this data fits with the observation made by some of us,[10] that the heterozygous forms seem to be quite common in the general population. In North Carolina, U.S., the prevalence of congenital FX deficiency in the heterozygous form has been estimated to be 2 per 10,000[11] but the homozygous forms appear much less common, as only about 50 families have been reported.[12,13] Inherited deficiencies of prothrombin have been described,[14] but so far only in about 50 patients.

IV. GENETICS

Hemophilia B is, with rare exceptions, a disease of males, the defective gene being located on chromosome X, in its Xq2.7 subregion;[15,16] males are necessarily hemizygous for the normal allele and therefore manifest the disorder. All the sons of a hemophilia B patient will be normal, and all the daughters will be obligatory carriers. Because of the high mutation rate of the disease, up to one third of hemophiliacs have a mute family history;[17,18] it seems probable, however, that a more accurate diagnosis at the gene level will reduce this figure. In a recent case report, Mariani et al.[19] by studying multiple *restriction fragment length polymorphisms* (RFLPs) in 10 hemophilia B kindreds found two families with a mute history of hemophilia in whom it was likely that a mutation had occurred. The inheritance of FVII deficiency has been shown to be autosomally recessive, with intermediate expressivity;[20,21] the severe defect occurs only in homozygotes, whereas an intermediate deficiency is found in heterozygotes.[20-22]

The inherited trait for FX deficiency has been clearly shown to be transmitted by a highly penetrant, incompletely recessive autosomal mode of inheritance.

Congenital disorders of prothrombin appear to be transmitted in different ways, depending upon the nature of the defect. In fact, hypoprothrobinemias

TABLE 1
Prevalence of Bleeding Manifestations in Hemophilia

Site	Prevalence (%)	Hemarthrosis (joint)	Prevalence (%)
Hemarthrosis	60–70	Knee	35
		Ankle	25
Hematomas (muscle and subcutaneous)	20–25	Elbow	30
		Wrist	3
		Shoulder	3
		Hip	1
Mucous membrane	5	Other	3

are inherited as autosomal, recessive traits;[23,24] homozygotes for this condition have prothrombin coagulant (FIIC) activities varying from 2 to 25 U/dl, and heterozygotes have levels as high as, or higher than, 50 U/dl, with no discrepancy between FIIC and the levels of prothrombin antigen (FIIAg). On the other hand, the genetics of dysprothrombinemias is complex; this aspect will be discussed under *Molecular Variants* (see Section VIII).

V. CLINICAL FEATURES

A. HEMOPHILIA B

The clinical manifestations in hemophilia B are, in general, identical to those of hemophilia A and are summarized in Table 1.

It is incorrect to consider hemophilia B a less severe disease than hemophilia A: this misbelief may have been derived from the fact that FIX deficiency is, in general, more easily treatable than hemophilia A. It is beyond the purpose of this review, however, to detail the clinical features and the natural history of the disease.

B. FACTOR VII DEFICIENCY

On the basis of single and scattered clinical case reports, it first appeared that congenital deficiencies of FVII had a considerable clinical heterogeneity, even among patients with comparable levels of FVIIC. Mariani and Mazzucconi,[20] re-examined this question by analyzing data from eight institutions in Europe concerning 40 homozygotes, and found that the incidence of menorrhagia and hemarthrosis is much higher in patients with severe (<3 U/dl) and moderate (3 to 5 U/dl) FVII deficiency, than in those with mild disease, and that postoperative bleeding occurs, regardless of the FVIIC level, if no replacement therapy is given. Moreover, a clinical-radiological study revealed that most of the severely affected patients (ca. 70%) had grade 3 or 4 changes, a pattern which is the same as that found in hemophilia. Triplett et al.,[25] in their study, observed that bleeding seldom occurs when FVIIC levels exceed 10 U/dl (measured by assays using human thromboplastin). Ragni et al.[26] in a review of the literature, noted a high incidence (12/75 = 16%) of bleeding from the central nervous system; most of these episodes (9/12) occurring within the first year of life. Hematuria, gastrointestinal bleeding, splenic hematomas, pulmonary hemorrhage, blood tears,[27] and subarachnoid hemorrhage have been reported, but are rare. Congenital FVII deficiency does not seem to protect from thrombotic complications, as evidenced by a severely affected patient who died of pulmonary embolism following an inferior vena cava thrombosis.[27a] In addition FVII congenital deficiency does not protect from atheroma, as suggested by the observations of Lefrere et al.[28] and Zacharski et al.[29]

C. FACTOR X DEFICIENCY

Bleeding manifestations may occur at any age, but more severely affected patients will have already exhibited severe symptoms in childhood. Less severely affected patients may bleed only following severe challenges to the hemostatic system, such as trauma or surgery. Menorrhagia, hemarthrosis, peri- and post-operative bleeding, as well as hemorrhage in the central nervous system, have all been described, mainly in severely affected patients with levels of FXC < 2 U/dl.

D. HYPO- AND DYSPROTHROMBINEMIAS

The clinical picture correlates well with the levels of FIIC, mainly when measured with the two-stage assay: patients with levels >40 U/dl do not have bleeding problems, whereas those who have levels <10 U/dl frequently exhibit easy bruising, epistaxis, menorrhagia, and hemorrhage following surgery or trauma. Hemarthroses are rarely observed.

VI. DIAGNOSIS AND DIFFERENTIAL DIAGNOSIS

The initial diagnostic clotting tests and results expected in single or combined deficiencies of the vitamin K-dependent clotting factors are summarized in Table 2. The reagents of choice for this preliminary screening must be sensitive to the relevant factor, especially when intermediate levels of the factor are expected, such as in heterozygotes. With regard to the prothrombin time (PT), this test should be performed using a tissue thromboplastin with a low ISI (international sensitivity index). The importance of using sensitive reagents has been stressed by some of us in a study[10] in which we evaluated the sensitivity of different tissue thromboplastins towards intermediate FVII levels (Table 3). The Thrombotest is a useful screening reagent with an ISI close to unity, which allows both the screening for FVII deficiencies and the detection of B_m variants in hemophilia B; the bleeding time may occasionally be found borderline in FVII and FX deficiencies, usually when the levels of the missing factor are very low.

After the screening evaluation, specific assays of the relevant factors need to be performed in order to define the diagnosis more precisely. For further

TABLE 2
Screening Tests for Vitamin K-Dependent Clotting Factors

Deficiency	APTT	PT	Thrombotest	Bleeding time
FIX	Prolonged	Normal	Normal[a]	Normal
FX	Prolonged	Prolonged	Prolonged	Normal
FII	Prolonged	Prolonged	Prolonged	Normal
FVII	Normal	Prolonged	Prolonged	Normal
Combined FII, FVII, FIX and FX	Prolonged	Prolonged	Prolonged	Normal

[a] Except for B_m variants.

specificity, activators sensitive to the presumed deficiencies should also be used. The presence/absence of antigens to the relevant factor is also referred to as CRM. The evaluation of the CRM (cross-reacting material or antigen) status in congenital deficiencies is important: first, to give a preliminary characterization of a variant; and second, to increase the power of detection of heterozygotes belonging to CRM$^+$ kindreds. The most sensitive factor antigen assays are those based upon radioimmunoassay (RIA) or immunoradiometric (IRMA) methods, but very sensitive and practical enzyme-linked immunoabsorbent assays (ELISAs) are available today, which allow the detection of levels <1 U/dl. Electroimmunoassays (EIA) and inhibitor neutralization assay (INA), cannot detect levels <5 to 10 and <10 to 15 U/dl, respectively. Further immunochemical evaluation can be carried out by crossed electrophoresis, SDS-page electrophoresis or immunoblotting. To characterize the variants from the functional angle, specific reagents for the relevant deficiencies are needed: e.g., *Stypven* (Russell's viper), *Echis carinatus,* Tiger snake, *Dispholidus typus venoms,* tissue factors of different animal origin, amydolitic reagents, and staphylocoagulase.

VII. COMBINED CONGENITAL DEFICIENCIES OF FACTORS II, VII, IX, AND X

To date, six patients with a combined deficiency of all the vitamin K-dependent clotting factors have been reported. The first case[30] concerned a girl with a significant bleeding disorder, very prolonged APTT (activated partial thromboplastin time) and PT and very low to undetectable levels of FII, FVII, FIX, and FX. There was no evidence of liver disease, malabsorption, or coumarin drug intake.

This patient who has been followed for 15 years,[14] responded partially to high doses of parenteral vitamin K, with reduction of the bleeding symptoms, and shortening of the screening test coagulation times, though without ever reaching normalization. A modest increase in the activities of individual

TABLE 3

Relationship Between Prothrombin Times[a] Carried out with Tissue Thromboplastin of Different Origin and FVIIC Levels[10]

FVIIC (U/dl)	Human thromboplastin			Rabbit lung and brain			Thrombotest			Ox-brain		
	n	x	SEM	n	x	SEM	n	x	SEM	n	x	SEM
50–60	11	1.15	0.05	5	1.02	0.02	11	1.25	0.05	5	1.07	0.08
40–50	11	1.15	0.06	15	1.07	0.01	12	1.33	0.03	9	1.12	0.03
30–40	11	1.29	0.05	7	1.11	0.03	6	1.34	0.02	—	—	—
20–30	9	1.32	0.05	9	1.15	0.02	8	1.49	0.06	—	—	—
63–124[b]	0.83–1.11[b]			0.77–1.10[b]			0.86–1.19[b]					

a   Values expressed as mean ratios (± SEM).
b   Range of normality.

vitamin K-dependent clotting factors was seen and with markedly higher levels of the relevant antigens. The other five patients with combined deficiencies of FII, FVII, FIX, and FX presented with mild to severe bleeding disorders;[31-35] in one case, protein C was also found to be decreased.[34]

The underlying defect of this composite deficiency may be attributed to a post-translational change involving all factors, rather than to a gene defect: indeed a single defect at the gene level can be excluded because the related genes are not tandemly arranged on the same chromosome, and also because the phenotypic expression mimics that found in patients with vitamin K deficiency or treated with coumarin anticoagulants: in both these conditions abnormal precursor molecules (des-γ-carboxy factors or PIVKAs [proteins induced by vitamin K antagonist]) accumulate in the liver and are released into the circulation. Therefore this combined disorder could be due to a lack (partial or total) of the Gla residues, which may in turn be due to abnormalities in the transport system for vitamin K or to some enzymatic defect in the vitamin K-epoxide cycle. This hypothesis is in keeping with the findings of Goldsmith et al.,[35] who noted a normal thrombin generation by the abnormal factors when nonphysiological activators, not requiring calcium for activation, were used.

VIII. MOLECULAR VARIANTS

A. HEMOPHILIA B

In 1968, Roberts et al.[36] proposed a nomenclature for FIX variants which is still used today. This nomenclature is based upon the evaluation of the following laboratory features:

1. The FIXC activity concentration
2. The FIXAg concentration
3. The ratio between FIXC and FIXAg
4. The ox-brain PT (Table 5)

The immunochemical variants of hemophilia B are illustrated in Table 4. Based on the numerous case reports published to date, it has been estimated[37] that 30 to 50% of all hemophilia B patients are of type B$^+$, characterized by the synthesis of an abnormal FIX molecule with a reduced coagulant activity; this type may be detected from the FIXC/FIXAg ratio which is less than 0.5 (i.e., the antigenic activity greatly exceeds the coagulant activity). In the group of hemophilia B$^-$/B^{red}, 4 subgroups can be identified:

1. Patients with no detectable synthesis of FIXAg; these patients have an increased risk for developing FIX antibodies (see Molecular Biology, Section IX)
2. Patients with a reduced synthesis (or a reduced half-life) of a normal FIX molecule[38]

TABLE 4
Classification[a] of Hemophilia B

	CRM⁻	CRMred		CRM⁺
FIXC	<1%	red	<1%–red	<1%–red
FIXAg	<1%	red	red	normal
FIXC/Ag	—	1	<0.5	<0.5
	No synthesis reduced synthesis reduced half-life (B⁻; B Leyden)		Synthesis of abnormal molecule (B⁺; B_m)	

[a]   Modified from Bertina.[37]

3.   Patients with a reduced synthesis of a variant FIX molecule with normal coagulant activity[39]
4.   Hemophilia B Leyden, characterized by a severe FIX deficiency before puberty, while after puberty FIXC and FIXAg increase at an average yearly rate of 4 to 5%[40,41]

The group of patients comprising the subgroups 2 and 3 is referred to as hemophilia Bred.

In the group of patients with hemophilia B⁺, the defect is associated with very low levels of FIXC and with normal levels of an abnormal variant FIX molecule. A subclassification of hemophilia B⁺ is based on the results of the oxbrain PT: Hougie and Twomey[42] reported that in some patients with hemophilia B, the ox-brain PT is markedly prolonged. Later, Denson et al.,[43] demonstrated that this prolongation was sensitive to the addition of an antiserum to FIX to the plasma. This type of hemophilia, currently referred to as hemophilia B_m, is a subtype of hemophilia B⁺, and accounts for about 5% of the patients with hemophilia B; it is also characterized by <1% of FIXC and normal to high FIXAg levels. Table 5 shows how hemophilia B⁺ patients can be subdivided by using the ox-brain PT. The "B⁺/non-B_m" subgroup can be further subdivided according to a normal or a mildly prolonged oxbrain PT but is probably more heterogeneous with respect to the underlying gene defect which consists of different point mutations (see Chapter 9, Section 1).

In the other patients of the B⁺ subgroup, the ox-brain PT can be very markedly prolonged (>4-fold) or markedly (2- to 4-fold), (Table 5). In some patients of the latter group the prolonged ox-brain PT is unaffected by the addition of the FIX antibody and hence cannot be included in the B_m variant group: in these patients, Mazzucconi et al.,[44] demonstrated that a combined mild FVII deficiency is the cause of the PT prolongation.

Table 6 summarizes current knowledge of the precise biochemical defects responsible for various FIX variants and how the respective defect affects

TABLE 5
Subclassification[a] of Hemophilia B$_m$

HEMOPHILIA B$^+$
Ox-brain prothrombin time

Normal	Mildly prolonged	Markedly prolonged	Very markedly prolonged
	Mild FVII deficiency		
Non-B$_m$			B$_m$

Modified from Bertina.[37]

their functional activity. Following the recommendations of the ICTH sub-committee on nomenclature, these FIX variants are identified by the toponym corresponding to the place of birth of the proband.

Hemophilia B Leyden deserves particular mention: these patients are severely affected from birth to puberty with FIXC and FIXAg levels <1%. At the age of puberty FIXC and FIXAg start to rise reaching normal or subnormal levels later in life.[40,41]

With some of the variants described above, more information has been obtained from molecular biology studies (see Section IX and Chapter 9, Section 1).

B. FACTOR X DEFICIENCY

The evaluation of FX congenital deficiency variants is based on the following laboratory features:

1. Partial thromboplastin time (PTT);
2. Prothrombin time (PT);
3. Stypven clotting time;
4. FX coagulant activity (FXC);
5. FX antigen (FXAg);
6. Ratio FXC/FXAg.

Denson et al.[57] have demonstrated a heterogeneity in congenital FX deficiency in six unrelated patients. These authors showed that FX deficiency, like hemophilia B, can be divided into three groups, according to their levels of FX antigen: a CRM$^+$ group in whom normal levels of antigen can be detected; a CRM$^-$ group in whom no antigen can be demonstrated; and, finally, a CRM^{red} group with intermediate levels of antigen. Subsequently, Fair et al.,[58] using a RIA for FXAg, found seven of eight of their patient group had normal levels of the antigen. A peculiar FX variant has been described by Girolami et al.[59,60] These authors described a large kindred with an abnormal FX molecule which, in contrast to previously discovered variants,

TABLE 6
FIX B⁺ Variants in Greater Detail

Toponym	FIXC	FIXAg	Biochemical feature	Functional features	Ref.
FIX Alabama	10	100	Asp to Gly(47)	Reduced activation in presence of Ca^{2+} FVIII and phospholipids	45, 46
FIX Lake Elsinor	<1	Normal	?	Reduced activating activity toward FX and no reactivity with AT III	47, 48
FIX Eindhoven	<1	80	?	Activity not increased by FVIIIa	49
FIX Chapel Hill	5	100	Arg to His (145)	Impaired activation by FXIa or FVIIa/TF	50, 51
FIX Deventer	<1	130	Possible Arg (180); substitution	Impaired activation by XIa/Ca^{2+}, FVII/TF or RVV/FX	52
FIX Long Beach	<1	Normal	?	Reduced FX activating activity; reactivity with AT III	53
FIX Lisse	25	130	?	Reduced affinity for heparin	54
FIX Los Angeles	<1	Normal	?	Reduced FX activating activity; normal reactivity with AT III	53
FIX Zutphen	<1	80	increased MW	Reduced activation by FXI/Ca^{2+} and by FVIIa/TF/Ca^{2+}; abnormal electrophoretic mobility with Ca^{2+}	55, 56

Note: TF = tissue factor; RVV = Russel's Viper Venon.

TABLE 7
Laboratory Features of FX Congenital Deficiency and FX Variants

Variant	APTT	PT	Stypven time	FXC TF	FXC Stypven	CRM status	Ref.
Patient GS	Prolonged	Slightly prolonged	Slightly prolonged	Low	Low	Negative	57
Stuart	Prolonged	Prolonged	Prolonged	Low	Low	Negative	61
Prower	Prolonged	Prolonged	Prolonged	Low	Low	Positive	61
Patient GF	Prolonged	Normal	Normal	?	?	Positive	62
Friuli	Prolonged	Prolonged	Normal	Low	Normal	Positive	59

could be directly activated by Russell's viper venom (i.e., the patients showed a normal Stypven time, see Table 7). All the patients also had normal levels of FXAg (CRM⁺). This variant is known as FX Friuli, from the region where this kindred originated.

The laboratory features of FX variants are shown in Table 7. Recently, a new case has been found outside the Friuli region[63] and there is evidence that this represents a new mutation. Fair et al.[64] have performed structural studies on the FX Friuli variant, and suggest that the defect may be attributed to an abnormal activation peptide. Another variant described by Parkin et al.,[62] is characterized by a normal PT and a normal Stypven time (see Table 7, Patient GF).

C. PROTHROMBIN DEFICIENCY

Congenital deficiencies of prothrombin represent some of the rarer hereditary clotting disorders and are divided into two groups: the "true" deficiencies (hypoprothrombinemias), and the variants (dysprothrombinemias).

Hypoprothrombinemias are inherited as autosomal recessive disorders; homozygotes are symptomatic and have corresponding levels of FIIC and FIIAg ranging from 2 to 25%. Heterozygotes are asymptomatic with FII levels of 50% or greater.

The characteristics of dysprothrombinemias, which represent the expression of abnormal molecular variants of prothrombin, are summarized in Table 8. Their mode of inheritance appears to be complex. From the analysis of the published cases of dysprothrombinemias it has been suggested that these disorders can be transmitted as a single locus or may represent the phenotypic expression of different genes encoding for two prothrombins. Where different genes are involved it has been postulated that these may encode for two different abnormal prothrombins (as suggested for prothrombin San Juan) or that one gene may encode for an abnormal prothrombin and the other for "true" hypoprothrombinemia (as suggested for prothrombins Houston, Quick, Molise, Metz, and Habana). If correct, the latter hypothesis is of interest in postulating that both parents possess abnormalities resulting in a compound (double) heterozygosity for dys- and hypoprothrombinemia in the propositus.

TABLE 8
Characteristics of Hereditary Dysprothrombinemias

Toponym/ eponym	Genotype	Prothrombin levels (U/dl)		Symptoms	Molecular defect	Ref.
		FIIC	FIIAg			
Cardeza	Heterozygous	50	100	No	Prothrombin 2 region	65
Madrid	Homozygous	3	103	Yes	FXa-catalyzed cleavage site between pro-fragment and thrombin region	66, 67
Barcelona	Homozygous	12	100	Yes	?	68, 70
Houston	Compound heterozygous	5–9	51	Yes	?	71
San Juan	Compound heterozygous	20	93	Yes	Calcium binding sites in one of the two defects	23
Padua	Heterozygous	50	100	Yes	FX specificity site	72
Brussels	Heterozygous	46	88	Yes	?	73
Quick	Compound heterozygous	<2	34	Yes	Thrombin region	74–76
Molise	Compound heterozygous	11	45	Yes	FXa-sensitive region	77
Metz	Compound heterozygous	10	50	Yes	Thrombin region	78, 79
Denver	Homozygous	<1	13	Yes	?	80
Gainsville	?	34	71	Yes	?	81
Salakta	?	15	100	No	Thrombin region of prothrombin molecule (?)	82
Poissey	Homozygous	2	50	Severe	?	83
Habana	Compound heterozygous	10	50	Yes	?	84

Most of the patients with dysprothrombinemias suffer from a significant bleeding diathesis (with the exception of prothrombin Cardeza and prothrombin Salakta): this feature seems to be independent of the levels of prothrombin coagulant activity, which can range from <1 to 50 U/dl. In some of these hereditary dysprothrombinemias, functional tests (carried out with appropriate activators) and preliminary biochemical evaluations, have allowed the probable structural defects to be pinpointed. These are listed briefly in Table 8.

D. FACTOR VII DEFICIENCY

The existence of phenotypic heterogeneity in congenital FVII deficiency was first documented by Goodnight et al.[85] Subsequently Denson et al.,[86] by using a more specific antibody to FVII, confirmed that there was a considerable divergence between activity and antigen. More recently, Mariani et al.,[21] reported their studies on 21 patients from 16 kindreds, and found that

TABLE 9
Variants of FVII Congenital Deficiency

Variant	FVIIC (U/dl)	FVIIAg (U/dl)	CRM status	FVIIC with various thromboplastins				Ref.
				Rabbit	Human	Simian	Ox	
Denson								86
Family 1	2–10	8–13	Red					86
Family 2	13–15	40–50	Red					
Family 3	1	2	Neg					
Family 4	<1	0	Neg					
Family 5	<1	18	Red					
Goodnight								85
B.C	2–5	7	Neg		2–5			
D.D	2–5	7	Neg		2–5			
G.A	5	12	Red		5			
M.Y	10	35	Red		10			
Mariani								21
19 Patients	≤3	14	Neg					
		2	Red					
		3	Pos					
2 Patients	3, 7	2	Red					
FVII Verona								87, 90
Propositus	20	50	Red	25	22	24	40	
Father	36–50	100	—					
FVII Padua 1								88
Propositus	9	95	Pos	9	38	40	105	
FVII Padua 2								89
Propositus		50	Red	40	40	46	20	

14 patients had no detectable antigen (CRM$^-$), four had reduced levels of antigen (CRM^{red}), while the remaining three had normal levels of antigen (CRM$^+$). Later, Mariani and Mazzucconi[20] in reviewing the literature concluded that of the three immunological patterns the most common was CRM$^-$ (50%), followed by CRM^{red} (39.5%) and CRM$^+$ (10.5%). Triplett et al.[25] reported that FVIIC levels correlated better with clinical bleeding when tissue factor of human origin was employed in the assay.

Specific FVII variants have been reported by Girolami et al.[87-90] One of them, denominated Verona,[87] appeared to be a compound heterozygote for the gene for the "true" deficiency and the gene for an abnormal FVII. Another variant[88] (Padua 1), described by the same author, is characterized by a different FVII activation when tissue extracts from different animal sources were used; slightly different from the latter was a variant subsequently described by Girolami et al.[89] (Padua 2), characterized by a normal pattern of activation with a rabbit thromboplastin. Later, Girolami et al.[90] reexamined the pattern of activation of FVII Verona and found that this variant too had a different pattern of activation which could be demonstrated by using different tissue thromboplastins. The laboratory features of the FVII variants described above are summarized in Table 9.

Recently, new observations have confirmed most of the observations previously reported: a new case of FVII Verona has been reported in Spain[91] and a new case of FVII Padua 1 has been reported in Japan.[92] In addition, Pardo et al.[93] have carried out studies on a large number of FVII deficient patients belonging to nine families from Spain. Interestingly, these authors found a different prevalence of the immunological variants, 69.5% being CRM$^+$, 26% CRM^{red} and 4.5% CRM$^-$; moreover, two new cases of the FVII variant Padua 2 and another Padua 1 variant, were observed.

IX. MOLECULAR BIOLOGY

Molecular biology has provided a new and very fruitful approach to the study of the structure, function, and biosynthesis of clotting factors including the vitamin K-dependent factors. Such studies are also revealing important information on the location and organization of the genes for these factors both in normal subjects and in patients with related clotting defects. The genes of most of the clotting factors have been cloned to a greater or lesser extent. In some cases a partial cDNA has been isolated, and in others the whole gene has been sequenced. With regard to the vitamin K-dependent procoagulant clotting factors, all the genes have been now fully sequenced and cloned. In this section, the technique of linkage analysis with RFLPs, associated with each clotting disorder and the specific gene defects, are examined.

Linkage analysis is important for carrier detection and prenatal diagnosis since it overcomes the difficulties related to the evaluation of phenotypic expressions of the relevant clotting factors. In fact, linkage analysis with intragenic RFLPs allows carrier detection and prenatal diagnosis with 99.9% reliability when a kindred gives an "informative" result for one or more RFLPs.[94]

A. HEMOPHILIA B
1. Linkage Analysis with RFLPs
So far, only six RFLPs, all of them intragenic, are known; the assessment of carriership is possible in approximately 70% of the potential carriers.[19,94-97] The features of the described RFLPs are summarized in Table 10. In particular,[94] the *Taq*I polymorphic site is located at the 5' side of intron d, *Xmn*I at the 5' side of intron c, *Dde*I/*Hinf*I in the intervening sequence of the gene 5' of exon b. The polymorphic site location for RFLP/*Msp*I is, at present, unknown. Two RFLP/*Bam*HI have been described: the first[97] is located 2 *Kbp* downstream of the *Bam*HI site in the 5' flanking sequence of the gene, the second[98] within 500 basepairs 5' to the *Xmn*I site in the second intron or in exon b.

All polymorphisms are point mutations except *Dde*I, which is a 50 bp insertion/deletion polymorphism. Most of the described polymorphisms (*Taq*I, *Xmn*I, *Dde*I/*Hinf*I, and possibly, *Msp*I) are located within an 11-Kb region of DNA and are in linkage disequilibrium in the white population. This partly

TABLE 10
Restriction Fragment Length Polymorphisms for FIX Locus

Restriction enzyme	Probe	Allelic bands (Kb) (−/+)	Frequency (%)	Heterozygosity (%)
*Xmn*I	cDNA(VIII)	11.5/6.5	72/28[a]	40[a]
*Taq*I	cDNA(VIII)	1.8/1.3	68/32[a]	44[a]
*Dde*I	cDNA(XIII)	1.7/1.75	24/76[a]	36[a]
*Msp*I	cDNA	2.4/5.8	80/20[b]	32[b]
5'*Bam*HI	cDNA	15/13	52/48[c]	23[c]
*Bam*HI	cDNA(VIII)	25/23	94/6[d]	11[d,e]

[a]   Ethnic variation reported among whites.[19,99,103]
[b]   See Reference 96.
[c]   See Reference 98.
[d]   See Reference 97.
[e]   Higher heterozygosity rate in blacks.[98]

restricts their clinical usefulness: thus assuming a heterozygosity rate of about 80% for at least one of the RFLPs, the combined rate of usefulness is only 66% because most of the described polymorphic sites are situated very close together.

The RFLPs so far described have revealed different heterozygosity rates among different populations. In fact, in Japanese[100] and other Asiatic populations (Chinese and Filipinos),[101] no heterozygosity was found when DNA was restricted with the endonucleases *Dde*I, *Msp*I, *Taq*I, or *Xmn*I. The presence of racial differences has been confirmed by Lubahn et al.[99] who found, compared to white Americans, a decreased heterozygosity in black Americans, East Indians, and Chinese and absence of heterozygosity in Malaysians. Recently Driscoll et al.[98] demonstrated that the heterozygosity for both *Bam*HI polymorphisms is higher in American Blacks as compared to Whites, and found that the *Bam*HI/RFLP is not in linkage disequilibrium with the 5' one.

In addition to the six FIX intragenic RFLPs reported above, one site has been described by McGraw et al.[102] at amino acid position 148, in the activation peptide (ACT or CGT codon) 3' to the *Msp*I site; this was detected by the enzyme *Mnl*I and subsequently identified by Winship and Brownlee[103] by an oligonucleotide probe. Moreover, two additional *Taq*I/RFLP dimorphic sites, located in exon VIII, have been identified.[104] These newly described *Taq*I sites can improve carrier detection in hemophilia B, since they do not appear to be in linkage disequilibrium with the "classical" 5' *Taq*I site. Finally, a linked extragenic site recognized by probe *DXS*99 with a heterozygosity of 50% has been recently identified,[105] this may allow for the DNA diagnosis of hemophilia B in Orientals.

With the availability of chorionic villi sampling from the 8th to the 12th week of pregnancy, prenatal diagnosis is now possible by the use of linkage

TABLE 11
Point Mutations in Hemophilia B

Toponym	Point mutation	Amino acid substitution	Position	FIXC (U/dl)	CRM status	Ref.
—	A to G	Unexpressed[a]	—	<1	Neg	116
IX Alabama	A to G	gly to asp	148	10	Pos	117
IX Chapel Hill	G to A	arg to his	145	5	Pos	51
IX Leyden	A to T	Unexpressed	—	<1[b]	Neg[b]	118
IX London 2	G to A	arg to gln	333	<1	Pos	119
IX Hilo	A to G	arg to glu	180	<1	Pos[c]	120

[a] Mutation occurred at a donor splice junction.
[b] Before puberty.
[c] B_m variant.

analysis through RFLPs. This was not possible from phenotype analysis because of the difficulties met in assessing the levels of FIX in cord blood and the presence of FIXAg in the amniotic fluid.[106]

2. Specific Gene Defects

Initially, much attention was focused on the study of those rare hemophilia B patients who developed inhibitors to FIX. Of the eight patients with such inhibitors studied from 1983 to 1987, seven showed gene deletions of varying extent.[108-110] Subsequently, Matthews et al.[111] evaluated FIX loci in nine patients with FIX antibodies, and found deletions in four patients (two of them were brothers), and an apparently normal gene in the remaining five patients. Of the 16 hemophilia B inhibitor patients thus far reported, (one[108] was also included in the Matthews' series[111]), 10 showed a detectable deletion of the FIX gene. Other observations demonstrated[112-116] that gene deletions can also be detected in hemophilia B in the absence of an inhibitor to FIX.

Point mutations, although representing the probable cause in the majority of hemophilia B variants, are extremely difficult to detect, unless they result in a change in a restriction site. Most of the documented point mutations represent the underlying cause of a rare FIX abnormality which had been already detected by functional and biochemical methods. Those point mutations which have been fully characterized are reported in Table 11.

The analysis of point mutations in hemophilia B variants provide an important opportunity for understanding the complex relationship between the protein structure of FIX and its functional role in blood coagulation. When a specific mutation in one of these variants is identified, and related to the aberrant function, the relationship between structure and function becomes better understood. For instance, the analysis of the first unnamed variant[116] reported in Table 11, suggests that the gene alteration located at the donor splice junction, impares the normal splicing of pre-mRNA to mRNA, resulting in the lack of FIX synthesis. On the other hand, FIX Alabama is characterized by a point mutation which results in the substitution of aspartic acid by glycine; this amino acid substitution could change the charge of the protein and might account for the moderate loss of specific activity.[117] In hemophilia B Leyden the reported defect involves the promoter region and it has been suggested that the increase in protein synthesis occurring after puberty is somehow influenced by testosterone.[118] In FIX London 2, the point mutation is responsible for an amino acid substitution causing the loss of a positive charge in a region of the catalytic domain which is highly conserved in human and bovine FIX, FX, and prothrombin; this change is considered consistent with the observed loss of activity.[119] A similar argument was used to explain the mild hemophilia caused by FIX Vancouver.[121] Finally in FIX Hilo, the point mutation causes an amino acid substitution which alters the Arg-Val cleavage site of the activation peptide which is also highly conserved among different mammalian species.[120] A similar point mutation (C to T) has been observed in the same codon in hemophilia B Deventer[122] while a B_m variant also has a substitution in the same position (Arg 180).

From the analysis of the variants so far described some conclusions can be drawn: the CRM$^-$ variants include splice junction and promoter region mutations, as well as gross deletions of the gene; the latter are more frequently observed in patients with FIX inhibitors (10 out of 16 of those reported thus far). The gene defects causing the CRM$^+$ phenotype, comprise intragenic deletions which do not alter the reading frame of RNA processing signals and amino acid substitutions affecting the cleavage site at the amino terminal end of the activation peptide, the first epidermal growth factor (EGF) domain, the serine protease domain and the propeptide. Since the gene of FIX in CRM^{red} variants has not been characterized yet, the underlying gene defects can only be putatively ascribed to mutations which interfere with some step in the normal pathway of gene expression, such as mutations in the regulatory regions (intron-exon boundaries), which may affect the stability of the mRNA or eventually influence the interaction of mRNA with the ribosome.

The analysis of further variants will contribute to a better understanding of the functional meaning of the single protein structures.

B. FACTOR X AND FACTOR VII DEFICIENCIES: LINKAGE ANALYSIS WITH RFLPS AND SPECIFIC GENE DEFECTS

Many different polymorphic sites associated with the FX gene have been observed. Hassan et al.,[123] recently analyzed the structure of the gene and assessed the allelic frequency of five intragenic RFLPs in Caucasians (Table 12); two of them have been previously described.[124,125]

The two *Eco*RI sites were found to be located within exons c and h, whereas the two *Pvu*II sites are both within exon h, 5' to the second *Eco*RI site.[125]

Linkage analysis with FX RFLPs can also be used for the identification of heterozygotes in FVII congenital deficiency since the FVII locus is located on the same chromosome 13[126,127] a few Kb from the FX locus.[128]

TABLE 12
Restriction Fragment Length
Polymorphisms for FX Locus[123]

Enzyme	Polymorphic bands (Kb)	Allele frequency (mean ± SEM)
*Eco*RI	7.5	0.90 ± 0.03
	7.2	0.10 ± 0.03
*Hind*III	7.3	0.95 ± 0.03
	7.6	0.05 ± 0.03
*Pvu*II	2.7	0.72 ± 0.05
	3.1	0.13 ± 0.04
	3.3	0.09 ± 0.03
	2.6	0.06 ± 0.03
*Pst*I	2.9	0.91 ± 0.04
	2.5	0.09 ± 0.04
*Taq*I	1.6	0.82 ± 0.04
	1.25	0.18 ± 0.04

Given the rarity of congenital FX deficiency, it has been possible to analyze the FX gene in only a few families;[123] no gross gene deletions or rearrangements have been found; in addition, available RFLPs were found to be useful for the identification of the abnormal allele in one family.

C. PROTHROMBIN DEFICIENCY

Although significant progress has been made in the characterization and cloning of the gene for human prothrombin,[129,130] no RFLPs have been described and no specific gene defects have been characterized for any of the known molecular variants which have been identified and analyzed from the biochemical and functional standpoints.

X. INHIBITORS

Of the patients with hemophilia B, 2 to 4% develop inhibitors to FIX.[131,132] These antibodies have a restricted specificity, and in one case a monoclonal type of antibody could be demonstrated.[133]

The titer of these antibodies may vary widely, from <1 to >1000 Bethesda Units and most of them belong to the IgG4 subclass, though in some IgG1 and IgG2 could also be found.[134-139] In patients with a high titer of inhibitor, all the IgG subclasses, except the IgG3, are likely to be present, whereas in low titer inhibitor patients, the IgG subclass is less heterogeneous suggesting that a stronger anamnestic response occurs when heterogeneity is less marked.[131]

To our knowledge no inhibitors to factors II, VII, and X have been described in the respective congenital deficiencies; this is not surprising given the rarity of these disorders.

XI. CARRIER DETECTION

The detection of carriers is a classical problem in the clinical management of hemophilia; this is also true for most of the other congenital deficiencies, whatever their mode of inheritance.

The average levels of clotting factors in heterozygotes for inherited clotting deficiencies is about one half that in the normal population. However, only some heterozygotes (20 to 30%) have levels so low that they can be detected unambiguously from their phenotypic expression.[10,140-142] The main problem is that there is such a large variation in factor levels that there is an overlap between the distribution of values between normal and heterozygote populations. A possible solution to this problem is to increase the precision of the bioassays and to utilize more powerful statistical methods to increase the probability of detecting the carrier status. With respect to the X-linked mode of inheritance there is an additional uncertainty due to the fact that heterozygotes may have a completely normal phenotype as a result of the random X chromosomal inactivation (lyonization). However, according to Graham[143] it is possible to "normalize" all the variables affecting the probabilistic evaluation, thus minimizing the misclassification rate to <10%.

In CRM$^+$ variants, an additional advantage is provided by the assay of the relevant antigen; in this case the two populations of normals and heterozygotes can be discriminated by using the ratio of factor activity to factor antigen. Such measurements can indeed reduce the error rate, although this cannot be entirely eliminated.

In contrast to the probabilistic detection of heterozygotes by evaluating their phenotypic expression of factor levels, the new technologies of genotype detection at the DNA level have the potential of giving "all or none" answers. Carrier detection can be performed through the so-called linkage analysis, based upon the identification of RFLPs associated with the gene. However, carrier detection through RFLPs requires appropriate circumstances: first, a given family must be "informative" for at least one of the polymorphic sites; and second, key individual members of the family must be available to the study. A further limitation for linkage analysis is represented by the presence of a homozygosity for the relevant intragenic RFLPs; in this case extragenic RFLPs can be used, but a 3 to 5% error rate should be taken into account due to the possibility of DNA recombinations.

With specific regard to hemophilia B, at the present time the informativity rate of RFLPs in Caucasians approaches 70% of the subjects; in a recent study by Mariani et al.,[19] in which three polymorphic sites were evaluated in 10 hemophilia B kindreds, linkage analysis allowed a diagnosis in 19 out of 20 potential carriers belonging to 9 out of 10 of the studied families.

Another substantial advantage of linkage analysis for hemophilia B is the fact that using this technique, prenatal diagnosis from the 8th to the 12th week of pregnancy is now possible. In fact, prenatal diagnosis was not possible before, since the phenotypic assessment of the fetus was hindered by the low

TABLE 13
Strategy for prenatal diagnosis

1. Draw the pedigree
2. Identify key individuals: Proband, parents, female(s) at risk (in childbearing age), at least one unaffected member
3. Assess the phenotype: a. Factor coagulant activity
   b. Factor antigen
   c. (Coagulant activity/antigen ratio)
   d. Perform statistical analysis for the calculation of the risk odds
4. Assess the genotype: RFLPs of the key individuals; identify sites suitable for linkage analysis; select one or two of them, possibly intragenic
5. Carry out DNA analysis on the villi from the 8th to the 12th week of pregnancy in women already evaluated to be at risk (items 1 to 4)

levels of FIX in the cord blood and by the presence of FIXAg in the amniotic fluid.[106]

The description of multiple polymorphic sites within the FX locus, has now provided the opportunity for detecting heterozygotes in FX and in FVII deficiencies; in fact, the FVII locus is so close to that of FX, that the risk of DNA recombination is very low (less than 0.1%).

We believe that a possible strategy for prenatal diagnosis in congenital factor deficiencies should be based on a careful evaluation of the pedigrees, on the identification of the carriers and individuals at risk through a precise phenotypic evaluation and, finally, on the linkage analysis with RFLPs in key members of the family (Table 13).

XII. TREATMENT

The treatment of vitamin K-dependent clotting factor deficiencies is based on the transfusion of plasma or plasma fractions. The only exception is represented by the combined deficiency of FII, FVII, FIX, and FX where high doses of vitamin K induce an increase of the factors, reducing clinical bleeding consistently.[14]

For many years the treatment of FII, FVII, FIX, and FX deficiencies was based on the use of concentrates containing all these factors. The simple reason for this was that the biochemical homologies of the vitamin K-dependent proteins facilitated their concentration from human plasma as a single fraction. The first four-factor concentrate was developed by Larrieu et al.[144] and Soulier et al.[145] by absorbing vitamin K-dependent factors with tricalcium phosphate. This preparation was named PPSB, after the initials of the trivial names of the factors present in the concentrate. Bidwell et al.[146] prepared an enriched four-factor concentrate by alcohol fractionation of the plasma. These four-factor concentrates have been used for years in France and the U.K. with good clinical results. Their potency, however, was low (both contained

TABLE 14

Recommended Initial Doses of FIX Concentrate in Hemophilia B[153]

Indications	Desired FIXC level (U/dl)	Does of infusate (IU/kg bw)
Mild bleeding episodes	20	20
Early hemarthrosis, early hematomas, epistaxis, gum bleeding		
Major bleeding episodes	40	40
Hemarthrosis and hematomas with swelling, head traumas without neurological symptoms, severe trauma without evidence of actual bleeding, GI bleeding		
Life-threatening episodes	60–80	60–80
Intracranial hemorrhage, major trauma with actual bleeding, surgery		

<20 IU FIX/ml). With the introduction of chromatographic procedures[147-149] more potent four-factor concentrates were produced (up to 30 to 60 IU FIX/ml) and it became possible to separate FVII from the other factors.[149]

These kinds of concentrates, produced mostly by industry, had been used for about 15 years, with good results, when it became apparent that some of them could cause thrombotic complications,[150-152] possibly due to the presence of factors in the activated form. This has stimulated the development and production of purer FIX concentrates, which have also resulted in safer products from the point of view of viral contamination, an issue which has become of paramount importance in recent years. Today, FIX concentrates are more potent (the FIX concentration may be as high as 100 to 200 IU/mg of protein) and contain lesser amounts of FX and prothrombin, no FVII and small amounts of protein C and protein S. Most importantly, all FIX concentrates are today submitted to viral inactivation procedures, so that the risk of transmission of blood-borne viruses is drastically reduced, if not completely abolished.

Infused FIX has a half-life of 18 to 24 h, and an *in vivo* recovery of 40 to 50%; this makes the treatment of hemophilia B easier than hemophilia A, since single daily infusions of concentrate are sufficient to keep the factor at safe levels for protracted treatments, such as those needed to avoid bleeding during and after surgery. The dose of FIX concentrate given to the patient depends on the clinical situation which in turn dictates the desired plasma level. It is essential to keep in mind that for each unit of FIXC infused per kilogram of body weight a yield of 1 IU/dl of plasma is expected. The recommended doses of FIX concentrate for a variety of clinical situations associated with bleeding of various severity are summarized in Table 14.

With the progress in plasma fractionation techniques, other factor concentrates have been developed. The first was a FVII concentrate.[149] Some FVII concentrates are now commercially available: they are all treated for viral inactivation. Since the half-life of FVII is very short (from 2 to 5 h), the corresponding dose of FVII concentrate to correct a bleeding episode in FVII deficient patients needs to be three to five times higher than the dose of FIX concentrate required in patients with hemophilia B. If FVII concentrates are not available, transfusion with fresh frozen plasma (FFP) is the treatment of choice: a loading dose of 10 to 20 ml/kg body weight, followed by 10 ml/kg on the subsequent days is usually sufficient to maintain hemostasis. Care should be taken to avoid blood volume overload which, considering the short FVII half-life and hence the need for repeated infusions, is a potential danger.

Although FX specific concentrates are not yet available, a deficiency of FX can be corrected by using FIX concentrates taking into account the specific FX potency of the concentrate; this should be recorded on the product label. Alternatively, FFP can be used, but again care should be taken not to overload the blood volume: the dose of FFP needed to ensure normal hemostasis is in the range of 10 to 20 ml/kg body weight. The half-life of FX is long, ranging from 24 to 40 h. This simplifies the treatment of FX deficiency. Since one death has been reported after the rapid administration of a FIX concentrate in a FX deficient patient,[149] the infusion should be done slowly. The recommended dosages to ensure hemostasis are the same as for hemophilia B.

The same considerations also hold with regard to replacement therapy in hypo- and dysprothrombinemias. The half-life of prothrombin is about 60 to 70 h; there is, therefore, little risk of blood volume overload since infusions may be given every second day.

As a general recommendation for the treatment of hereditary FII, FVII, and FX deficiencies, FFP is the material of choice when factor replacement therapy is needed to correct mild hemorrhagic symptoms or indicated as a prophylactic measure. The use of FFP is obviously more effective in those deficiencies where the missing factor has a long half-life (FII, FX). Such a therapeutic regime reduces the risk related to the use of commercial concentrates, which is higher in patients who seldom receive blood derivatives.

REFERENCES

1. **Pavlovsky, A.,** Contribution to the pathogenesis of hemophilia, *Blood,* 2, 185, 1947.
2. **Aggeler, P. M., White, S. G., Glendenning, M. B., Page, E. W., Leake, T. B., and Bates, G.,** Plasma thromboplastin component (PTC) deficiency: a new disease resembling hemophilia, *Proc. Soc. Exp. Biol. Med.,* 79, 692, 1952.
3. **Biggs, R., Douglas, A. S., and MacFarlane, R. G.,** Christmas disease: a condition previously mistaken for hemophilia, *Br. Med. J.,* 2, 1378, 1952.
4. **Alexander, B., Goldstein, R., Landwehr, G., and Cook, C. D.,** Congenital STPA deficiency: a hitherto unrecognized coagulation defect with hemorrhage rectified by serum and serum fractions, *J. Clin. Invest.,* 30, 596, 1952.

5. **Hougie, C., Barrow, E. M., and Graham, J. B.,** Stuart clotting defect. I. Segregation of an hereditary hemorrhagic state from the heterogeneous group heretofore called "stable factor" (SPCA, proconvertin, factor VII) deficiency, *J. Clin. Invest.,* 36, 485, 1957.

6. **Seegers, W. H., Brinkhous, K. M., Smith, H. P., and Warner, E. D.,** The purification of thrombin, *J. Biol. Chem.,* 126, 91, 1938.

7. **Larsson, S. A.,** Hemophilia in Sweden, Ph.D. thesis, University of Lund Medical Writing, Malmo, 1984.

8. **McKee, P. A.,** Hemostasis and disorders of blood coagulation, in *The Metabolic Basis of Inherited Disease,* 5th ed., Stanbury, J. B., Wyngaarden, J. B., Fredrickson, D. S., Goldstein, J. L., and Brown, M. S., Eds., McGraw-Hill, New York, 1983, 1531.

9. **Hougie, C.,** Disorders of hemostasis-congenital disorders of blood coagulation factors, in *Hematology,* 3rd ed., Williams, W. J., Beutler, E., Erslev, A. J., Lichtman, M. A., Eds., McGraw-Hill, New York, 1983, chap. 152.

10. **Mazzucconi, M. G., Mariani, G., Chistolini, A., Pasquali Lasagni, R., Motta, M., Ghirardini, A., Altieri, D., Mannucci, P. M., and Mandelli, F.,** Evaluation of the nature of mildly prolonged prothrombin times, *Am. J. Hematol.,* 24, 37, 1987.

11. **Graham, J. B., Barrow, E. M., and Hougie, C.,** Stuart clotting defect II: genetic aspects of a "new" hemorrhagic state, *J. Clin. Invest.,* 36, 497, 1957.

12. **Mammen, E. F.,** Factor X abnormalities, *Semin. Thromb. Hemost.,* 9, 31, 1983.

13. **Mori, K., Sakai, H., and Nakano, N.,** Congenital factor X deficiency in Japan, *Tohoku J. Exp. Med.,* 133, 1, 1981.

14. **Roberts, H. R. and Foster, P. A.,** Inherited disorders of prothrombin conversion, in *Hemostasis and Thrombosis,* 2nd ed., Colman, R. W., Hirsh, J., Marder, V. J., and Salzman, E. W., Eds., J. B. Lippincott, Philadelphia, 1987, chap. 11.

15. **Boyd, Y., Bukle, V. J., Munro, E. A., Choo, K. H., Migeon, B. R., and Craig, I. W.,** Assignment of the hemophilia B (factor IX) locus to the q26.qter region of the Xchromosome, *Ann. Hum. Genet.,* 48, 145, 1984.

16. **Camerino, G., Grzeschik, K. H., Jaje, M., de la Salle, H., Tolstoshev, P., Lecocq, J. P., Heilig, R., and Mandel, J. L.,** Regional localization on the human X-chromosome and polymorphism of the coagulation factor IX gene (hemophilia B locus), *Proc. Natl. Acad. Sci. U.S.A.,* 81, 498, 1984.

17. **Ramgren, O., Nilsson, I. M., and Blombak, M.,** Hemophilia in Sweden. IV. Hereditary investigations, *Acta Med. Scand.,* 171, 759, 1962.

18. **Barrai, I., Cann, H. M., Cavalli, T., Sforza, L. L., and De Nicola, P.,** The effect of parental age on rates of mutation for hemophilia and evidence for different mutation rates for hemophilia A and B, *Am. J. Human Genet.,* 20, 175, 1968.

19. **Mariani, G., Chistolini, A., Hassan, H. J., Gallo, E., Xigen, G., Papacchini, M., Di Paolantonio, T., and Fantoni, A.,** Carrier detection for hemophilia B: evaluation of multiple polymorphic sites, *Am. J. Hematol.,* 33, 1, 1990.

20. **Mariani, G. and Mazzucconi, M. G.,** Factor VII congenital deficiency, *Haemostasis,* 13, 169, 1983.

21. **Mariani, G., Mazzucconi, M. G., Hermans, J., Ciavarella, N., Faiella, A., Hassan, H. J., Mannucci, P. M., Nenci, G. G., Orlando, M., Romoli, D., and Mandelli, F.,** Factor VII deficiency: immunological characterization of genetic variants and detection of carriers, *Br. J. Haematol.,* 48, 7, 1981.

22. **Mariani, G., Hermans, J., Orlando, M., Mazzucconi, M. G., Ciavarella, N., Faiella, A., Berrettini, M., Chistolini, A., Di Nucci, G. D., Mannucci, P. M., and Mandelli, F.,** Carrier Detection in factor VII deficiency, *Br. J. Haematol.,* 60, 687, 1985.

23. **Shapiro, S. S. and McCord, I. S.,** Prothrombin, in *Haemostasis and Thrombosis,* Vol. 4, Spaet, T. H., Ed., Grune & Stratton, New York, 1978, 177.

24. **Kattlove, H. E., Shapiro, S. S., and Spivack, M.,** Hereditary prothrombin deficiency, *N. Engl. J. Med.,* 282, 57, 1970.

24a. **Mariani, G.,** Le Emofilie (Emofilia A e B), in *Trattato Italiano di Medicina Interna,* Introzzi, P., Ed., USES Edizioni Scientifiche, Firenze, Italy, 1988, 4418.

25. **Triplett, D. A., Brandt, J. T., Batard, M. A., McGann-Batard, M. A., Shaeffer Dixon, J. L., and Fair, D. S.,** Hereditary factor VII deficiency heterogeneity defined by combined functional and immunochemical analysis, *Blood,* 66, 1284, 1985.
26. **Ragni, M. V., Lewis, J. H., Spero, J. A., and Hasiba, V.,** Factor VII deficiency, *Am. J. Hematol.,* 10, 79, 1981.
27. **Slem, G. and Kumi, M.,** Bloody tears due to congenital factor VII deficiency, *Ann. Ophtalmol.,* 10, 593, 1978.
27a. **Shifter, T., Machtey, I., Creter, D.,** Thromboembolism in congenital factor VII deficiency, *Acta Haematol.,* 71, 60, 1984.
28. **Lefrere, J. J., Chaunu, M. P., Conard, J., Horellou, M. H., and Samama, M.,** Congenital factor VII deficiency and cerebrovascular stroke, *Lancet,* ii, 1006, 1985.
29. **Zacharski, L. R., DelPrete, S. A., Kisiel, W., Hunt, J., Cornell, C. J., and Marrin, C. A.,** Atherosclerosis and coronary bypass surgery in hereditary factor VII deficiency, *Am. J. Med.,* 84, 955, 1988.
30. **McMillan, C. W. and Roberts, H. R.,** Congenital combined deficiency of coagulation factors II, VII, IX and X, *N. Engl. J. Med.,* 274, 1313, 1966.
31. **Chung, K. S., Bezeaud, A., Goldsmith, J. C., McMillan, C. W., Menache, D., and Roberts, H. R.,** Congenital deficiency of blood clotting factors II, VII, IX, X, *Blood,* 53, 776, 1979.
32. **Johnson, C. A., Chung, K. S., McGrath, K. M., Bean, P. E., Roberts, H. R.,** Characterization of variant prothrombin in a patient deficient in factors II, VII, IX, X, *Br. J. Haematol.,* 44, 461, 1980.
33. **Vicente, V., Maia, R., Alberca, I., Tamagnini, G. P. T., and Lopez Borrasca, A.,** New patient congenitally deficient in factors II, VII, IX, X, *Thromb. Haemost.,* 50, 272, 1983.
34. **Samama, M., Bertina, R. M., Conrad, J., and Horellou, M. H.,** Combined congenital deficiency in protein C and in factors II, VII, IX, X, *Thromb. Haemost.,* 50, 359, 1983.
35. **Goldsmith, G. H., Pence, R. E., and Ratnoff, O. D.,** Studies of a family with combined functional deficiencies of vitamin K dependent coagulation factor, *J. Clin. Invest.,* 69, 1253, 1982.
36. **Roberts, H. R., Grizzle, J. E., McLester, W. D., and Penick, G. D.,** Genetic variants of hemophilia B: detection by means of a specific PTC inhibitor, *J. Clin. Invest.,* 47, 360, 1968.
37. **Bertina, R. M.,** Factor IX variants, in *Haemostasis and Thrombosis,* 2nd ed., Bloom, A. L., Thomas, D. P., Eds., Churchill Livingstone, London, 1987, chap. 24.
38. **Ljung, R. and Holmberg, L.,** Genetic variants of hemophilia B detected by immuno-radiometric assay: implications for prenatal diagnosis, *Pediatr. Res.,* 16, 195, 1982.
39. **Thompson, A. R.,** Monoclonal antibodies to an epitope on the heavy chain of factor IX missing in three hemophilia B patients, *Blood,* 62, 1027, 1983.
40. **Veltkamp, J. J., Meilof, J., Remmelts, H. G., van der Vlerke, D., and Loeliger, E. A.,** Another genetic variant of hemophilia B: hemophilia B Leyden, *Scand. J. Haematol.,* 7, 82, 1970.
41. **Briet, E., Bertina, R. M., Tilburg, N. H., and van Veltkamp, J. J.,** Hemophilia B Leyden. A sex-linked hereditary disorder that improves after puberty, *N. Engl. J. Med.,* 306, 788, 1982.
42. **Hougie, C. and Twomey, J. J.,** Hemophilia Bm: a new type of factor FX deficiency, *Lancet,* i, 698, 1967.
43. **Denson, K. W., Biggs, R., and Mannucci, P. M.,** An investigation of three patients with Christmas disease due to an abnormal type of factor IX, *J. Clin. Pathol.,* 21, 160, 1968.
44. **Mazzucconi, M. G., Bertina, R. M., Romoli, D., Orlando, M., Avvisati, G., and Mariani, G.,** Factor VII activity and antigen in hemophilia B variants, *Thromb. Haemost.,* 43, 16, 1980.

45. **Davis, L. M., McGraw, R. A., Graham, J. B., Roberts, M. R., and Stafford, D. W.,** Identification of the genetic defect in factor EX Alabama: DNA sequence analysis reveals a Gly substitution for Asp[47], *Blood,* 64, 262, 1984.

46. **Briet, E., Griffith, J., Braunstein, K. M., and Roberts, H. R.,** Determination of the relative activities of 2 factor IX variants — factor IX Alabama and factor IX Chapel Hill — in a purified factor X activating system, *Fed. Proc.,* 41, 656, 1982.

47. **Osterud, B., Kasper, C. K., Lavine, K. K., Prodanos, C., and Rapaport, S. I.,** Purification and properties of an abnormal blood coagulation factor IX (factor IX B_m)/kinetics of its inhibition of factor X activation by factor VII and bovine tissue factor, *Thromb. Haemost.,* 45, 55, 1981.

48. **Usharani, P., Warn-Cramer, B. J., Kasper, C. K., and Bajaj, S. P.,** Characterization of three abnormal factor IX variants (B_m Lake Elsinor, Long Beach, and Los Angeles) of hemophilia B. Evidence for defects affecting the latent catalytic site, *J. Clin. Invest.,* 75, 76, 1985.

49. **Mertens, K., Cupers, R., van der Linden, I. K., and Bertina, R. M.,** The functional defect of factor IX Eindhoven, a genetic variant of factor IX, *Thromb. Haemost.,* 50, 249, 1983.

50. **Griffith, M. J., Breitkreutz, L., Trapp, H., Briet, E., Noyes, C. M., Lundblad, R. L., and Roberts, H. R.,** Characterization of the clotting activities of structurally different forms of activated factor IX. Enzymatic properties of normal human factor IXa-alfa, factor IXa-beta and activated factor IX Chapel Hill, *J. Clin. Invest.,* 75, 4, 1985.

51. **Noyes, C. M., Griffith, M. J., Robert, H. R., Lundblad, R. L.,** Identification of the molecular defect in factor IX Chapel Hill: substitution of histidine for arginine at position 145, *Proc. Natl. Acad. Sci. U.S.A.,* 80, 4200, 1983.

52. **Bertina, R. M. and van der Linden, I. K.,** Factor IX Deventer. Evidence for the heterogeneity of hemophilia B_m, *Thromb. Haemost.,* 47, 136, 1982.

53. **Osterud, B., Kasper, C. K., Lavine, K. K., and Prodanos, C.,** Factor IX variants of hemophilia B. The effect of activated factor XI in the reaction product of factor VII and tissue factor on the abnormal factor IX molecules, *Thromb. Res.,* 15, 235, 1979.

54. **Bertina, R. M. and Veltkamp, J. J.,** The abnormal factor IX of hemophilia B + variants, *Thromb. Haemost.,* 40, 335, 1978.

55. **Bertina, R. M. and Veltkamp, J. J.,** A genetic variant of factor IX with decreased capacity for Ca^{2+} binding, *Br. J. Haematol.,* 62, 623, 1979.

56. **Bertina, R. M. and van der Linden, I. K.,** Factor IV Zutphen. A genetic variant of blood coagulation factor IX with an abnormally high molecular weight, *J. Lab. Clin. Med.,* 100, 695, 1982.

57. **Denson, K. W. E., Lurie, A., De Cataldo, F., and Mannucci, P. M.,** The factor X defect: recognition of abnormal forms of factor X, *Br. J. Haematol.,* 18, 317, 1968.

58. **Fair, D. S., Plow, E. F., and Edgington, T. L.,** Combined functional and immuno-chemical analysis of normal and abnormal factor X, *J. Clin. Invest.,* 64, 884, 1979.

59. **Girolami, A., Molaro, G., Lazzarin, M., Scarpa, R., and Brunetti, A.,** A new congenital hemorrhagic condition due to the presence of an abnormal factor X (Factor X Friuli), *Br. J. Haematol.,* 19, 179, 1971.

60. **Girolami, A., Lazzarin, M., Scarpa, R., and Brunetti, A.,** Further studies on the abnormal factor X (factor X Friuli) coagulation disorder: a report of another family, *Blood,* 37, 534, 1971.

61. **Bachmann, F., Duckert, F., and Koller, K.,** The Stuart-Prower factor assay and its clinical significance, *Thromb. Diath. Haemorrh.,* 2, 24, 1958.

62. **Parkin, J. D., Madarus, F., Sweet, B., and Castaldi, P. A.,** A further inherited variant of coagulation factor X, *Aust. N. Z. J. Med.,* 4, 561, 1974.

63. **Girolami, A., Lazzarin, M., Procidano, M., and Luzzato, G.,** A family with heterozygous factor X defect outside Friuli, *Blut,* 46, 149, 1983.

64. **Fair, D., Revak, D., Edgington, T., and Girolami, A.,** Structural studies on the factor X Friuli variant, *Thromb. Haemost.,* 50, 279, 1983.

65. **Shapiro, S. S., Martinez, J., and Holburn, R. R.,** Congenital dysprothrombinemia: an inherited structural disorder of human prothrombin, *J. Clin. Invest.,* 48, 2251, 1969.
66. **Bezeaud, A., Guillin, M. C., Olmeda, F., Quintana, M., and Gomez, N.,** Prothrombin Madrid: a new familial abnormality of prothrombin, *Thromb. Res.,* 16, 47, 1979.
67. **Guillin, M. C. and Bezeaud, A.,** Characterization of a variant of human prothrombin: prothrombin Madrid, *Ann. N.Y. Acad. Sci.,* 320, 414, 1981.
68. **Josso, F., Monasterio de Sanchez, J., Lavergne, J. M., Menache, D., and Soulier, J. P.,** Congenital abnormality of the prothrombin molecule (factor II) in four siblings: prothrombin Barcelona, *Blood,* 38, 9, 1971.
69. **Rabiet, M. J., Elion, J., Benarous, R., Labie, D., and Josso, F.,** Activation of prothrombin Barcelona: evidence for active high molecular weight intermediates, *Biochim. Biophys. Acta,* 584, 66, 1979.
70. **Rabiet, M. J., Benarous, R., Labie, D., and Josso, F.,** Abnormal activation of a human prothrombin variant: prothrombin Barcelona, *FEBS Lett.,* 87, 132, 1978.
71. **Weinger, R. S., Rudy, C., Moake, J. L., Olson, J. D., and Cimo, P. L.,** Prothrombin Houston: a dysprothrombin identifiable by crossed immunoelectrofocusing and abnormal *Echis carinatus* venom activation, *Blood,* 55, 811, 1980.
72. **Girolami, A., Bareggi, G., Brunetti, A., and Sticchi, A.,** Prothrombin Padua: a "new" congenital dysprothrombinemia, *J. Lab. Clin. Med.,* 84, 654, 1974.
73. **Kahn, M. J. P. and Gouaerts, A.,** Prothrombin Brussels; a new congenital defective protein, *Thromb. Res.,* 5, 141, 1974.
74. **Owen, C. A., Henriksen, R. A., McDuffie, F. C., and Mann, K. G.,** Prothrombin Quick: a new identified dysprothrombinemia, *Mayo Clin. Proc.,* 53, 29, 1978.
75. **Henriksen, R. A., Owen, W. G., Nesheim, M. E., and Mann, K. G.,** Investigation of the catalytic properties of the dysthrombin, thrombin Quick, *Thromb. Haemost.,* 42, 57, 1979.
76. **Henriksen, R. A., Owen, W. G., Nesheim, M. E., and Mann, K. G.,** Identification of a congenital dysthrombin: thrombin Quick, *J. Clin. Invest.,* 66, 934, 1980.
77. **Girolami, A., Coccheri, S., Palareti, G., Poggi, M., Burul, A., and Cappellato, G.,** Prothrombin Molise: a "new" congenital dysprothrombinemia, double heterozygosis with an abnormal prothrombin and true prothrombin deficiency, *Blood,* 52, 115, 1978.
78. **Rabiet, M. J., Elion, J., Labie, D., and Josso, F.,** Prothrombin Metz: purification and characterization of a variant of human prothrombin, *Thromb. Haemost.,* 42, 57, 1979.
79. **Josso, F., Rio, Y., and Beguin, S.,** A new variant of human prothrombin: prothrombin Metz, demonstration in a family showing double heterozygosity for congenital hypo-prothrombinemia and dysprothrombinemia, *Haemostasis,* 12, 309, 1982.
80. **Montgomery, R. R., Corrigan, J. J., Clarke, S., and Johnson, J.,** Prothrombin Denver: a new dysprothrombinemia, *Circulation,* 62, 279, 1980.
81. **Smith, L. G., Coone, L., and Kitchens, C. S.,** Prothrombin Gainesville: a new dys-prothrombinemia in a pair of identical twins, *Am. J. Hematol.,* 11, 223, 1981.
82. **Bezeaud, A., Soria, C., Drouet, L., and Guillin, M. C.,** Prothrombin Salakta: pro-thrombin variant with an abnormal thrombin activity, *Thromb. Haemost.,* 50, 250, 1983.
83. **Dumont, M. D., Fisher, A. M., Bros, A., Chassevet, J., and Aufevre, J. P.,** Pro-thrombin Poissey: a new variant of human prothrombin, *Thromb. Haemost.,* 50, 250, 1983.
84. **Rubio, R., Almagro, D., Cruz, A., and Corral, J. F.,** Prothrombin Habana: a new disfunctional molecule of human prothrombin associated with a true prothrombin defi-ciency, *Br. J. Haematol.,* 54, 553, 1983.
85. **Goodnight, S. H., Feinstein, D. I., Osterud, B., and Rapaport, S. I.,** Factor VII antibody-neutralizing material in hereditary and acquired factor VII deficiency, *Blood,* 38, 1, 1971.
86. **Denson, K. W., Conrad, J., and Samama, M.,** Genetic variants of factor VII, *Lancet,* 1, 1234, 1972.

87. **Girolami, A., Falezza, G., Patrassi, G., Stenico, M., and Vettore, L.,** Factor VII Verona coagulation disorder: double heterozygosis with an abnormal factor VII and heterozygous factor VII deficiency, *Blood,* 50, 603, 1977.

88. **Girolami, A., Fabris, F., Dal Bo Zanon, R., Cella, G., and Toffanin, F.,** Factor VII Padua: a congenital disorder due to an abnormal factor VII with a peculiar activation pattern, *J. Lab. Clin. Med.,* 91, 387, 1977.

89. **Girolami, A., Cattarozzi, G., Dal Bo Zanon, R., Cella, G., and Toffanin, F.,** Factor VII Padua 2: another factor VII abnormality with defective ox brain thromboplastin activation and a complex hereditary pattern, *Blood,* 54, 46, 1979.

90. **Girolami, A.,** The congenital variants of prothrombin complex factors, *Acta Haematol.,* 63, 339, 1980.

91. **Fernandez Pavon, A., Cuesta Garcia, M. V., Garcia Munoz, M. S., Lopez Pastor, A., Torreblanca, J., Fernandez Chacon, J. L.,** Factor VII Verona: presentation of a new family, *Sangre,* 31, 489, 1986.

92. **Takamiya, O., Funahashi, S., Kinoshita, S., Yoshioka, A., and Ikawa, H.,** Factor VII activity and antigen in a patient with abnormal factor VII, *Clin. Lab. Haematol.,* 10, 159, 1988.

93. **Pardo, A., Oteyza, J. P., Blanco, L., Correa, J., Steegman, J. L., Tamayo, M., Fernandez, I., Escribano, L., and Navarro, J. L.,** Study of different factor VII deficiency variants in nine families from Spain, *Haemostasis,* 17, 268, 1987.

94. **Winship, P. R., Anson, D. S., Rizza, C. R., and Brownlee, G. G.,** Carrier detection in hemophilia B using two further intragenic restriction fragment length polymorphism, *Nucl. Acid Res.,* 12, 8861, 1984.

95. **Giannelli, F., Choo, K. H., Winship, P. R., Rizza, C. R., Anson, D. S., Rees, D. J. G., Ferrari, N., and Brownlee, G. G.,** Characterization and use of an intragenic polymorphic marker for detection of carriers of hemophilia B (factor IX deficiency), *Lancet,* i, 239, 1984.

96. **Camerino, G., Oberle, I., Drayna, D., and Mandel, J. L.,** A new MspI restriction fragment length polymorphism in the hemophilia B locus, *J. Hum. Genet.,* 71, 79, 1985.

97. **Hay, C. W., Robertson, K. A., Yong, S. N., Thompson, A. R., Growe, G. H., and MacGillivray, R. C. A.,** Use of a *Bam*HI polymorphism in the factor IX gene for the determination of hemophilia B carrier status, *Blood,* 67, 1508, 1986.

98. **Driscoll, M. C., Dispenzieri, A., Tobias, E., Miller, C. H., and Aledort, L. M.,** A second *Bam*HI DNA polymorphism and haplotype association in the factor IX gene, *Blood,* 72, 61, 1988.

99. **Lubahn, D. B., Lord, S. T., Bosco, J., Kirshtein, J., Jeffreis, O. J., Parker, N., Levtzow, C., Silverman, L. M., and Graham, J. B.,** Population genetics of coagulant factor IX: frequencies of two DNA polymorphism in five ethnic groups, *Am. J. Hum. Genet.,* 40, 527, 1987.

100. **Kojima, T., Tanimoto, M., Kamiya, T., Obata, Y., Takahashi, T., Ohno, R., Kurachi, K., and Saito, H.,** Possible absence of common polymorphism in coagulation factor IX gene in Japanese subjects, *Blood,* 69, 349, 1987.

101. **Chen, S. H. and Kurachi, K.,** unpublished data, 1987, see Reference 100.

102. **McGraw, R. A., Davis, L. M., Noyes, C. M., Graham, J. B., Roberts, H. R., and Stafford, D. W.,** Evidence for a prevalent dimorphism in the activation peptide of human coagulation factor IX, *Proc. Natl. Acad. Sci. U.S.A.,* 82, 2847, 1985.

103. **Winship, P. R. and Brownlee, G. G.,** Diagnosis of hemophilia B carriers using intragenic oligonucleotide probes, *Lancet,* i, 218, 1986.

104. **Poon, M. C., Chul, D. H. K., Patterson, M., Starozik, D. M., Dimnik, L. S., and Hoar, D. I.,** Hemophilia B (Christmas disease) variants and carrier detection analyzed by DNA probes, *J. Clin. Invest.,* 79, 1204, 1987.

105. **Mulligan, L., Holden, J. J. A., and White, B. W.,** A DNA marker closely linked to the factor IX (hemophilia B) gene, *Hum. Genet.,* 75, 381, 1987.

106. **Thompson, A. R.**, Factor IX and prothrombin in amniotic fluid and fetal plasma: constraints on prenatal diagnosis of hemophilia B and evidence of proteolysis, *Blood,* 64, 867, 1984.
107. **Giannelli, F., Choo, K. H., Rees, D. J. G., Boyd, Y., Rizza, C. R., and Brownlee, G. G.**, Gene deletions in patients with hemophilia B and anti-factor IX antibodies, *Nature,* 303, 181, 1983.
108. **Peake, I. R., Furlong, B. L., and Bloom, A. L.**, Carrier detection by direct gene analysis in a family with hemophilia B (factor IX deficiency), *Lancet,* i, 242, 1984.
109. **Hassan, H. J., Leonardi, A., Guerriero, R., Chelucci, C., Cianetti, L., Ciavarella, N., Ranieri, P., Pilolli, D., and Peschle, C.**, Hemophilia B with inhibitor: molecular analysis of the subtotal deletion of the factor IX gene, *Blood,* 66, 728, 1985.
110. **Bernardi, F., Del Senno, L., Barbieri, R., Buzzoni, D., Gambari, R., Marchetti, G., Conconi, F., Panicucci, F., Positano, M., and Pitruzzello, S.**, Gene deletion in an Italian hemophilia B subject, *J. Med. Genet.,* 22, 305, 1985.
111. **Matthews, R. J., Anson, D. S., Peake, I. R., and Bloom, A. L.**, Heterozygeneity of the factor IX locus in nine hemophilia B inhibitor patients, *J. Clin. Invest.,* 79, 746, 1987.
112. **Chen, S. H., Yoshitake, S., Chance, P. F., Bray, G. L., Thompson, A. R., Scott, C. R., and Kurachi, K.**, An intragenic deletion of the factor IX gene in a family with hemophilia B, *J. Clin. Invest.,* 76, 2161, 1985.
113. **Bray, G. L. and Thompson, A. R.**, Partial factor IX antigen (IXAg) in urines from normal subjects and patients with hemophilia B due to partial gene deletions, *Clin. Res.,* 33, 544, 1985.
114. **Taylor, S. A. M., Lillicrap, D. P., Blanchette, V., Giles, A. R., Holden, J. J. A., and White, B. N.**, A complete deletion of the factor IX gene and new *Taq*I variant in hemophilia B kindred, *Hum. Genet.,* 79, 273, 1988.
115. **Vidaud, M., Chabret, C., Gazengel, C., Grunebaum, L., Cazenave, J. P., and Goossens, M.**, A de novo intragenic deletion of the potential EGF domain of the factor IX gene in a family with severe hemophilia B, *Blood,* 68, 961, 1986.
116. **Rees, D. J., Rizza, C. R., and Brownlee, G. G.**, Hemophilia B caused by a point mutation in a donor splice junction of the human factor IX gene, *Nature,* 316, 643, 1985.
117. **Davis, L. M., McGraw, R. A., Ware, J. L., Roberts, H. R., and Strafford, D. W.**, Factor IX$_{Alabama}$: a point mutation in a clotting protein results in hemophilia B, *Blood,* 69, 140, 1987.
118. **Reitsma, P. H., Bertina, R. M., Ploos van Amstel, J. K., Riemens, A., Briet, E.**, The putative factor IX gene promoter in hemophilia B Leyden, *Blood,* 72, 1074, 1988.
119. **Tsang, T. C., Bentley, D. R., Mibashan, R. S., and Giannelli, F.**, A factor IX mutation, verified by direct genomic sequencing, causes hemophilia B by a novel mechanism, *EMBO J.,* 7, 3009, 1988.
120. **Huang, M. N., Kasper, C. K., Roberts, H. R., Stafford, D. W., and High, K. A.**, Molecular defect in factor IX$_{Hilo}$, a hemophilia B$_m$ variant: Arg ---- Gln at the carboxyterminal cleavage site of the activation peptide, *Blood,* 73, 718, 1989.
121. **Geddes, V. A., Louie, G. V., Brayer, G. D., and MacGillivray, R. T. A.**, Molecular basis of hemophilia B: identification of the defect in factor IX Vancouver, *Thromb. Haemost.,* 58, 294, 1987.
122. **Reitsma, P., Bertina, R. M., and Briet, E.**, Personal communication, 1989, see Reference 120.
123. **Hassan, H. J., Guerriero, R., Chelucci, C., Leonardi, A., Mattia, G., Leone, G., Mariani, G., Mannucci, P. M., and Peschle, C.**, Multiple polymorphic sites in factor X locus, *Blood,* 71, 1353, 1988.
124. **Jaye, M., Ricca, G., Kaplan, R., Howk, R., Mudd, R. Go, Y., Fair, D. S., and Drohan, W.**, Polymorphism associated with the human coagulation factor X (F10) gene, *Nucl. Acids Res.,* 13, 8286, 1985.

125. **Hay, C. W., Robertson, K. A., Fung, M. R., and MacGillivray, R. T. A.,** RFLPs for Pst I and Eco RI in the human blood clotting factor X gene, *Nucl. Acids Res.,* 14, 5118, 1986.

126. **Royle, N. J., Fung, M. R., MacGillivray, R. T. A., and Hamerton, J. L.,** The gene for clotting FX is mapped to 13q32, *Cytogenet. Cell Genet.,* 41, 185, 1986.

127. **Antonarakis, S. A.,** Diagnosis of genetic disorders at the DNA level, *N. Engl. J. Med.,* 320, 153, 1989.

128. **Davie, E.,** personal communication, 1988.

129. **Friezner Degen, S. J., MacGillivray, R. T. A., and Davie, E. W.,** Characterization of the complimentary deoxyribonucleic acid and gene coding for human prothrombin, *Biochemistry,* 22, 2087, 1983.

130. **Freizner Degen, S. J. and Davie, E.,** The prothrombin gene and serine protease evolution, *Ann. N.Y., Acad, Sci.,* 485, 66, 1986.

131. **Orstavik, K. H. and Miller, C. H.,** IgG subclass identification of inhibitors to factor IX in hemophilia B patients, *Br. J. Haematol.,* 68, 451, 1988.

132. **Rizza, C. R. and Spooner, R. J. D.,** Treatment of hemophilia and related disorders in Britain and Northern Ireland during 1976–1980: report on behalf of the directors of hemophilia centres in the United Kingdom, *Br. Med. J.,* 286, 929, 1983.

133. **Pike, I. M., Yount, W. J., Puritz, E. M., and Roberts, H. R.,** Immunochemical characterization of a monoclonal gammaG4lambda human antibody to factor IX, *Blood,* 40, 1, 1972.

134. **Reisner, H. M., Roberts, H. R., Krumholz, S., and Yount, W. J.,** Immunochemical characterization of a polyclonal human antibody to factor IX, *Blood,* 50, 11, 1977.

135. **Allain, J. P. and Frommel, D.,** Failure of immunosuppression in a hemophilia B patient with specific antibody, *Thromb. Haemost.,* 36, 86, 1976.

136. **Nilsson, I. M., Hedner, U., and Bjorlin, G.,** Suppression of factor IX antibody in hemophilia B by factor IX and cyclophosphamide, *Ann. Intern. Med.,* 78, 91, 1973.

137. **Nilsson, I. M., Jonsson, S., Sundqvist, S. B., Ahlberg, A., and Bergentz, E.,** A procedure for removing high titer antibodies by extra-corporeal protein-A-sepharose absorption in hemophilia: substitution therapy and surgery in a patient with hemophilia B and antibodies, *Blood,* 58, 38, 1981.

138. **Hedner, U. and Nilsson, I. M.,** Induced intolerance in hemophilia patients with antibodies against IX:C, *Acta Med. Scand.,* 214, 191, 1983.

139. **Miller, C. H., Orstavik, K. H., and Hilgartner, M. W.,** Characterization of an occult inhibitor to factor IX in a hemophilia B patient, *Br. J. Haematol.,* 61, 329, 1985.

140. **Simpson, N. E. and Biggs, R.,** The inheritance of Christmas factor, *Br. J. Haematol.,* 8, 191, 1962.

141. **Holmberg, L., Nilsson, I. M., Henriksson, P., and Orstavik, K. H.,** Homozygous expression of hemophilia B in a heterozygote, *Acta Med. Scand.,* 204, 231, 1978.

142. **Kasper, C. K., Osterud, B., Minami, J. Y., Shonick, W., and Rapaport, S. I.,** Hemophilia B: characterization of genetic variants and detection of carriers, *Blood,* 50, 351, 1977.

143. **Graham, J. B.,** Genetics of haemostasis, in *Haemostasis and Thrombosis,* Bloom, A. L., and Thomas, D. P., Eds., Churchill Livingstone, London, 1987, chap. 28.

144. **Larrieu, M. J., Caen, J., Soulier, J. P., and Bernard, J.,** Treatment of hemophilia B with a plasma fraction rich in antihemophilic B factor (PPSB), *Pathol. Biol.,* 7, 2507, 1959.

145. **Soulier, J. P., Blatrix, C., and Steinbuch, M.,** Fractions "coagulantes" contenant les facteurs de coagulation adsorbables par le phosphate tricalcique, *Press Med.,* 72, 1233, 1964.

146. **Bidwell, E., Booth, J. M., Dike, G. W. R., and Denson, K. W. E.,** The preparation for therapeutic use of a concentrate of factor IX containing also factor II, VII, and X, *Br. J. Haematol.,* 13, 568, 1967.

147. **Tullis, J. L., Melin, M., and Jurgian, P.,** Clinical use of human prothrombin complexes, *N. Engl. J. Med.,* 273, 667, 1965.
148. **Tullis, J. L.,** Clinical experience with factor IX concentrates, in *Hemophilia and New Hemorrhagic States,* Brinkhous, K. M., Ed., University of North Carolina Press, Chapel Hill, 1970, 35.
149. **Dike, G. W. R., Bidwell, E., and Rizza, C. R.,** The preparation and clinical use of a new concentrate containing factor IX, prothrombin, and factor X and of a separate concentrate containing factor VII, *Br. J. Haematol.,* 22, 469, 1972.
150. **Kasper, C. K.,** Post-operative thromboses in hemophilia B, *N. Engl. J. Med.,* 289, 160, 1973.
151. **Blatt, P. M., Lundblad, R. L., Kingdon, H. S., McLean, G., and Roberts, H. R.,** Thrombogenic materials in prothrombin complex concentrates, *Ann. Intern. Med.,* 81, 766, 1974.
152. **Cederbaum, A. L., Blatt, P. M., and Roberts, H. R.,** Intravascular coagulation of human prothrombin complex concentrates, *Ann. Intern. Med.,* 84, 683, 1976.
153. **Levine, P.,** Clinical manifestations and therapy of hemophiliacs A and B in *Hemostasis and Thrombosis,* 2nd ed., Colman, R. W., Hirsh, J., Marder, V. J., and Salzmann, E. W., Eds., J. B. Lippincott, Philadelphia, 1987, chap. 6.

Chapter 9

RECENT ADVANCES IN THE MOLECULAR AND FUNCTIONAL PATTERNS OF CONGENITAL DEFICIENCIES OF THE VITAMIN K-DEPENDENT CLOTTING FACTORS

Guglielmo Mariani and M. Papacchini

TABLE OF CONTENTS

0-8493-6423-X/93/$0.00 + $.50
© 1993 by CRC Press, Inc.

I. HEMOPHILIA B

Since the factor (F)IX gene contains only eight exons totaling about 3 Kb, it is possible to amplify the exon-containing regions from the genomic DNA of hemophilia B patients and screen for mutations in the amplified DNA; such a strategy has led to the identification and characterization of numerous mutations. In a recent publication Koeberl et al.[1] were able to identify mutations in 61 of the 65 patients studied. It is noteworthy that most mis-sense mutations described in the study tend to alter amino acids conserved in other related coagulation factors (FX, FVII, and protein C): this means that the conserved residues are important for the protein function. Also Green et al.[2] were able to detect the mutations in the factor IX gene from all the hemophilia B cases (45) registered at Malmo hemophilia center.

Almost 400 hemophilia B gene defects have now been discovered: practically every kind of mutation has been identified, including frameshifts and splicing defects. In the second edition of the remarkable database held by Giannelli et al.[3] (Table 1), of the 388 mutants, 206 were unique mutations (53.1%), the others (182) repeats; of these repeats, 132 (72.5%) were shown to occur at CG doublets consisting of CG → TG or CG → CA change. Among the whole database, the overall prevalence of the mutations involving a CG doublet is 39% (151/388 mutations). This modified cytosine is among the most unstable residues and the resulting mutation, as has been pointed out by Giannelli,[3] has to be considered a true "hot spot". The remaining 50 "repeat mutations" not involving the CG doublet occur, as repeated events, more rarely (2 or 3 times), compared to the CGs which has been reported in the database on at least ten occasions, up to the 19 reports for mutations at nucleotide 31,008.

Very recently, Taylor et al.[4] reported on the molecular characterization of the original Christmas Disease mutation: they identified a mutation residing at nucleotide 30,070 where a guanine was replaced by a cytosine, altering the amino acid encoded at position 206 in the FIX protein from a cysteine to a serine. This was the index case of Christmas Disease, as described by Biggs in 1952; the mutation which causes a phenotype characterized by the absence of both FIX activity and antigen is very rare, since this is the only mutation of this kind reported to the hemophilia B database.[3]

Little information is given in the hemophilia B database[3] on the severity of the defects and on the functional changes caused by the single mutations. However, it is clear that the B_m variant may derive from the expression of different mutations (C → G; C → A; G → T; G → E; G → A; C → A; C → T; T → C) occurring in different areas of the gene (nucleotides 20,518 → 20,524; 31,053; 31,221 → 31,223; 31,290), suggesting that the activation of FIX by $FVII_a$ or FX_a requires the integrity of different polypeptide regions which probably reside in adjacent but functionally related loops.

Another Registry has been set up by Peake[5] for the FVIII/FIX Scientific Standardization Committee of the International Society for Hemostasis and

TABLE 1
Mutation in FIX Locus[3]

Location[a]	Exon	Nucleotide number	Number of mutants[b]	Unique molecular events[b]
Signal peptide (-46 to -18)	a	30–116	1	1
Propeptide (-17 to -1)	b	6,323–6,375	28	4
Gla (1 to 46)	b	6,326–6,373	32	22
	c	6,678–6,701		
EGF (1st) (47 to 84)	d	10,392–10,505	31	18
EGF (2nd) (85 to 127)	e	17,669–17,797	13	12
Activation (128 to 195)	f	20,363–20,565	47	22
Catalytic (196 to 415)	g	30,039–30,153	196	98
	h	30,822–31,372		
Subtotal			348	177
Promoter			12	8
Donor splice sites			17	13
Acceptor splice sites			7	6
Cryptic splice			4	2
Poly(A) site			0	0
Totals			388	206

[a] Amino acid numbers used (Anson et al., 1984).
[b] Excluding normal variants within double mutants.

Thrombosis (ISTH). The Registry provides information on DNA polymorphisms within or close to the FIX locus. In addition to the *restricted fragment-length polymorphisms* (RFLPs) described in Chapter 8 (Table 10), two additional polymorphisms have been identified: an *Hha*I and a *Mnl*I which can be screened by PCR analysis. The first is located in the 3' flanking region displaying a heterozygosity in approximately 50% of the studied population; the second has been identified in the locus 148 (threonine/alanine dimorphism), with a 45% heterozygosity.

The *Hha*I/PCR polymorphism is equally informative in American blacks and whites, but is less informative (about 30%) in Asian populations; the *Mnl*I/PCR polymorphism, instead, is less informative in American blacks (21% of heterozygosity) and scarcely informative (10% of heterozygosity) in Asian populations.[5]

TABLE 2
Described Point Mutations within the FVII Locus

Variant (toponym)	Amino acid substitution	FVII:C (activator) (U/dl)	FVII:Ag (U/dl)
FVII$_{Nagoya}$	Arg304 → Tryptophan	5 (rabbit, simian) 60 (ox)	?
FVII$_{Padual}$	Arg304 → Glutamine	28 (human) 0 (rabbit)	104

II. FACTOR VII

New interesting data is available concerning the analysis of the polymorphic sites within the FVII locus. To our knowledge, the first FVII intragenic polymorphism has been described by Green et al.,[6] and is detected after digestion of PCR amplified genomic DNA; the frequency of the allele representing the loss of the cutting site is 10% and the rare individuals homozygous for the mutation are positioned in the low percentiles of FVII activity and antigen; the heterozygous subjects for this mutation have FVII levels 22% lower, on average, than the mean of the "normal" population. The base change giving rise to this polymorphism is a G to A substitution in the codon for the amino-acid 353. Since it is known from prospective studies that high FVII levels are associated with risk of arterial thrombosis and myocardial infarction, the absence of this cutting site could be interpreted as protective with regard to this very common type of thrombosis.

Subsequently, Marchetti et al.[7] identified through PCR amplification a polymorphism in intron 7 of the FVII gene. This polymorphism, located in one of the five regions of tandem repeats, has an estimated frequency of the two alleles (480 and 443 bp) of 0.3 and 0.7.

The evaluation of the repeat polymorphism analysis in FVII congenital deficiencies has allowed the identification of a condition of double heterozygosity in 2/6 severe FVII deficiencies examined.[8] This finding indicates that in these two patients, two independent gene lesions have been inherited and that, as demonstrated for other factors, FVII congenital deficiencies can also be due to a variety of mutations.

Mutations causing disease have also been recently characterized from molecular biology studies: independently described mutations have been localized in exon VIII and deal with the same amino-acid substitution (Arg 304); their features are detailed in Table 2. Two groups independently[9,10] identified the point mutation which is responsible for the so-called Padual defect, a CRM$^+$ variant characterized by low FVII levels when the factor is activated by a rabbit brain thromboplastin and intermediate levels when human tissue factor is used as activator. The Padual defect results from the abolition of a positive charge in a position of the catalytic domain of FVII which is important for the interaction between the enzyme and its activator, tissue

TABLE 3
Described Point Mutations within the FX Locus

Variant (toponym)	Amino acid substitution	FX:C (U/dl)	FX:Ag (U/dl)	Functional patterns
FX$_{Vorarlberg}$	Gla^{14} → Lys	<10 (extr)^a 25 (intr)^b	20	Very low activation by TF^c; low by FIX$_a$
FX$_{Malmo4}$	Gla^{26} → Asp.ac	43 (intr)^b	—	Low activation by FIX$_a$/VIII$_a$ and normal by TF/FVII$_a$
FX$_{Santo Domingo}$	Arg → Glycine (Signal peptide)	<1	5	Altered cellular secretion

^{a} Extrinsic pathway activation-based assay.
^{b} Intrinsic pathway activation-based assay.
^{c} TF = tissue factor.

factor. In FVII$_{Nagoya}$ a slightly different mutation (Table 2) has been described,[11] with respect to the same codon. The functional features are similar, if not identical, to these of FVII Padua1.

III. FACTOR X

For FX, two mutations have been recently described by the same group[12,13] with respect to the Gla region. Interestingly, it seems that mutations involving codons responsible for different Gla residues yield different activation patterns by the complexes IX$_a$/VIII$_a$ or TF/VII$_a$ (Table 3).

A new FX variant has been recently and independently described by Watzke et al.[14] and Racchi et al.[15] — FX$_{Santo Domingo}$. In this case the mutation was localized by both groups in the signal peptide (G → A in exon I, codon-20) (Table 3). This defect of the signal sequence was demonstrated to exert its effect posttranscriptionally, at the level of translation. This FX variant was shown to be translated, but failed to be secreted and was slowly destroyed intracellularly.[14]

IV. PROTHROMBIN

Two new mutants concerning prothrombin have been recently reported: for one (Prothrombin Segovia)[16] the functional assays only were given, consisting in a different activation pattern with different activators (i.e., normal activation being obtained with the Taipan venom, a very defective one using the *Echis Carinatus* venom). In the second mutant,[17] the molecular defect has been fully described: two gene mutations were found, one characterized by a nucleotide deletion in exon VIII (-G, codon 249–250), the second consisting of a point mutation in exon X (C → T = Tryptophan 340 →

Arginine). The first mutation results in frameshift and premature translation termination, the second, occurring within the active B chain of thrombin, results in a marked alteration of hydrophobicity pattern.

V. CONCLUSIONS

As the number of described mutations increases, it is becoming clear that a correlation exists between certain types of mutations and the levels of lacking factor, the clinical severity and the type of functional alteration. It is now possible to categorize the defects: for instance, deletions, stop codon mutations and frameshifts almost invariably account for the underlying physiopathological event of a severe hemophilia.

With the possibility of precisely defining the mutations it is now much easier to investigate the origin of the mutations in sporadic cases, to assess the frequency of a given mutation in a given population of hemophiliacs and finally to improve the quality of the diagnostic procedures with regard to the carrier status assessment and prenatal diagnosis.

REFERENCES

1. **Koeberl, D. D., Bottema, C. D. K., Ketterling, R. P., Bridge, P. J., Lillicrap, D. P., and Sommer, S. S.,** Mutations causing hemophilia B: direct estimate of the underlying rates of spontaneous germ-line transitions, and deletions in human gene, *Am. J. Hum. Genet.,* 47, 202, 1990.
2. **Green, P. M., Montadon, A. J., Ljung, R., Bentley, D. R., Nilsson, I. M., Ling, S., and Giannelli, F.,** Hemophilia B mutations in a complete Swedish population sample. A test of new strategy for the genetic councelling of disease with high mutational heterogeneity, *Br. J. Haematol.,* 78, 390, 1991.
3. **Giannelli, F., Green, P. M., High, K. A., Sommer, S., Lillicrap, D. P., Ludwig, M., Olek, K., Reitsma, P. H., Goossens, M., Yoshioka, A., and Brownlee, G. G.,** Hemophilia B: database of point mutations and short additions and deletions-second edition, *Nucl. Acid Res.,* 19, 2194, 1991.
4. **Taylor, S. A. M., Duffin, J., Cameron, C., Teitel, J., Garvey, B., and Lillicrap, D. P.,** Characterization of the original Christmas disease mutation (Cysteine 206 → Serine): from clinical recognition to molecular pathogenesis, *Thromb. Haemost.,* 67, 63, 1992.
5. **Peake, I.,** Registry of DNA polymorphisms within or close to the human Factor VIII and Factor IX genes, minutes (appendix one) of the FVIII/FIX Standardization Committee of the Int. Soc. Hemostasis and Thrombosis, 1991.
6. **Green, F., Kelleher, C., Wilkes, H., Temple, A., Meade, T., and Humphries, S.,** A common polymorphism of the Factor VII gene determines coagulation factor VII levels in healthy individuals, *Thromb. Haemost.,* 65, 667, 1991.
7. **Marchetti, G., Gemmati, D., Patracchini, P., Pinotti, M., and Bernardi, F.,** PCR detection of a repeat polymorphism within the F7 gene, *Nucl. Acids Res.,* 19, 4570, 1991.
8. **Bernardi, F.,** personal communication.

9. **O'Brien, D. P., Gale, K., Anderson, J. S., McVey, J. H., Meade, T., Miller, G., and Tuddenham, E. D.,** FVII-304 GLN: a dysfunctional FVII molecule with reduced affinity for tissue factor, *Thromb. Haemost.,* 65, 769 (Abstr.), 1991.

10. **James, H. L., Kumar, A., Girolami, A., Hunnard, J. G., and Fair, D. S.,** Variant coagulation factors X and VII with point mutations in a highly conserved motif in the substrate binding pocket. Comparative molecular modelling, *Thromb. Haemost.,* 65, 937 (Abstr.), 1991.

11. **Matsushita, T., Emi, N., Takamatsu, J., and Saito, H.,** Identification and in vitro expression analysis of a single amino acid substitution in blood clotting factor VII$_{Nagoya}$. *Blood,* 78, 181a (Abstr.), 1991.

12. **Watzke, H. H., Lechner, K., Roberts, H. R., Sakamuri, V. R., Welsch, D. J., Friedman, P., Mahr, G., Jagadeeswaran, P., Monroe, D. M., and High, K. A.,** Molecular defect (Gla^{+14} → Lys) and its functional consequences in a hereditary factor X deficiency (factor X "Vorarlberg"), *J. Biol. Chem.,* 265, 11,982, 1990.

13. **Wallmark, A., Larson, P., Ljiung, R., Monroe, D., and High, K.,** Molecular defect (Gla^{25} → Asp) and its functional consequences in a hereditary factor X deficiency (Factor X "Malmo4"), *Blood,* 78, 60a, 1991.

14. **Watzke, H. H., Wallmark, A., Hamaguchi, N., Stafford, D. W., and High, K. A.,** Molecular analysis and in vitro expression of a hereditary factor X deficiency with a severe bleeding disorder, *Thromb. Haemost.,* 65, 809 (Abstr.), 1991.

15. **Racchi, M., Stanfiled-Oakley, S., Lively, M., and High, K.,** Factor X "Santo Domingo": intracellular accounting for failure of secretion, *Blood,* 78, 277a (Abstr.), 1991.

16. **Collados, M., Fernandez, J., Paramo, J. A., Pinacho, A., Prosper, F., and Rocha, E.,** Functional study of a congenital dysprothrombinemia: prothrombin Segovia, *Thromb. Haemost.,* 65, 1261 (Abstr.), 1991.

Chapter 10

VITAMIN K-DEPENDENT PROTEINS IN MALIGNANCY

John L. Francis

TABLE OF CONTENTS

0-8493-6423-X/93/$0.00 + $.50

203

I. INTRODUCTION

The death rate from cancer in many parts of the Western world is second only to that from coronary heart disease. Most cancers are solid tumors, and death usually results from secondary spread (metastasis), rather than the primary tumor itself. A thorough understanding of the factors affecting the metastatic process is essential for the development of appropriate forms of anticancer treatment.[1] Some types of treatment (e.g., surgery, radiotherapy, and certain forms of chemotherapy) are only aimed at controlling the primary tumor, and therefore anything which also inhibits metastasis may improve the efficacy of current therapy.[2] The involvement of hemostatic mechanisms with aspects of malignant growth and spread has long been recognized because of the higher incidence of thromboembolic complications in patients with cancer.[3] Metastasis is a multistep process and there is now evidence that hemostatic components may be involved at several of these stages (Table 1). Discussion of all the possible roles of these pathways in malignant disease, particularly those of platelets and the fibrinolytic system, are outside the scope of this review and have been reviewed elsewhere.[4-7] Evidence that the vitamin K-dependent coagulation factors may play a role in malignant spread, or may otherwise be altered in patients with cancer, has been provided by a variety of biochemical, histological, and pharmacological experiments. Elucidation of the role of these factors would increase our understanding of the malignant process and may also improve current cancer therapy through pharmacological modulation of hemostatic pathways.

TABLE 1

Possible Mechanisms of Hemostatic Involvement, and Corresponding Pharmacological Approaches to Treatment, at Different Stages of the Metastatic Process[1]

Stage of metastasis	Possible mechanisms involved	Potential treatments
Detachment from primary tumor	Plasminogen activators	Antifibrinolytics
Migration into circulation	Heparanase	Heparin
	Plasminogen activators	Antifibrinolytics
Cellular interactions in circulation	Platelet aggregation	Antiplatelet drugs
	By direct mechanisms	Antiplatelet Gp
	By tumor-derived thrombin	Heparin
	or other procoagulants	Oral anticoagulants
Arrest of tumor cells	Platelet thrombi	Antiplatelet drugs
	Fibrin thrombi	Heparin
		Oral anticoagulants
Invasion and growth	Heparanase	Heparin
	Plasminogen activators	Antifibrinolytics
	PDGF	Antiplatelet drugs
	Peritumor fibrin	Oral anticoagulants

Note: Gp = glycoproteins, PDGF = platelet-derived growth factor.

II. PLASMA VITAMIN K-DEPENDENT PROTEINS IN PATIENTS WITH MALIGNANT DISEASE

A. QUANTITATIVE CHANGES

Although clinically obvious thrombosis or bleeding affect relatively few patients with malignant disease, many more have a hemostatic defect detectable by laboratory tests.[8] The exact incidence depends on the sensitivity of the laboratory techniques employed. Thus, when more sophisticated tests for hemostatic activation are applied, the detection of subclinical disseminated intravascular coagulation (DIC) in patients with cancer may be more readily achieved. Some laboratory evidence of intravascular activation of the coagulation and/or fibrinolytic mechanisms can be found in most cancer patients,[9] although variations in the criteria for laboratory diagnosis have made it difficult to determine the incidence of acute DIC in patients with malignant disease.

The prothrombin time, which is widely used as an indicator of the levels of the vitamin K-dependent factors, is prolonged in approximately 14% of patients with malignant disease,[9,10] although the proportion is greater in those with established DIC.[11] The incidence of a prolonged activated partial thromboplastin time (APTT) is rather more variable,[9,10] but is certainly higher in individuals with overt DIC.[11] Although these abnormalities may reflect deficiencies in factors II, VII, and X, (FII, FVII, and FX, respectively) they may also be due to low levels of factors V and VIII (FV and FVIII, respectively) which may be degraded in subjects with DIC. Overall, routine screening tests are of only limited value in detecting subclinical intravascular clotting activation, as 50% of unselected patients give normal results.[11]

B. QUALITATIVE CHANGES

The normal hepatic synthesis of coagulation factors II, VII, IX, and X requires the presence of vitamin K. When these factors are synthesized in the absence of vitamin K, their des-γ-carboxy (precursor) forms are released into the plasma. Lacking their γ-carboxyglutamic acid (Gla) residues, these proteins cannot bind calcium ions and therefore cannot participate in the clotting process. These proteins are known as *proteins induced by vitamin K absence or antagonism* (PIVKA) and the most extensively studied form is the precursor of prothrombin (factor II), referred to as PIVKA II. In 1984, Liebman et al.[12] reported that plasma levels of PIVKA II measured by radioimmunoassay were increased in two thirds of patients with hepatocellular cancer. Subsequent studies, also by immunological assay for PIVKA II, have largely agreed with this frequency,[13,14] although a slightly higher figure (74%) was obtained with a novel type of coagulation assay.[15] In hepatoma cells cultured without vitamin K, PIVKA II production can be blocked by adding vitamin K to the culture medium.[13] In patients with hepatocellular carcinoma, however, elevated PIVKA II is not related to low plasma vitamin K levels, and vitamin K administration results in only a small reduction in PIVKA II concentrations.[14] Elevation of PIVKA II levels is reasonably specific to hepatoma (in the absence of other evidence of vitamin K deficiency or antagonism) since most other types of parenchymatous liver disease, metastatic liver cancer and tumors of other organs have normal levels.[13,14,16] PIVKA II levels appear to be related to tumor size, falling after tumor resection[14,16] and rising again following disease recurrence.[14] Thus, the measurement of PIVKA II seems to be diagnostically useful, especially when combined with measurement of α-fetoprotein levels. Indeed, the use of both markers improves the detection rate of hepatoma by some 20% over each method alone.[16]

III. THE EFFECT OF ORAL ANTICOAGULANTS ON THE GROWTH AND SPREAD OF MALIGNANT DISEASE

The presence of fibrin in association with intravascular tumor deposits was first observed over a century ago.[17] Fibrin appears to be an integral part of the tumor stroma in a wide variety of animal and human malignancies, combination with cyclophosphamide inhibited both primary and secondary and is essential for significant tumor growth to occur.[18] For this reason, many investigators have tried various anticoagulant agents in attempts to stop tumor growth by interfering with peritumor fibrin formation. Although heparin has been used, it has generally been ineffective, and most work has therefore concentrated on the use of oral anticoagulants for this purpose. In general, these drugs are well absorbed and are taken up from the plasma into tissues, particularly the liver. Because of the ease of administration of oral anticoagulants, and the considerable clinical experience of their use, this class of drugs has been extensively used in attempts to treat experimental and human malignancies. The results of such studies have given the greatest support to the theory that vitamin K-dependent proteins are involved in the malignant process.

A. ANIMAL STUDIES

Tumor cells are deposited in organs despite anticoagulation.[19] This suggested that the initial deposition or lodgement of malignant cells is not affected by oral anticoagulants, and therefore most studies have concentrated on the effect of these drugs on the subsequent growth and spread of the tumor. The most commonly used animal model for the study of antihemostatic therapy in malignant disease has been the Lewis Lung (3LL) carcinoma. This tumor develops spontaneously in the lungs of C57BL mice, and has several features which make it a useful model for this purpose. The properties and characteristics of the 3LL tumor, and their similarities to human small-cell carcinoma of the lung, have been reviewed elsewhere.[20] Oral anticoagulation, initiated at the same time as tumor implantation, inhibits primary tumor growth in the 3LL model, and also reduces the number of spontaneous lung metastases.[21-23] Intermittent anticoagulation does not inhibit metastasis, but still retards primary tumor growth. Warfarin inhibited the development of spontaneous metastases from rat intestinal carcinomas induced by azoxymethane (AOM).[24] In a later study using a similar model, Goeting et al.[25] found that warfarin reduced the number of preneoplastic lesions (microadenomas) in the descending colon and rectum of AOM-treated animals. Thus, it seemed that warfarin either prevented microadenoma formation or reversed the process. Since previous studies by this group showed that warfarin had no effect on the cell kinetics of this tumor model,[26] they suggested that the action of warfarin was partly targeted on preneoplastic or early neoplastic cells. Interestingly, as noted later in this review, the antitumor effect was evident at "nonanticoagulating" doses of warfarin.[25]

Warfarin has not always been successful in reducing metastatic spread in experimental tumor systems. For example, this anticoagulant had no effect on the metastatic capacity of a benzopyrene-induced fibrosarcoma in C57BL/6J mice.[27] However, as discussed later, this failure may be related to the nonvitamin K-dependent type of procoagulant expressed by this particular tumor. Combinations of warfarin with a cytotoxic agent may be more effective in decreasing tumor growth. For example, both warfarin alone, and in growth of a transplanted tumor in mice,[28] and, in mice foot pad tumors, warfarin plus adriamycin resulted in fewer lung metastases than either agent alone.[29] Furthermore, oral anticoagulants may improve the results of cyclophosphamide or 5-fluorouracil treatment, and exhibit distinct signs of synergism with bleomycin.[22] Not all workers have found the combination of warfarin and conventional chemotherapy to be effective.[30] However, as the latter study used an animal model which was inappropriate to the human situation, the results may not reflect the potential value of oral anticoagulant therapy.

Dietary vitamin K deficiency also reduces metastatic spread.[21,31] Although this is good evidence that the antitumor effect of oral anticoagulants is due to their anti-vitamin K properties rather than to some other property, dietary deprivation does not provide a realistic therapeutic approach in humans.

B. HUMAN STUDIES

1. Early Trials

The inhibitory effects of oral anticoagulants on experimental tumor models have stimulated a number of clinical trials in human cancer. Warfarin may potentiate the effect of conventional chemotherapy in various malignancies, and once the disease is under control, may be adequate for maintenance therapy by itself.[32] In the 67% of cancer patients who did not respond, death occurred within 6 months. In a controlled trial comparing warfarin and chemotherapy with chemotherapy only in a variety of advanced malignancies, overall survival at 2 years was significantly better in the combination therapy group.[33] Furthermore, patients who responded to chemotherapy were likely to benefit from addition of warfarin, and once again, anticoagulation alone was adequate for maintenance therapy in patients controlled by chemotherapy. Patients may also require lower doses of chemotherapeutic drugs for adequate disease control after starting oral anticoagulants.[34] The combination of warfarin and chemotherapy significantly prolonged survival in patients with advanced cancer,[34,35] but ovarian cancers, breast tumors and lymphosarcomas seemed to be particularly responsive.[35]

A further clinical study worthy of comment was that conducted by Hoover et al.[36] in patients undergoing amputation for osteosarcoma. Subjects were placed in a control group (n = 21) or received anticoagulation (n = 9). Although the numbers were small, significantly more (56%) anticoagulated patients survived 5 to 8 years compared to the controls (14%). In another small (n = 24) study of small-cell carcinoma of the bronchus, the combination of warfarin and chemotherapy did not improve survival compared to chemotherapy alone.[37] In later studies, Thornes and co-workers[38] showed that warfarin decreased the recurrence rate in malignant melanoma following surgical resection, and the combination of warfarin and chemotherapy in recurrent colon cancer resulted in significantly lower mortality and greater survival than chemotherapy alone.[39] Preliminary results in a controlled trial of oral anticoagulants in advanced breast cancer involved low numbers of patients, but at least encouraged continuation of the trial.[40]

2. Retrospective Studies

An alternative way to determine the value of anticoagulants in cancer is to study the morbidity and mortality rates from malignant disease in individuals on longterm anticoagulant therapy. Ries et al.[41] followed patients with cervical carcinoma who had been treated with anticoagulants (heparin and warfarin) to prevent thromboembolism. The recurrence rate was decreased from 22.9 to 12.6% in the anticoagulated group and survival was said to be improved. Interestingly, the occurrence of peritumor fibrin in the treated group was markedly decreased (see later). A retrospective approach was also taken by Michaels[42] and later by Annegers and Zacharski.[43] However, although these two studies followed 918 patients for a total of 5110 person-years, they failed to find significant differences between the number of new malignancies and that expected for the general population.

3. Major Controlled Clinical Trials

It should be emphasized that most early studies of the antitumor effect of oral anticoagulants were conducted on small numbers of patients, and the benefits, if any, of such an approach have been difficult to assess. Furthermore, many of these trials were uncontrolled, or used historical control methods. However, in 1976, a team of investigators led by Dr. L. Zacharski, initiated the Veterans Administration Cooperative Study Program (CSP #75) to test the hypothesis that such drugs could modify the course of various human cancers. On the basis of earlier experimental work, sodium warfarin was chosen for this study. The rationale and experimental design for this study have been described by Zacharski et al.[44]

CSP #75 recruited 431 patients between April 1976 and March 1982. Subjects suffered from lung, colorectal, prostate, or head and neck cancer, and, based on clinical and histological criteria, were allocated to one of nine groups. Data were analyzed first for patients with small cell carcinoma of the lung (SCCL). The median survival for 25 control patients was 24 weeks, but this was extended to 50 weeks in the warfarin group.[45] The anticoagulated patients also took longer to exhibit signs of disease progression. However, when the final report of the trial was published,[46] no differences in survival between warfarinized and control patients were evident for the colorectal, prostate, head, and neck cancers and non-SCCL patients. Thus, the data suggested that warfarin may modify the course of at least some types of human cancer, including SCCL. Although these results undoubtedly provide a basis for further studies of warfarin treatment, particularly in SCCL, anticoagulation cannot yet be recommended as part of the standard treatment of this condition.[47]

4. On-Going Clinical Trials

Warfarin anticoagulation was used by Thornes[48] as the sole means of preventing recurrence of malignant melanoma. In 1981, warfarin was replaced by coumarin, the parent compound with little anticoagulant activity, without affecting the trend towards recurrence prevention.[48] Coumarin is well suited to clinical trials as it is relatively nontoxic and requires little laboratory control. Equally, melanoma is an ideal tumor model in which to study effects on recurrence rates, and a multicenter, controlled, randomized, and double-blind trial of coumarin (50 mg/d) in this disease is currently in progress. Several other trials are also on-going at present. The Cancer and Leukemia Group B (CALGB) have recently confirmed the beneficial effect of warfarin in disseminated SCCL[49] and an additional trial in subjects with limited extent disease is now underway. The International European phase III study of adjuvant urokinase and warfarin in Dukes' B and C colorectal cancer is randomizing in a two-tiered manner, giving rise to four treatment groups. In the first tier, patients will receive postoperative urokinase infusion or no treatment. After staging, all Dukes' B and C patients are allocated to warfarin or no treatment. The study will complete with a 5 year follow-up and reports on recurrence rates and survival. Finally, the Southeastern (U.S.) Cancer Study Group is conducting a multicenter trial of adjuvant warfarin in stage II and III colon cancer. In this study, all potentially curable and resectable subjects will be randomized to surgery alone, or warfarin therapy beginning 1-d preoperatively and continuing for 12 months. Thus, full anticoagulation would not be present during surgery; an attempt to provide a compromise between an unacceptable risk of bleeding, and lack of anticoagulant cover in a period thought to be critical in the establishment of metastases.

IV. MECHANISM OF THE ANTITUMOR ACTION OF ORAL ANTICOAGULANTS

The evidence reviewed in the previous sections suggests that oral anticoagulants might be a useful adjunct to the treatment of some types of primary and metastatic cancer. It also seems that while these agents are known primarily as anticoagulants, their antitumor effects cannot be entirely explained on these grounds. There are three major arguments for the antimetastatic effect being mediated by mechanisms other than a plasma anticoagulant effect. First, normalization of vitamin K-dependent clotting factor levels in anticoagulated animals did not reverse the antimetastatic effect in the 3LL model.[31] Second, the precise dose of warfarin does not seem to affect its antitumor action, and both high and low doses have comparable effects on the 3LL tumor.[21] Similarly, low, "nontherapeutic" doses of warfarin reduced primary tumor incidence in AOM-induced colorectal cancer in rats, but increasing the dose to achieve "therapeutic" anticoagulation did not further reduce the tumor incidence.[25] Third, although warfarin is a mixture of $R(+)$ and $S(-)$ enantiomers, the $R(+)$ form has much less anticoagulant activity. Both primary growth and spontaneous metastasis of the 3LL tumor were reduced by RS and $S(-)$ treatment, but not by treatment with $R(+)$ warfarin.[50] However, both enantiomers are effective inhibitors of microsomal vitamin K metabolism in 3LL tumors — which is qualitatively similar to that of liver cells.[51] This suggested that oral anticoagulants may act on some aspect of cellular, vitamin K-dependent metabolism, at doses lower than required for plasma anticoagulation. As discussed in detail below, there is now evidence that oral anticoagulants may act by interfering with a vitamin K-dependent, cellular pathway of blood coagulation, although the precise nature of such a pathway remains controversial. In order to understand the possible mechanisms by which such interference might take place it is necessary to consider the clotting process at the level of the malignant cell.

V. TUMOR CELL PROCOAGULANTS AND VITAMIN K-DEPENDENT CLOTTING FACTORS

The histological demonstration of fibrin around tumor deposits and the beneficial effects of oral anticoagulants on some tumors discussed above, have led to considerable interest in the ability of tumor cells to influence the coagulation process. In particular, the identification of vitamin K-dependent pathways of tumor-mediated coagulation would provide the biochemical basis for the clinical use of oral anticoagulants in cancer therapy. Indeed, cellular procoagulant pathways which might depend on vitamin K for their functional integrity have now been identified and are discussed in the following sections.

A. TISSUE FACTOR

Many normal tissues contain a powerful procoagulant which does not normally occur in plasma.[52] This activity was referred to as "tissue thromboplastin" for many years, but following more detailed biochemical characterization, is now usually known as tissue factor (TF). The TF-mediated pathway of blood coagulation is referred to as the "extrinsic" pathway, and, although TF itself is probably not vitamin K-dependent, most factors involved in this pathway (factors II, VII and X) do require vitamin K for full biological activity. In this pathway, TF acts as a cofactor, forming a complex with plasma factor VII, to greatly increase the protease activity of the latter. Although it was originally thought that the sole substrate for this enzyme was factor X, factor IX is also activated in this way, and the total amount of factor Xa thus generated is a function of these combined (vitamin K-dependent) pathways.

1. In Normal Cells

TF has been demonstrated in normal cells by several methods. Cell culture techniques have shown that TF activity is expressed on the cell surface[53] and TF has been demonstrated in the plasma membranes of most normal body tissues and atheromata[54,55] and saliva.[56] Interestingly, warfarin reduced salivary TF levels in the latter study, leading to the suggestion that TF may be a vitamin K-dependent protein,[57] although there is little other evidence to support this hypothesis. Normal human endothelial cells are capable of TF synthesis, and, of particular potential relevance to clotting activation in cancer patients, can be stimulated to express TF by tumor necrosis factor (TNF).[58] This process may be instrumental in the prothrombotic state associated with malignant disease, since enhanced endothelial procoagulant activity is accompanied by depression of the protein C anticoagulant pathway; possibly by TNF-induced suppression of the endothelial gene for thrombomodulin.[59] The cellular distribution of TF has been referred to as a hemostatic "envelope" ready to activate coagulation when vascular integrity is disrupted.[60] This presumably gives considerable scope for clotting activation during the infiltration of malignant tumor cells. Finally, "stimulated" normal monocytes and macrophages may also produce TF[61] as well as the vitamin K-dependent clotting factors,[62,63] and this potentially important source of cellular procoagulant activity in malignant disease is discussed in the following section.

2. In Malignant Tumor Cells

Given the wide distribution of TF in normal tissues, it is perhaps hardly surprising that various malignant tumors, of both human and animal origin, also produce TF. Among human tumors, TF activity has been described in gastric,[64,65] colon[65,66] ovarian,[67] and renal tumors.[68] Cell lines derived from human breast cancers have given variable results.[66,68] Some tumor cells, e.g., human teratocarcinoma, may shed vesicles which possess TF activity, as well as acting later in the coagulation cascade by providing a surface for prothrombinase generation.[68]

The occurrence of coagulation factors VII and X in the extravascular spaces around renal cell carcinoma (RCC) cells suggests that the extravascular fibrin deposition associated with this tumor could be initiated by TF.[69] Although direct immunohistochemical evidence for this is lacking in RCC, the presence of TF as well as prothrombin and factors VII and X,[69-71] have been demonstrated in SCCL. The fact that thrombin is generated around this tumor has been elegantly shown by the demonstration of thrombin-specific cleavage sites in fibrinogen surrounding viable tumor cells.[72]

Nevertheless, the possibility of an alternative, non-TF-dependent pathway of fibrin formation cannot be excluded, even though the presence of "cancer procoagulant" (CP) (see later), demonstrable by immunohistochemical methods, has not yet been reported.

Macrophages are an integral part of the lymphoreticular infiltrate of many tumor types, and it is clear that such cells may make important contributions to the local procoagulant activity. As mentioned above, monocytes and macrophages may be stimulated by various factors to express TF. A recent study has shown that tumor-associated macrophages may provide all the components necessary (except fibrinogen) for extrinsic pathway coagulation.[73] Whether these cells can actually synthesize all these factors for themselves, or whether they are simply absorbed during their earlier circulation as blood monocytes, has not yet been fully established. The presence and synthesis of factor VII in mature human macrophages has, however, been proven,[74] and it is likely that this capability is extended to the other vitamin K-dependent clotting factors—as has been found in cells of animal origin.[62,63] Thus, tumor-associated macrophages would be capable of initiating, propagating, and stabilizing the local fibrin network, and might therefore be an important target for vitamin K antagonist therapy.

B. DIRECT FACTOR X-ACTIVATING ACTIVITY
1. Cancer Procoagulant

A major landmark in tissue procoagulant research occurred with the demonstration that, while normal tissue contained a procoagulant with all the characteristics of TF, malignant tissue from the same histological source contained a quite different activity.[75] This procoagulant apparently activated factor X directly, since it was equally effective in normal and factor VII-deficient plasma, and was termed CP.

The diversity of human tumor types which apparently contain CP is remarkable, and include adenocarcinoma of colon and kidney, carcinoma of lung, breast, liver, and kidney, neuroblastoma, liposarcoma, and sarcoma,[75-77] malignant melanoma,[78] and acute leukemia.[79] CP is not confined to human malignancies, however, and has been demonstrated in the rabbit V2 carcinoma,[75] parietal yolksac carcinoma,[80] SV40-transformed hamster fibroblasts,[80,81] 3LL carcinoma[82-84] Ehrlich carcinoma and JW sarcoma,[82] and B16 melanoma cells.[81,85] Furthermore, the use of a polyclonal antibody to CP revealed that the procoagulant activities of the murine tumors 3LL, B16, and JWS are immunologically, as well as enzymatically, indistinguishable from the rabbit V2 procoagulant.[86] These are significant observations, as much of the work to suggest that tumor spread may be modulated by vitamin K antagonism comes from the study of these experimental tumors and their procoagulant activities.

The main characteristic which distinguishes CP from the rather more widespread TF, is the ability of the former to initiate coagulation in the absence of factor VII.[75] The procoagulant is inhibited by iodoacetamide and mercuric chloride, and reactivated by dithiothreitol;[87] classic properties of a cysteine proteinase. Although CP can activate factor X, it can also interfere with the thrombomodulin-protein S-protein C inhibitor pathway,[88] and it is not yet clear which is the more significant pathological role of this protein. CP has been purified from the rabbit V2 carcinoma to yield a homogenous preparation with a molecular weight of 68,000 Da and an isoelectric point of 4.8.[89] The protein had very low levels of hexose and sialic acid, and the predominant amino acids were serine, glycine, and glutamic acid. Thus, CP appeared to be different from other known activated clotting factors (which are mainly serine proteases), or other cysteine proteinases which may be secreted by malignant tumors. Preliminary analysis suggests that CP does contain some Gla residues — suggesting a dependence of vitamin K for expression of biological activity.[88] This might explain the reported effects, discussed above, of oral anticoagulants on tumors which express this type of procoagulant.

2. Tissue Factor-Factor VII Complex

It has recently become apparent that CP may not be the only factor X-activating activity (FXAA) in malignant tissue samples. Using a chromogenic substrate assay to measure the ability of tissue homogenates to generate factor Xa from purified factor X, we have shown that colorectal and breast tumor tissue contains significantly greater FXAA than normal colon mucosa from the same patients.[90-92] However, the characteristics of the human colorectal and breast procoagulant were distinct from both TF and CP.[93,94] Although like CP, the procoagulant activated factor X directly, it was inhibited by DFP and phospholipase C, was readily adsorbed on to aluminium hydroxide and barium citrate and was almost totally abolished by antibodies to human TF and factor VII. Furthermore, the activity was not blocked by cysteine protease inhibitors such as iodoacetamide or mercuric chloride. Taken together, these findings indicate that this procoagulant is most likely to be a TF-factor VII complex. This conclusion is supported by several independent observations. First, the procoagulant associated with 3LL cells, widely thought to be CP, may not be a single protein but may instead be composed of a cellular element, and a vitamin K-dependent serum factor, possibly factor VII.[95] Second, the procoagulant associated with mouse exudate macrophages appears to be a serine protease resulting from the complexing of membrane-bound TF and a factor VII-like substance.[96] Finally, the procoagulant activities of amniotic fluid,[97] which is immunologically identical to CP,[98] and bronchoalveolar lavage,[99,100] also have properties compatible with a stable TF-factor VII complex. This dependence on factor VII may also explain the sensitivity of this type of tissue procoagulant to vitamin K absence or antagonism, especially as both factors VII and X have been identified in the intercellular spaces between tumor cells.[69,71]

How might factor VII occur in the areas adjacent to malignant tumors? First, it seems likely that any changes in vascular permeability sufficient to allow extravasation of plasma fibrinogen will also permit egress of factor VII. Second, infiltrating macrophages may provide both factor VII and TF, and possibly other clotting factors, and thus a complete procoagulant activity.[62,63] Nevertheless, whether the TF-VII complex responsible for factor X activation in breast and colorectal tumors occurs *in vivo,* or is actually an artefact of the tissue homogenization process, is not clear. It is possible that the factor VII component is derived from contaminating blood during tissue homogenization and only binds to TF *in vitro*. This is supported by the finding of a significant correlation between tissue hemoglobin (as a measure of blood contamination) and FXAA in normal breast and colorectal tissue.[93] Such a correlation was not found in malignant tissue (Figure 1), and thus it is conceivable, although certainly not proven, that the TF-VII complex is an artefact of normal tissue preparation, but occurs *in vivo* in malignant tumors. It is also possible that the tumor itself produces the factors necessary for the local generation of thrombin. In SCCL, a tumor susceptible to oral anticoagulant

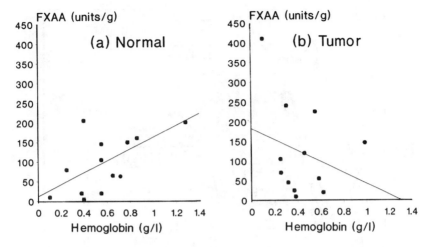

FIGURE 1. Correlation of hemoglobin levels with factor X-activating activity (FXAA) in (a) normal breast tissue and (b) malignant breast tumor homogenates.

therapy, immunohistochemical studies have revealed a complete extrinsic coagulation pathway, as well as the presence of proteins C and S.[101] As discussed below, vitamin K carboxylase activity may be common to many normal and malignant cell types.[102] Tumor cells may therefore be able to provide at least three out of the five factors required for local fibrin formation. Presumably, in the normal state, the procoagulant "trigger" for coagulation (TF and/or CP) and the "substrate" (fibrinogen) are not present. The possible pathways by which procoagulant activities may influence coagulation are illustrated in Figure 2.

There is much evidence to suggest that tumor-derived procoagulant activity plays a role in the metastatic process. As reviewed above, there is also evidence that vitamin K antagonism may influence this process, and because of the established role of vitamin K in the coagulation pathway, attention has focused on the effects of these agents on the ability of tumors to activate coagulation. The following section will consider the effect of vitamin K absence or antagonism on cellular procoagulant activity.

VI. THE ROLE OF CELLULAR VITAMIN K-DEPENDENT FACTORS IN METASTASIS

A. THE EFFECT OF VITAMIN K ABSENCE OR ANTAGONISM ON TUMOR PROCOAGULANT ACTIVITY

Both dietary deficiency of vitamin K[23,103,104] and treatment with oral anticoagulants[23,103,105] reduce the FXAA of the 3LL carcinoma. Administration of vitamin K to the treated animals reverses this effect. Normalization of the plasma levels of factors II, VII, IX, and X by infusion of clotting

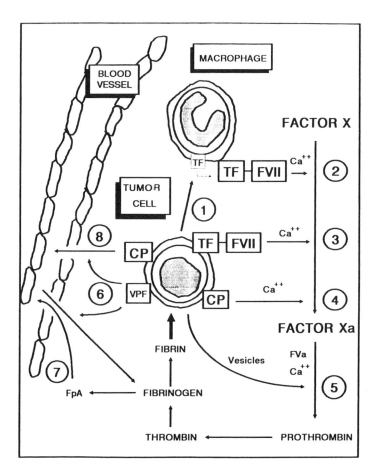

FIGURE 2. Current concepts of the interactions between malignant cells and stimulated mono-
cytes/macrophages and the blood coagulation system. Tumor cells can stimulate macrophages
(1) to express tissue factor (TF), which by complexing with factor VII (FVII), activates factor
X (2). The factor VII required for this reaction may be derived from the plasma or the macrophage
itself. Peripheral blood monocytes (not shown) may behave in a similar fashion. Tumor cells
may also express TF (3) or produce cancer procoagulant (CP) which can activate factor X directly
(4). The subsequent activation of prothrombin may be helped by vesicles shed from tumor cells
which act as a surface for prothrombinase generation (5). The source of factors V (FV) and
prothrombin are unclear, but may also be provided by macrophages. Thrombin then cleaves
fibrinogen, which is derived from plasma under the influence of vascular permeability factor
(VPF) (6). Fibrin is deposited around the tumor, while the liberated fibrinopeptide A (FpA) (7)
and CP (8) may leak back into the circulation. (Reproduced from Francis, J. L., *Med. Lab.
Sci.,* 46, 331, 1989. With permission.)

factor concentrates however, does not correct cellular procoagulant activity.[23] Heparin on the other hand, has no effect on the procoagulant activity of this tumor.[23] The FXAA of the JW sarcoma and B16 melanoma cells is also reduced by warfarin administration.[106]

In many of these studies, it has not always been clear whether the FXAA expressed by the tumor cells has been due to CP or other types of activity (e.g., TF-factor VII interaction). The 3LL and rabbit V2 procoagulants however, have been characterized as CP (see above), and are apparently depressed by warfarin anticoagulation.[107] This raises the possibility, alluded to earlier, that CP is a vitamin K-dependent protein. The biochemical basis for this might be the presence of γ-glutamyl carboxylase in the microsomal fraction of these and other (JW sarcoma and B16 melanoma) tumors.[51,107] As the procoagulant activities of all four tumors are immunologically identical,[86] it is possible that CP could represent at least one of the substrates for γ-glutamyl carboxylase in these tissue. There is little doubt that various tumor cells are capable of vitamin K-dependent protein carboxylation and produce Gla-containing proteins.[102,108] Vitamin K carboxylase activity has been reported in lung epidermoid carcinoma, melanoma, and adenocarcinomas of breast and lung and these cells synthesize a family of vitamin K-dependent proteins.[102] Although the exact identity of these proteins remains to be established, one of them was positively identified as protein S. As this ability is shared with many normal cells,[108] the possibility must be considered that tumor-derived γ-carboxylated proteins may differ from their normal counterparts and/or that they might confer some sort of selective advantage on the malignant cell. However, experimental support for this theory is presently lacking.

The effect of vitamin K absence or antagonism on TF is less well defined. As mentioned above, warfarin apparently reduced salivary TF activity,[56] but had no effect on monocyte TF expression.[109] Furthermore, warfarin did not affect the TF activity of murine fibrosarcoma cells,[27] which is evidence against TF being a vitamin K-dependent protein.[57]

B. PROCOAGULANT ACTIVITY IN NORMAL TISSUES

In human cancer, the site of early metastatic growth is largely the result of hemodynamic factors. Thus, tumors with a portal venous drainage spread initially to the liver, while those with a systemic drainage progress to the lungs.[110] The later patterns of spread and tumor dissemination in animal systems are not explained by this simple model. As Paget,[111] over 100 years ago, first noted, not all tissues are similarly receptive to metastatic tumor growth. Indeed, given a dose of viable tumor in proportion to their percentage of cardiac output, some organs are unexpectedly frequent sites of tumor growth.[112,113] In this way, a ranking of "fertility" for tumor growth can be

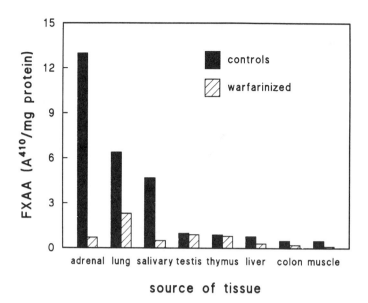

FIGURE 3.   Factor X-activating activity (FXAA) in various normal rat organs and the effect of warfarin treatment.

constructed.[114] Thus, adrenal and lung are good ''soils,'' while colon and liver are relatively poor. The ability of the latter organs to support tumor growth can, however, be enhanced by trauma.[115,116]

In a recent study in this laboratory, we demonstrated a correlation between the FXAA of various normal rat tissues and their predilection for tumor growth.[117] Very similar results were obtained from fresh human tissues obtained at post-mortem. The procoagulant activity could be blocked by anti-factor VII, suggesting that it was of the TF-factor VIIa complex type. The ranking of the procoagulant activity of these organs parallels their predilection for metastatic tumor growth, derived from earlier experiments in which tumor cells were injected intra-arterially.[114,118,119] In addition, oral anticoagulation, which as discussed above, reduces metastatic tumor growth in some experimental models,[22,50,120] was associated with a parallel reduction in FXAA of these organs (Figure 3).

VII. THE ROLE OF PLASMA VITAMIN K-DEPENDENT FACTORS IN METASTASIS

Several recent studies may force a reevaluation of the hypothesis that the antimetastatic effect of warfarin is due to inhibition of *cellular* procoagulant pathways.

First, 3LL cells grown in the presence of warfarin, or in vitamin K-deficient media, activate factor X to similar extents, but culturing the cells in the presence of serum from warfarin-treated animals, or administration of warfarin to tumor-bearing animals, reduces procoagulant activity.[95] More recently, the same group[104] showed that 3LL cells grown in vitamin K-deficient conditions lose both FXAA and metastatic competence, while exposure to normal serum restores these properties.

Second, Smith et al.[121] conducted a careful dose-response study in two independent rat models — a chemically-induced arterial thrombosis, and a spontaneously metastasizing prostatic carcinoma — and clearly showed that the degree of anticoagulation is directly correlated with both antithrombotic and antimetastatic effects. In this study, the therapeutic index of chronic warfarin therapy in rats was very narrow, and the authors concluded that the difficulties of maintaining anticoagulation within this range in man may limit the success of this approach in human cancers.

Third, the antimetastatic effect of warfarin in the Mtln3 tumor, a tumor with properties close to those of human breast cancer, was totally abolished by restoration of plasma-clotting factor levels.[122] In these experiments, restoration of plasma-clotting factor levels for 12 h immediately before tumor injection abolished the antitumor effect of warfarin. This effect was not seen if normalization of clotting factor levels was delayed until 12 h after tumor injection. Thus, it appears that the major role of coagulation in metastasis occurs in the first 12 h after tumor cells enter the blood. This suggests a mechanism involving processes such as tumor cell survival or endothelial adhesion, supporting the conclusions reached rather earlier by others.[36,123]

The differences between the results of McCulloch and George[122] and those of Hilgard and Maat[31] may be due to the difference in the type of tumor used, or in the clotting factor concentrates used to normalize blood coagulation. Thus, the concentrate used by Hilgard and Maat[31] contained relatively little factor VII, although subsequent work by McCulloch and George[124] suggested that factor VII alone is not implicated in the metastatic process. However, the *complex* of coagulation factors II, IX, and X does appear to contain a component which greatly enhances experimental metastasis.[124] This may help to explain the antimetastatic effect of warfarin, although reduction in the fibrin-forming capacity of the blood (by arvin-induced defibrination) did not affect the tumor-promoting property of the coagulation complex. Although the authors point to a mechanism which involves specific clotting factors, rather than coagulation as a whole, the defibrination process still left some 30% of the original fibrinogen levels. Thus, the possibility of fibrin-mediated enhancement of metastasis cannot be completely excluded. Furthermore, although producing supranormal plasma levels of factor VII did not enhance metastasis in this model, this does not necessarily exclude a major role for factor VII in this process. Indeed, recent studies in this laboratory have shown that the number of pulmonary metastases following injection of the MC28 fibrosarcoma was decreased by warfarin, but was restored following injection of a factor VII concentrate at the time of, and 4 h after, tumor injection to the anticoagulated animals.[125] These data appear to be at variance with the findings of McCulloch and George,[124] although the factor VII concentrate used in our study was not completely free of the other vitamin K-dependent clotting proteins. The role(s) of *individual* vitamin K-dependent coagulation proteins in the metastatic process clearly requires further study.

Taken together, the data from the studies mentioned above suggest:

1.   Inhibition of malignant cell vitamin K function does not affect factor X activation.
2.   The cellular procoagulant activity is not a vitamin K-dependent protein.
3.   FXAA depends on a warfarin-sensitive (vitamin K-dependent) protein which is found in serum, *and* a cellular component.
4.   The vitamin K-dependent serum protein plays a major role in metastasis.
5.   There is a direct correlation between primary tumor FXAA and metastatic spread.

VIII. OTHER EXPLANATIONS FOR THE ANTIMETASTATIC EFFECT OF WARFARIN

Several workers have looked beyond the coagulation mechanism for the antimetastatic effect of oral anticoagulants. For example, Chang and Hall[126] suggested that warfarin has a cytotoxic effect *in vitro,* probably by preventing DNA and RNA synthesis. Depletion of cytoribosomal RNA by warfarin was also reported by Kirsch et al.,[127] who additionally noted that the drug affected the tissue distribution and plasma clearance of 5-fluorouracil. Immunological mechanisms may also be involved. Coumarin drugs stimulate macrophage activity and therefore stimulate the reticuloendothelial system, while selective inhibition of macrophage function abolishes the antimetastatic effect of warfarin.[128] General stimulation of macrophage activity could increase protein lysis and assist the host to defend itself against tumor invasion.[129] Another possible mechanism is suggested by the report that warfarin inhibits movement of tumor cells, but not normal cells.[130] This might reduce the number of cells shed from the primary tumor, or impede tumor cell movement through vessel walls. There is an increasing volume of evidence that natural killer (NK) lymphocytes play an important role in controlling metastatic growth and spread, possibly by eliminating circulating tumor cells. NK cells can recognize and destroy tumor cells without prior sensitization or activation. It is also possible that NK cells are essential for the antimetastatic effect of warfarin, that coating of tumor cells with platelet and/or fibrin thrombi protects against NK cell recognition, and that anticoagulants increase the susceptibility of tumor cells to destruction by NK cells.[131] The possible cytotoxic or immunological mechanisms by which warfarin might influence tumor cell spread have been reviewed in greater detail elsewhere.[132]

IX. CLOSING REMARKS

Available data shows that tumor cells are capable of vitamin K-dependent carboxylation, that they may synthesize various vitamin K-dependent clotting factors and that they can also express proteins capable of initiating the extrinsic coagulation pathway. Other clinical and experimental evidence points to a role for these factors in the growth and spread of malignant disease, yet the results of trials of oral anticoagulant therapy remain confusing. Thus, for almost every study which documents a beneficial effect for a given agent in a particular tumor, there is another which contradicts these findings. It is possible that hemostatic manipulation is effective in some tumors but not others, that certain tumors may be able to "bypass" an antihemostatic attack, or that the degree of hemostatic blockade needed to exert an antimetastatic effect would itself be injurious to the host.[133] It is also clear that human trials are generally never as successful as preliminary studies in experimental animals. This may be due to differences in tumor biology, but it is more probably due to the fact that most animal models allow hemostatic modulation *at the time* of metastatic spread, while in the human disease, this has often already occurred at the time of presentation.[2] Other factors which may cloud the issue include the study design (particularly the types of controls used), the stage of disease being treated, and the criteria for tumor response. It is to be hoped that much better designed studies, such as those undertaken by the Veterans Administration Study Group,[45,46] and others currently in progress, coupled with improved studies of tumor-related clotting activities, will clarify the role of vitamin K-dependent factors and vitamin K antagonist therapy in the treatment of human cancer.

REFERENCES

1. **Bastida, E.,** The metastatic cascade: potential approaches for the inhibition of metastasis, *Sem. Thromb. Hemost.,* 14, 66, 1988.
2. **Crissman, J. D.,** Is there clinical relevance for therapies which disrupt the metastatic cascade? in *Hemostatic Mechanisms and Hemostasis,* Honn, K. V. and Sloane, B. F., Eds., Martinus Nijhoff, Boston, 1984, 1.
3. **Trousseau, A.,** *Clinique Medicale de l'Hotel de Paris,* Vol. 3, 5th ed., J. B. Balliere et Fils, Paris, 1865, 94.
4. **Dvorak, H. F.,** Thrombosis and cancer, *Human Pathol.,* 18, 275, 1987.
5. **Dvorak, H. F.,** Abnormalities of hemostasis in malignancy, in *Hemostasis and Thrombosis, Basic Principles and Clinical Practice,* Colman, R. W., Hirsh, J., Marder, V., and Salzman, E. W., Eds., J. B. Lippincott, Philadelphia, 1987, 1143.
6. **Muszbek, L.,** Ed., *Hemostasis and Cancer,* CRC Press, Boca Raton, FL, 1987.
7. **Francis, J. L.,** Haemostasis and cancer, *Med. Lab. Sci.,* 46, 331, 1989.

8. **Bick, R. L.**, Alterations of haemostasis associated with malignancy. Etiology, patho-physiology, diagnosis and management, *Sem. Thromb. Haemost.*, 5, 1, 1978.

9. **Sun, N. C. J., McAfee, W. M., Hum, G. J., and Weiner, J. M.**, Haemostatic abnormalities in malignancy, a prospective study of one hundred eight patients. I. Co-agulation studies, *Am. J. Clin. Pathol.*, 71, 10, 1979.

10. **Edwards, P. L., Rickles, F. R., Moritz, T. E., Henderson, W. G., Zacharski, L. R., Forman, W. B., Cornell, C. J., Forcier, R. J., O'Donnell, J. F., Headley, E., Kim, S-H., O'Dell, R., Tornyos, K., and Kwaan, H. C.**, Abnormalities of blood coagulation tests in patients with cancer, *Am. J. Clin. Pathol.*, 88, 596, 1987.

11. **Kies, M. S., Posch, J. J., Giolma, J. P., and Rubin, R. N.**, Hemostatic function in cancer patients, *Cancer*, 46, 831, 1980.

12. **Liebman, H. A., Furie, B. C., Tong, M. J., Blanchard, R. A., Kwang-Juei, L., Shou-Dong, L., Coleman, M. S., and Furie, B. S.**, Des-γ-carboxy (abnormal) pro-thrombin as a serum marker of primary hepatocellular carcinoma, *N. Engl. J. Med.*, 310, 1427, 1984.

13. **Okuda, H., Obata, H., Nakanishi, T., Furukawa, R., and Hashimoto, E.**, Production of abnormal prothrombin (des-γ-carboxy prothrombin) by hepatocellular carcinoma, *J. Hepatol.*, 4, 357, 1987.

14. **Fujiyama, S., Morishita, T., Hashiguchi, O., and Sata, T.**, Plasma abnormal pro-thrombin (des-γ-carboxy prothrombin) as a marker of hepatocellular carcinoma, *Cancer*, 61, 1621, 1988.

15. **Soulier, J-P., Gozin, D., and Lefrere, J-J.**, A new method to assay des-γ-carboxy-prothrombin. Results obtained in 75 cases of hepatocellular carcinoma, *Gastroenterology*, 91, 1258, 1986.

16. **Hattori, N., Ohmizo, R., Unoura, M., Tanaka, N., Kobayashi, K., and the PIVKA-II Collaborative Working Group,** Abnormal prothrombin measurements in hepatocel-lular carcinoma, *J. Tumour Marker Oncol.*, 3, 207, 1988.

17. **Billroth, T.**, *Lectures in Surgical Pathology and Therapeutics*, translated from the 8th edition, New Sydenham Society, 1878.

18. **Dvorak, H. F.**, Tumors: wounds that do not heal, *N. Engl. J. Med.*, 315, 1650, 1986.

19. **Fisher, B. and Fisher, E. R.**, Anticoagulants and tumor cell lodgement, *Cancer Res.*, 27, 421, 1967.

20. **Zacharski, L. R.**, Basis for selection of anticoagulant drugs for therapeutic trials in human malignancy, *Haemostasis*, 16, 300, 1986.

21. **Hilgard, P.**, Experimental vitamin K deficiency and spontaneous metastases, *Br. J. Cancer*, 35, 891, 1977.

22. **Hilgard, P., Schulte, H., Wetzig, G., Schmitt, G., and Schmidt, C. G.**, Oral anti-coagulation in the treatment of a spontaneously metastasizing murine tumor (3LL), *Br. J. Cancer*, 35, 78, 1977.

23. **Colluci, M., Delaini, F., de Bellis Vitti, G., Locati, D., Poggi, A., Semeraro, N., and Donati, M. B.**, Warfarin inhibits both procoagulant activity and metastatic capacity of Lewis Lung carcinoma cells, *Biochem. Pharmacol.*, 32, 1689, 1983.

24. **Williamson, R. C. N., Lyndon, P. J., and Tudway, A. J. C.**, Effects of anticoagulation and ileal resection on the development and spread of experimental intestinal carcinomas, *Br. J. Cancer*, 42, 85, 1980.

25. **Goeting, N. L. M., Trotter, G. A., and Taylor, I.**, Effect of warfarin on formation and growth of pre-neoplastic lesions in chemically-induced colorectal cancer in the rat, *Br. J. Surg.*, 73, 487, 1986.

26. **Goeting, N. L. M., Trotter, G. A., Cooke, T., Kirkham, N., and Taylor, I.**, Effect of warfarin on cell kinetics, epithelial morphology and tumor incidence in induced co-lorectal cancer in the rat, *Gut*, 26, 807, 1985.

27. **Lorenzet, R., Bottazzi, B., Locati, D., Colucci, M., Mantovani, A., Semeraro, N., and Donati, M. B.**, Failure of warfarin to affect the tissue factor activity and the metastatic potential of murine fibrosarcoma cells, *Eur. J. Cancer Clin. Oncol.*, 21, 263, 1985.

28. **Berkada, F. B., d'Souza, J. P., and Bakemier, R. F.,** The effect of anticoagulants on tumor growth and spread in mice, *Proc. Am. Assoc. Cancer,* 15, 99, 1974.

29. **Hoover, H. C. and Ketcham, A. S.,** Reducing experimental metastasis formation with anticoagulation and chemotherapy, *Surg. Forum,* 26, 173, 1975.

30. **Higashi, H. and Heidelberger, C.,** Late effect of warfarin alone or in combination with 5FU on primary and metastatic adenocarcinoma 755, *Cancer Chemother. Rep.,* 55, 29, 1971.

31. **Hilgard, P. and Maat, B.,** Mechanism of lung tumor colony reduction caused by coumarin anticoagulation, *Eur. J. Cancer,* 15, 183, 1979.

32. **Thornes, R. D.,** Anticoagulant therapy in patients with cancer, *J. Irish Med. Ass.,* 62, 426, 1969.

33. **Thornes, R. D.,** Warfarin as maintenance therapy for cancer, *J. Irish Coll. Phys. Surg.,* 2, 41, 1972.

34. **Thornes, R. D.,** Oral anticoagulant therapy of human cancer, *J. Med.,* 5, 83, 1974.

35. **Thornes, R. D.,** Adjuvant therapy of cancer via the cellular immune mechanism or fibrin induced by fibrinolysis and oral anticoagulants, *Cancer,* 35, 91, 1975.

36. **Hoover, H. C., Ketcham, A. S., Millar, R. C., and Gralnick, H. R.,** Osteosarcoma: improved survival with anticoagulation and amputation, *Cancer,* 41, 2475, 1978.

37. **Standford, C. F.,** Anticoagulants in the treatment of small cell carcinoma of the bronchus, *Thorax,* 34, 113, 1979.

38. **Thornes, R. D., Lynch, G., and Sheehan, M. V.,** Cimetidine and coumarin therapy of melanoma, *Lancet,* 2, 328, 1982.

39. **Chlebowski, R. T., Gota, C. H., Chan, K. K., Weiner, J. M., Block, J. B., and Bateman, J. R.,** Clinical and pharmokinetic effects of combined warfarin and 5FU in cancer, *Cancer Res.,* 42, 4827, 1982.

40. **Sagripanti, A., Carpi, A., Baicchi, U., Nicolini, A., Ferdeghini, M., and Grassi, B.,** Oral anticoagulants in breast cancer patients, (abstract), *Thromb. Hemost.,* 58, 236, 1987.

41. **Ries, J., Ludwig, H., and Appel, W.,** Anticoagulants in the radiation treatment of carcinoma of the female genetalia, *Med. Welt.,* 38, 2042, 1968.

42. **Michaels, L.,** The incidence of course of cancer in patients receiving anticoagulant therapy. Retrospective and prospective studies, *J. Med.,* 5, 98, 1974.

43. **Annegers, J. F. and Zacharski, L. R.,** Cancer morbidity and mortality in previously anticoagulated patients, *Thromb. Res.,* 18, 399, 1980.

44. **Zacharski, L. R., Henderson, W. G., Rickles, F. R., Forman, W. B., Cornell, C. J., Forcier, R. J., Harrower, H. W., and Johnson, R. O.,** Rationale and experimental design for the VA Cooperative Study of anticoagulation (warfarin) in the treatment of cancer, *Cancer,* 44, 732, 1979.

45. **Zacharski, L. R., Henderson, W. G., Rickles, F. R., Forman, W. B., Cornell, C. J., Forcier, R. J., Edwards, R., Headley, E., Kim, S-H., O'Donnell, J. R., O'Dell, R., Tornyos, K., and Kwaan, H. C.,** Effect of warfarin on survival in small cell carcinoma of the lung. Veterans Administration Study No. 75, *JAMA,* 245, 831, 1981.

46. **Zacharski, L. R., Henderson, W. G., Rickles, F. R., Forman, W. B., Cornell, C. J., Forcier, R. J., Edwards, R. L., Headley, E., Kim, S-H., O'Donnell, J. F., O'Dell, R., Tornyos, K., and Kwaan, H. C.,** Effect of warfarin anticoagulation on survival in carcinoma of the lung, colon, head and neck, and prostate. Final report of VA Cooperative Study #75, *Cancer,* 53, 2046, 1984.

47. **Rickles, F. R., Hancock, W. W., Edwards, R. L., and Zacharski, L. R.,** Antimetastatic agents. I. Role of cellular procoagulants in the pathogenesis of fibrin deposition in cancer and the use of anticoagulants and/or antiplatelet drugs in cancer treatment, *Semin. Thromb. Hemost.,* 14, 88, 1988.

48. **Thornes, R. D.,** Prevention of the spread and recurrence of cancer by coumarins and fibrinolytic agents, in *Hemostasis and Cancer,* Muszbek, L., Ed., CRC Press, Boca Raton, FL, 1987, 47.

49. **Chahinian, A. P., Propert, K. J., Ware, J. H., Zimmer, B., Perry, M. C., Hirsh, V., Skarin, A., Kopel, S., Holland, J. F., Cornis, R. L., and Green, M. R.,** A randomized trial of anticoagulation with warfarin and alternating chemotherapy in extensive small-cell lung cancer by the Cancer and Leukemia Group B, *J. Clin. Oncol.,* 7, 993, 1989.

50. **Poggi, A., Mussoni, L., Kornblihtt, L., Ballabio, E., de Gaetano, G., and Donati, M. B.,** Warfarin enantiomers, anticoagulation, and experimental tumor metastasis, *Lancet,* i, 163, 1978.

51. **Wilson, A. C. and Fasco, M. J.,** Vitamin K-dependent proteins in microsomes of primary Lewis Lung tumors, *Int. J. Cancer,* 38, 877, 1986.

52. **Nemerson, Y.,** Tissue factor and hemostasis, *Blood,* 71, 1, 1988.

53. **Maynard, J. R., Heckman, C. A., Pitlik, F. A., and Nemerson, Y.,** Association of tissue factor activity with the surface of cultured cells, *J. Clin. Invest.,* 55, 814, 1975.

54. **Zeldis, S. M., Nemerson, Y., Pitlick, F. A., and Lentz, T. L.,** Tissue factor (thromboplastin): localization to plasma membranes by peroxidase-conjugated antibodies, *Science,* 175, 766, 1972.

55. **Wilcox, J. N., Smith, K. M., Schwartz, S. M., and Gordon, D.,** Localization of tissue factor in the normal vessel wall and in the atherosclerotic plaque, *Proc. Natl. Acad. Sci. U.S.A.,* 86, 2839, 1989.

56. **Zacharski, L. R. and Rosenstein, R.,** Reduction of salivary tissue factor (TF) by warfarin therapy, *Blood,* 53, 366, 1979.

57. **Zacharski, L. R., Rosenstein, R., and Phillips, P. G.,** Tissue factor: a vitamin K-dependent clotting factor, *Ann. N.Y. Acad. Sci.,* 370, 311, 1981.

58. **Nawroth, P. P. and Stern, D. M.,** Modulation of endothelial cell hemostatic properties by tumor necrosis factor, *J. Exp. Med.,* 163, 740, 1986.

59. **Conway, E. M. and Rosenberg, R. D.,** Tumor necrosis factor suppresses transcription of the thrombomodulin gene in endothelial cells, *Mol. Cell. Biol.,* 8, 5588, 1988.

60. **Drake, T. A., Morrissey, J. H., and Edgington, T. S.,** Selective cellular expression of tissue factor in human tissues, *Am. J. Pathol.,* 134, 1087, 1989.

61. **Edwards, R. L. and Rickles, F. R.,** Macrophage procoagulants, in *Progress in Thrombosis and Hemostasis,* Spaet, T. H., Ed., Grune and Stratton, Orlando, FL, 1981, 183.

62. **Østerud, B., Lindahl, U., and Seljelid, R.,** Macrophages produce blood coagulation factors, *FEBS Lett.,* 120, 41, 1980.

63. **Muller, A. D., van Dam-Mieras, M. C. E., and Hemker, H. C.,** Measurement of macrophage cellular procoagulant activity, *Haemostasis,* 15, 108, 1985.

64. **Sakuragawa, N., Takahashi, K., Hoshiyama, M., Jimbo, C., Ashizawa, K., Matsuoka, M., and Ohnishi, Y.,** The extract from the tissue of gastric cancer as procoagulant in disseminated intravascular coagulation syndrome, *Thromb. Res.,* 10, 457, 1977.

65. **Szczepanski, M., Bardadin, K., Zawadzki, J., and Pypno, W.,** Procoagulant activity of gastric, colorectal and renal cancer is factor VII-dependent, *J. Cancer Res. Clin. Oncol.,* 114, 519, 1988.

66. **Cajot, J-F., Kruithof, E. K. O., Scleuning, W-D., Sordat, B., and Bachmann, F.,** Plasminogen activators, plasminogen activator inhibitors and procoagulant analyzed in twenty human tumor cell lines, *Int. J. Cancer,* 38, 719, 1986.

67. **Mussoni, L., Conforti, G., Gambacorti-Passerini, C., Alessio, G., Pepe, S., Vaghi, M., Erba, E., Amato, G., Landoni, F., Mangioni, C., Morasca, L., Semeraro, N., and Donati, M. B.,** Procoagulant and fibrinolytic activity of human ovarian carcinoma cells in culture, *Eur. J. Cancer Clin. Oncol.,* 22, 373, 1986.

68. **Dvorak, H. F., van der Water, L., Bitzer, A. M., Dvorak, A. M., Anderson, D., Harvey, V. S., Bach, R., Davis, G. L., DeWolf, W., and Carvalho, A. C. A.,** Procoagulant activity associated with plasma membrane vesicles shed by cultured tumor cells, *Cancer Res.,* 43, 4334, 1983.

69. **Zacharski, L. R., Memoli, V. A., and Rousseau, S. M.,** Coagulation-cancer interaction in situ in renal cell carcinoma, *Blood,* 68, 394, 1986.

70. **Zacharski, L. R., Schned, A. R., and Sorenson, G. D.**, Occurrence of fibrin and tissue factor antigen in human small cell carcinoma of the lung, *Cancer Res.*, 43, 3963, 1983.
71. **Zacharski, L. R., Memoli, V. A., Rousseau, S. M., and Kisiel, W.**, Occurrence of blood coagulation factors in situ in small cell carcinoma of the lung, *Cancer*, 60, 2675, 1987.
72. **Zacharski, L. R., Memoli, V. A., and Rousseau, S. M.**, Thrombin-specific sites of fibrinogen in small cell carcinoma of the lung, *Cancer*, 62, 299, 1988.
73. **Adany, R., Kappelmayer, E., Szegedi, A., Fabian, E., and Muszbek, L.**, Factors of the extrinsic pathway of blood coagulation in tumor associated macrophages, *Thrombos. Haemostas.*, 62, 850, 1989.
74. **Chapman, H. A., Allen, L. C., Stone, O. L., and Fair, D. S.**, Human alveolar macrophages synthesize factor VII in vitro. Possible role in interstitial lung disease, *J. Clin. Invest.*, 75, 2030, 1985.
75. **Gordon, S. G., Franks, J. J., and Lewis, B.**, Cancer procoagulant A: a factor X-activating procoagulant from malignant tissue, *Thromb. Res.*, 6, 127, 1975.
76. **Gordon, S. G., Franks, J. J., and Lewis, B. J.**, Comparison of procoagulant activities in extracts of normal and malignant human tissue, *J. Natl. Cancer Inst.*, 62, 773, 1979.
77. **Gordon, S. G.**, Cancer procoagulant, in *Hemostasis and Cancer*, Muszbek, L., Ed., CRC Press, Boca Raton, FL, 1987, 19.
78. **Donati, M. B., Gambacorti-Passerini, C., Casali, B., Falanga, A., Vannotti, P., Fossati, G., Semeraro, N., and Gordon, S. G.**, Cancer procoagulant in human tumor cells: evidence from melanoma patients, *Cancer Res.*, 46, 6471, 1986.
79. **Falanga, A., Alessio, M. G., Donati, M. B., and Barbui, T.**, A new procoagulant in acute leukemia, *Blood*, 71, 870, 1988.
80. **Gordon, S. G. and Lewis, B. J.**, Comparison of procoagulant activity in tissue culture medium from normal and transformed fibroblasts, *Cancer Res.*, 38, 2467, 1978.
81. **Gordon, S. G., Gilbert, L. C., and Lewis, B. J.**, Analysis of procoagulant activity of intact cells from tissue culture, *Thromb. Res.*, 26, 379, 1982.
82. **Curatolo, L., Colucci, M., Cambini, A. L., Poggi, A., Morasca, L., Donati, M. B., and Semeraro, N.**, Evidence that cells from experimental tumors can activate coagulation factor X, *Br. J. Cancer*, 40, 228, 1979.
83. **Hilgard, P. and Whur, P.**, Factor X-activating activity from Lewis Lung Carcinoma, *Br. J. Cancer*, 41, 642, 1980.
84. **Colucci, M., Curatolo, L., Donati, M. B., and Semeraro, N.**, Cancer cell procoagulant: evaluation by an amidolytic assay, *Thromb. Res.*, 18, 589, 1980.
85. **Gilbert, L. C. and Gordon, S. G.**, Relationship between cellular procoagulant activity and metastatic capacity of B16 mouse melanoma cells, *Cancer Res.*, 43, 536, 1983.
86. **Falanga, A., Dalessandro, A. P. B., Casali, B., Roncaglioni, M. C., and Donati, M. B.**, Several murine metastasizing tumors possess a cysteine proteinase with cancer procoagulant characteristics, *Int. J. Cancer*, 39, 774, 1987.
87. **Gordon, S. G. and Cross, B. A.**, A factor X-activating cysteine protease from malignant tissue, *J. Clin. Invest.*, 67, 1665, 1981.
88. **Gordon, S. G.**, Personal communication, 1990.
89. **Falanga, A. and Gordon, S. G.**, Isolation and characterisation of cancer procoagulant: a cysteine protease from malignant tissue, *Biochemistry*, 24, 5558, 1985.
90. **Dover, R., Goeting, N. L. M., Taylor, I., Roath, O. S., and Francis, J. L.**, Factor X-activating activity in patients with colorectal carcinoma, *Br. J. Surg.*, 74, 1122, 1987.
91. **Francis, J. L., El-Baruni, K., Roath, O. S., and Taylor, I.**, Factor X-activating procoagulant activity in breast tumors (abstr.), *Br. J. Haematol.*, 69, 124, 1988.
92. **Francis, J. L., El-Baruni, K., Roath, O. S., and Taylor, I.**, Factor X-activating activity in normal and malignant colorectal tissue, *Thromb. Res.*, 52, 207, 1988.
93. **El-Baruni, K., Taylor, I., Roath, O. S., and Francis, J. L.**, Factor X-activating procoagulant in normal and malignant breast tissue, *Haematol. Oncol.*, 8, 323–332, 1990.

94. **Francis, J. L.,** Unpublished data, 1989.

95. **Fasco, M. J., Wilson, A. C., Lincoln, D., and Gierthy, J.,** Evidence for a warfarin-sensitive serum factor that participates in factor X activation by Lewis Lung tumor cells, *Int. J. Cancer,* 39, 631, 1987.

96. **Shands, J. W.,** Macrophage factor X activator formation: metabolic requirements for synthesis of components, *Blood,* 65, 169, 1985.

97. **Pusey, M. L. and Mende, T. J.,** Studies on the procoagulant activity of human amniotic fluid II. The role of factor VII, *Thromb. Res.,* 39, 571, 1985.

98. **Gordon, S. G., Hasiba, U., Cross, B. A., Poole, M. A., and Falanga, A.,** Cysteine proteinase procoagulant from amnion-chorion, *Blood,* 66, 1261, 1985.

99. **Idell, S., Gonzalez, K., Bradford, H., MacArthur, C. K., Fein, A. M., Maunder, R. J., Garcia, J. G. N., Griffith, D. E., Weiland, J., Martin, T. R., McLarty, J., Fair, D. S., Walsh, P. N., and Colman, R. W.,** Procoagulant activity in bronchoalveolar lavage in the adult respiratory distress syndrome. Contribution of tissue factor associated with factor VII, *Am. Rev. Respir. Dis.,* 136, 1466, 1987.

100. **Hasday, J. D., Bachwich, P. R., Lynch, J. P., and Sitrin, R. G.,** Procoagulant and plasminogen activator activities of bronchoalveolar fluid in patients with pulmonary sarcoidosis, *Exp. Lung Res.,* 14, 261, 1988.

101. **Wojtukiewicz, M. Z., Zacharski, L. R., Memoli, V. A., Kisiel, W., Kudryk, B. J., Rousseau, S. M., and Stump, D. C.,** Abnormal regulation of coagulation/fibrinolysis in small cell carcinoma of the lung, *Cancer,* 65, 481, 1990.

102. **Al-Mondhiry, H. and Wallin, R.,** Synthesis of vitamin K-dependent proteins by cultured human tumor cells, *Thromb. Haemostas.,* 62, 661, 1989.

103. **Delaini, F., Colucci, M., De Bellis Vitti, G., Locati, D., Poggi, A., Semeraro, N., and Donati, M. B.,** Cancer cell procoagulant: a novel vitamin K-dependent activity, *Thromb. Res.,* 24, 263, 1981.

104. **Fasco, M. J., Eagan, G. E., Wilson, A. C., Gierthy, J. F., and Lincoln, D. L.,** Loss of metastatic and primary tumor factor X-activator capabilities by Lewis Lung carcinoma cells cultured in vitamin K-dependent protein deficient serum, *Cancer Res.,* 48, 6504, 1988.

105. **Poggi, A., Colucci, M., Delaini, F., Semeraro, N., and Donati, M. B.,** Reduced procoagulant activity of Lewis Lung Carcinoma cells from mice treated with warfarin, *Eur. J. Cancer,* 16, 1641, 1980.

106. **Donati, M. B., Semeraro, N., and Gordon, S. G.,** Relationship between procoagulant activity and metastatic capacity of tumor cells, in *Hemostatic Mechanisms and Metastasis,* Honn, K. V. and Sloane, B. F., Eds., Martinus Nijhoff, Boston, 1984, 84.

107. **Roncaglioni, M. C., Dalessandro, A. P. B., Casali, B., Vermeer, C., and Donati, M. B.,** γ-glutamyl carboxylase activity in experimental tumor tissues: a biochemical basis for vitamin K-dependence of cancer procoagulant, *Haemostasis,* 16, 295, 1986.

108. **Hauschka, P. V., Haroon, Y., Buchthal, S. D., and Bell, R. G.,** Vitamin K-dependent processes in tumor cells, *Haemostasis,* 16, 273, 1986.

109. **Zacharski, L. R. and Beck, J. R.,** Monocyte tissue factor activity in anticoagulated patients, *Thromb. Res.,* 29, 207, 1983.

110. **Viadana, E., Bross, I. D. J., and Pilkren, J. W.,** Cascade spread of blood-bourne Metastases in solid and non-solid cancers of humans, in *Pulmonary Metastasis,* Weiss, L. and Gilbert, H. A., Eds., G. K. Hall, Boston, 1979, 142.

111. **Paget, S.,** The distribution of secondary tumor growth in cancers of the breast. *Lancet,* 1, 571, 1889.

112. **Hart, I. R., Talmadge, J. E., and Fidler, I. J.,** Metastatic behavior of a murine reticulum cell sarcoma exhibiting organ-specific growth, *Cancer Res.,* 41, 1281, 1981.

113. **Nicolson, G. L.,** Organ preference of metastasis, in *Cancer Metastasis: Experimental and Clinical Strategies,* Alan R. Liss, 1986, 25.

114. **Murphy, P., Alexander, P., Senior, P. V., Flemming, J., Kirkham, N., and Taylor, I.,** Mechanisms of organ selective tumor growth by bloodbourne cancer cells, *Br. J. Cancer,* 57, 19, 1988.

115. **Alexander, J. W. and Altemeier, W. A.**, Susceptibility of injured tissue to haematogenous metastases: an experimental study, *Ann. Surg.*, 159, 933, 1964.
116. **Skipper, D., Jeffrey, M. J., Cooper, A. J., Taylor, I., and Alexander, P.**, Preferential growth of bloodbourne cancer cells in colonic anastomoses, *Br. J. Cancer*, 57, 564, 1988.
117. **Carty, N., Taylor, I., Roath, O. S., El-Baruri, K., and Francis, J. L.**, Tissue procoagulant activity may be important in sustaining metastatic tumor growth, *Clin. Exp. Metast.*, 10, 175–181, 1992.
118. **Proctor, J. W.**, Rat sarcoma model supports both "soil seed" and "mechanical" theories of metastatic spread, *Br. J. Cancer*, 34, 651, 1976.
119. **Hart, I. R.**, "Seed and Soil" revisited: mechanisms of site-specific metastasis, *Cancer Metast. Rev.*, 1, 1, 1982.
120. **Mooney, B., Serlin, M., and Taylor, I.**, The effect of warfarin on spontaneously metastasizing colorectal cancer in the rat, *Clin. Oncol.*, 8, 55, 1982.
121. **Smith, G. F., Neubauer, B. L., Sundboom, J. L., Best, K. L., Goode, R. L., Tanzer, L. R., Merriman, R. L., Frank, J. D. and Herrmann, R. G.**, Correlation of the *in vivo* anticoagulant, antithrombin and antimetastatic efficacy of warfarin in the rat, *Thromb. Res.*, 50, 163, 1988.
122. **McCulloch, P. and George, W. D.**, Warfarin inhibition of metastasis: the role of anticoagulation, *Br. J. Surg.*, 74, 879, 1987.
123. **Brown, J. M.**, A study of the mechanism by which anticoagulation with warfarin inhibits blood-borne metastases, *Cancer Res.*, 33, 1217, 1973.
124. **McCulloch, P. and George, W. D.**, Promotion of metastasis by a specific complex of coagulation factors may be independent of fibrin formation, *Br. J. Cancer*, 58, 158, 1988.
125. **Carty, N. and Francis, J. L.**, unpublished data, 1990.
126. **Chang, J. D. and Hall, T. C.**, *In vitro* effect of sodium warfarin on DNA and RNA synthesis in mouse L1210 leukemia cells and Walker tumor cells, *Oncology*, 28, 232, 1973.
127. **Kirsch, W. M., Schulz, D., van Buskirk, J. J., and Young, H. E.**, Effects of sodium warfarin and other carcinostatic agents on malignant cells: a study of drug synergy. *J. Med.*, 5, 69, 1974.
128. **Maat, B.**, Selective macrophage inhibition abolishes warfarin-induced reduction of metastasis, *Br. J. Cancer*, 41, 313, 1980.
129. **Thornes, R. D., Smyth, H., Brown, O., O'Gormal, M., Reen, D. J., Farrell, D., and Holland, P. D. J.**, Effects of proteolysis on the human immune mechanism in cancer, *J. Med.*, 5, 92, 1974.
130. **Thornes, R. D., Edlow, D. W., and Wood, S.**, Inhibition of locomotion of cancer cells *in vivo* by anticoagulant therapy, *John Hopkins Med. J.*, 123, 305, 1968.
131. **Gorelick, E., Bere, E., and Herberman, R. B.**, Mechanisms of the antimetastatic effects of anticoagulant drugs: dependence on natural killer (NK) cell activity, in *Hemostasis and Cancer*, Muszbek, L., Ed., CRC Press, Boca Raton, FL, 1987, 37.
132. **Zacharski, L. R.**, Mechanisms of inhibition of cancer dissemination by warfarin, in *Mechanisms of Cancer Metastasis. Potential Clinical Implications*, Honn, K. V., Powers, W. E. and Sloane, B. F., Eds., Martinus Nijhoff, Boston, 1986, 145.
133. **Kramer, B.**, Historical overview of clinical experience with anticoagulant therapy, in *Hemostatic Mechanisms and Metastasis*, Honn, K. V. and Sloane, B. F. Eds., Martinus Nijhoff, Boston, 1987, 355.

Chapter 11

VITAMIN K DEFICIENCY IN THE NEWBORN: HISTORICAL PERSPECTIVES, DIAGNOSIS, AND PREVENTION

William E. Hathaway

TABLE OF CONTENTS

0-8493-6423-X/93/$0.00 + $.50
© 1993 by CRC Press, Inc.

229

I. HISTORICAL PERSPECTIVES

The history of the association of a bleeding tendency in the newly born infant with a deficiency of vitamin K is fascinating and, as will be discussed later, a splendid example of the cyclical nature of discovery-rediscovery in Medical Science (see Table 1). For several centuries a neonatal bleeding disorder which could not be easily attributed to intercurrent disease had been recognized.[1,2] In 1894, Charles Townsend[3] described 50 cases of a generalized bleeding tendency in otherwise healthy infants which was limited to the first week of life. Townsend differentiated the majority of the cases from hemophilia or severe infection and indicated that the mortality rate was 62 to 79% (his report plus the literature). He named the syndrome "hemorrhagic disease of the newborn".[3] In 1910, Schwarz and Ottenberg[4] suggested that hemorrhagic disease of the newborn (HDN) was due to a failure of the recently described blood-clotting system and that transfusion therapy may be helpful. However, it was not until 1937 that Brinkhous et al.[5] described hypoprothrombinemia (blood level of prothrombin of less than 5% of the normal adult range) in an infant with HDN; an observation also made by Quick and others using the new prothrombin time (PT).[6]

In 1939, soon after the discovery of vitamin K by Henrik Dam, concentrates of vitamin K_1 became available for clinical use. In the same year, four groups reported on their experiences in giving such concentrates to normal newborn infants and infants with HDN.[7-10] Nygaard's studies[7] were the most extensive (54 infants) and showed that (1) the PT in the normal newborn becomes prolonged over the first 5 d and then returns to near normal; (2) this physiologic prolongation of the PT is not seen in infants given intramuscular vitamin K at birth; (3) vitamin K exhibited a therapeutic effect in 3 cases of HDN. In another study, Waddell and associates[8] reported "strikingly reduced" PT after oral administration of vitamin K concentrates to two infants with HDN. In a third study Dam and associates[9] showed that the administration of vitamin K concentrates to several infants with conditions associated with mild or severe jaundice brought about a pronounced reduction in the PT. Finally, Hellman and Shettles[10] showed improvements in the neonatal PT after oral vitamin K had been given to the mother before delivery (2 cases) and to preterm infants after delivery (2 cases). Investigations by Salomonsen[11] (published a year later) indicated that breast milk feeding was associated with hypoprothrombinemia in the newborn and that the previous incidence of HDN of 0.84% was reduced to zero by feeding all newborns cow's milk during the first 2 d of life. Thus, most of our currently accepted concepts regarding the perinatal use of vitamin K to prevent HDN were documented in these initial studies 50 years ago.

Studies published in the next few years highlighted a controversy regarding vitamin K prophylaxis which has waxed and waned to the present time. These studies were facilitated by the availability of *synthetic* vitamin K in the form of water-soluble salts of 2-methyl 1,4-naphthoquinone (vitamin

TABLE 1
Events and Opinions Regarding Neonatal Vitamin K Prophylaxis — The First 50 Years

Year	Increased Prophylaxis		Decreased Prophylaxis
1939	Vitamin K first used to prevent HDN		
1940s	Bohlender et al.[12] Poncher[1] Lehmann[17]	**Controversy** **Prevent HDN by maternal or infant vitamin K administration**	Parks et al.[15] Sanford et al.[16] Potter[18]
1950s	Dam et al.[20] study of 33,000 infants AAP recommends 5 mg K$_3$ analogs (I.M.) for all newborn[21]		Kernicterus in preterm infants after vitamin K$_3$ analogs
1960s	AAP[26] - recommends vitamin K$_1$ (1 mg I.M. or 2 mg oral) for all newborn Vest;[22] Aballi[24,25] Definition of role of vitamin K in neonatal bleeding		No vitamin K, lower socioeconomic groups, breast feeding — increased incidence HDN
1970s	Branchet et al.[33] — Recognition and definition of late HDN		
			Failure to find PIVKA in cord blood questions need for vitamin K
1980s	Research (tissue vitamin K and PIVKA-II measurements) suggest low or marginal reserves of vitamin K at birth: reconfirms need for prophylaxis for all newborn		Resurgence of HDN (esp late) associated with no prophylaxis (Japan, Europe, North America, Australia)

K$_3$ or menadione) but not as then of any of the naturally occurring forms vitamin K$_1$ (or phylloquinone) and vitamins K$_2$ (or menaquinones). Some pertinent findings are as follows. Synthetic vitamin K (1 mg) given intravenously to the mother prior to delivery prevented the hypoprothrombinemia which occurred in the normal infant.[12] The vitamin K requirement of the newborn infant was estimated at 1 μg of menadione per day[13] and the efficacy of oral vitamin K given to the mother 2 h prior to delivery or to the infant immediately after delivery in preventing the "physiologic" depression of the PT was confirmed.[14] Although these observations were repeatedly confirmed, the association of the prophylactic administration of vitamin K with prevention of neonatal bleeding was challenged by Parks and Sweet.[15] who showed that a single dose of oral vitamin K (5 mg) to mothers in labor had no evident effect in reducing the incidence of neonatal hemorrhages. Likewise, Sanford et al.[16] in a study of 1693 newborn babies found hemorrhagic manifestations to be approximately 6.6% whether the infants or their mothers were given vitamin K or not. However, in a study of 13,000 infants to whom 0.5 mg of a vitamin K analogue was given intramuscularly, Lehmann[17] found significantly less fetal hemorrhage in the treated group. In 1945, Potter[18] reviewed the controversy extensively and added a large "controlled" study from Chicago in which 3.2 mg of Hykinone® (2-methyl-1,4-naphthoquinone3-sodium sulfonate) was administered parenterally to mothers on admission to the labor rooms. Her study found no difference in control vs. treatment groups using neonatal deaths as the endpoint; in fact, no cases of HDN were documented in the 13,000 cases reported. In 1948, the American Academy of Pediatrics (AAP) Committee on Fetus and Newborn made the recommendation that the routine care of premature infants should include an intramuscular dose of 4.8 mg of menadione on admission of the infant.[19]

The initial reactions in the literature to prophylactic vitamin K for the newborn gradually subsided and was apparently laid to rest by the monumental study of over 33,000 infants by Dam and associates[20] in 1952. These authors concluded:

1. A mild vitamin K refractory physiologic hypoprothrombinemia is seen in all infants at birth but this gradually diminishes over the first year.
2. During the first few days of life a constant and pronounced vitamin K-dependent hypoprothrombinemia occurs in breast fed infants and occasionally in artificially fed infants.
3. Such hypoprothrombinemia can be prevented by administration of vitamin K to the mother (given between 24 and 4 h prior to delivery) or to the infant after delivery and will be associated with a decreased incidence of hypoprothrombinemic hemorrhages.
4. Extremely low prothrombin values may be seen at birth in asphyxiated infants; vitamin K given to the mother may partially prevent the decrease. In 1954, the AAP recommended that 5 mg of synthetic vitamin K should be given intramuscularly to all newborn infants.[21]

However, as reviewed by Vest in 1966,[22] the universal use of vitamin K for neonatal prophylaxis was being questioned because of possible toxic manifestations of synthetic vitamin K analogues based on menadione when these were given in large doses to immature infants. As early as 1955, Allison[23] reported on the occurrence of kernicterus and hemolytic anemia in premature infants given relatively high doses of a water soluble analogue Synkavit® (menadiol sodium diphosphate). Clinical reports and animal investigations confirmed that high (up to 30 mg) of menadione and its water soluble derivatives provoke Heinz body formation, hemolysis, anemia, and hyperbilirubinemia in preterm infants. These changes were not seen with large doses (10 mg) of vitamin K_1 (Konakion).

Both Vest[22] and Aballi et al.[24,25] emphasized the beneficial effects of even small (25 μg) doses of vitamin K in preventing HDN. Although the infant could be given prophylaxis by administration of vitamin K to the mother prenatally, the difficulty in the timing and delivery of an optimal dose via this indirect route plus the danger of giving too much synthetic vitamin K were real drawbacks which suggested that direct administration to the neonate would be preferable. These investigators also drew attention to the fact that other groups of newborns with bleeding diatheses did not respond to vitamin K. Many of these infants were frequently ill with infections and respiratory distress syndromes. The term "secondary hemorrhagic disease" was used to distinguish these infants from those with classical HDN. Most of the above information regarding HDN was reviewed by the Committee on Nutrition of the AAP in 1961 who concluded:[26] "vitamin K_1 is therefore the drug of choice. A single parenteral dose of 0.5–1.0 mg or oral dose of 1.0–2.0 mg is probably adequate for prophylaxis." This recommendation is still in effect today.

In the 1960's, reports of an increased incidence of HDN in lower socioeconomic populations where breast feeding was widely prevalent led the Cincinnati group[27,28] to reemphasize the role of breast feeding in the pathogenesis of the disorder. They demonstrated that a parenteral dose of 100 μg of menadione at birth was effective in prevention of classical HDN in breast fed infants. During the same period, several reports[29-32] noted that apparently healthy infants could present with a hemorrhagic diathesis due to vitamin K deficiency in the first few months of life; most of these infants were either breast fed or had evidence of a malabsorption syndrome. By the mid 1970s, a bleeding syndrome in 1 to 3-month-old exclusively breast-fed infants which was due to vitamin K deficiency without evidence of malabsorption had been described by Isarangkura (maiden name, Bhanchet) and coworkers.[33] The syndrome was called acquired prothrombin complex deficiency (APCD) and occurred in infants who had not received prophylactic vitamin K at birth. Other reports of APCD or "late" HDN soon appeared.[34-36]

Meanwhile, in Europe, several papers were published questioning the need for routine vitamin K prophylaxis for all newborn infants.[37-40] The reopening of this controversy was based mainly on the failure to find undercarboxylated species of prothrombin (des-γcarboxyprothrombin) in neonatal cord blood specimens (see Diagnosis below). Three of these papers or letters were published in the *Lancet* and their conclusions were challenged by Aballi[41] and Edson[42] while an editorial in the *Lancet* also addressed the issue.[43] The editorial concluded that the best solution would be to have a program of selective vitamin K prophylaxis (preterm and low birth weight infants), a solution that also would be more cost effective and might solve the dilemma facing clinicians. Others,[44] using indirect measurements of noncarboxylated prothrombin, suggested that infants with complications of labor and delivery were more susceptible to vitamin K deficiency.

For various reasons including the fear of neuromuscular complications from intramuscular injections, economic considerations, the growing influence of holistic medicine, and the failure to obtain unequivocal laboratory evidence of vitamin K deficiency in normal term infants at birth, the late 1970s and early 1980s saw a widespread abandonment of routine neonatal vitamin K prophylaxis. A flurry of reports of "resurgence" or "return" of

HDN soon followed.[45-51] Most of these hemorrhagic events occurred in term infants who had not received vitamin K prophylaxis and who had been breast fed. While a few cases could be ascribed to classical HDN and presented in the first few days of life, over 90% were infants with late HDN with a disturbingly high incidence of intracranial bleeding. With the great concern engendered by this trend, the pendulum has again swung to widespread acceptance of neonatal vitamin K prophylaxis.[52-54] Many questions, however, still remain. Some of these, such as the physiological significance of elevated levels of des-γ-carboxyprothrombin in infants, their relationship to vitamin K status as assessed from plasma and tissue concentrations of the vitamin and the most effective way to give prophylaxis for classical and late HDN are still controversial and will be discussed below.

II. DIAGNOSIS

The diagnosis of vitamin K deficiency in the newborn infant will be discussed from both the clinical and laboratory viewpoints. These issues have been reviewed in detail elsewhere.[52,55,56] The *clinical* bleeding syndromes due to vitamin K deficiency are described in Table 2 and are commented on briefly. Although idiophatic early (at birth) HDN is rarely seen;[55] several reports[5759] have suggested that infants born of mothers with convulsive disorders who received barbiturates or phenytoin are prone to develop early HDN. Occasionally other maternal medications (rifampicin and isoniazid) have been implicated. A recent prospective study noted that 25% of infants born to mothers taking anticonvulsants had increased plasma levels of des-γ-carboxyprothrombin.[60] The clinical manifestations of classical HDN (first week of life) are well known and may be differentiated from other bleeding syndromes as necessary.[55]

As noted above, late HDN or APCD is a syndrome of severe bleeding in 1 to 2 month old infants almost always involving the central nervous system and is often fatal. The syndrome occurs in breast fed infants who have usually not received prophylactic vitamin K. The apparent prevalence of late HDN ranges from 1:200 in England[61] to 1:1700 live births in Japan.[62] In the U.S., where practically all infants receive vitamin K parenterally at birth, late HDN is almost never observed.

The *laboratory* detection of mild or subclinical states of vitamin K deficiency in the neonatal period (as opposed to the detection of overt vitamin K deficiency which is characterized by bleeding due to severe depression of the vitamin K-dependent clotting factors) has been difficult and has resulted in the perpetuation of many of the controversies noted above. When tissues stores of vitamin K become depleted the glutamic acid residues on the vitamin K-dependent coagulation proteins (prothrombin and factors VII, IX, and X) become incompletely carboxylated and lose their ability to function as normal procoagulants. These abnormal proteins circulate as non- or partially carboxylated (des-γ-carboxy) precursors also known as *proteins induced in vitamin*

TABLE 2
Vitamin K Deficiency Hemorrhagic Syndromes in Infancy

	Age	Common bleeding sites	Cause	Prevention by vitamin K administration at birth	Comments
Early HDN	0–24 h	Cephalohematoma; scalp monitor; intracranial; intrathoracic; intra-abdominal	Maternal drugs: Warfarin Anticonvulsants Antituberculous chemotherapy Idiopathic	Not in all instances	Frequently life-threatening; guidelines for safe management of high-risk pregnancies needed
Classical HDN	1–7 d	Gastrointestinal; skin; nasal; circumcision	Idiopathic Maternal drugs	Yes	Incidence increased in breast-fed neonates and reduced by early formula feedings
Late hemorrhagic disease	1–3 months	Intracranial; skin; gastrointestinal	Idiopathic Secondary: Diarrhea Malabsorption (cystic fibrosis, α-1-antitrypsin deficiency, biliary atresia) Prolonged warfarin exposure	Probably yes No	Common cause of intracranial hemorrhage in breast-fed infants 1–3 months of age; may be aggravated by antibiotic administration

Note: HDN = hemorrhagic disease of the newborn.

From Hathaway, W. E., *Hematol. Oncol. Clin. N. Am.*, 1, 371, 1987. With permission.

K absence (PIVKA). Their presence is associated with an eventual reduction of clotting activity in specific factor assays or screening tests (prothrombin time or thrombotest).[63] The forgoing suggests that the vitamin K deficient state can be assessed either by: (1) direct measurement of circulating or tissue vitamin K levels and comparison to controls in the replete state; (2) detection of the undercarboxylated proteins in the plasma; or (3) determination of the clotting factor activity by direct assays of factors II, VII, IX, X, or global screening tests. Conventional clotting tests are easiest to perform but are the least specific because vitamin K-dependent clotting factor levels in the fetus and newborn show a characteristic physiologic depression and dependence on gestational age: clotting tests are also the least sensitive because of the overlap of normal and abnormal values. Assays for des-γ-carboxyprothrombin or PIVKA-II are more sensitive but may be less specific in the newborn because of the possible persistence of developmental alterations in the fetal proteins. Tissue assays for vitamin K (mainly phylloquinone) are probably the most specific and sensitive but are difficult to perform especially with the small amounts of samples usually available (see Chapter 3). Even the most insensitive and nonspecific test (i.e., the PT) is useful for confirming the diagnosis of HDN when used in conjunction with the clinical response to vitamin K therapy including the return of the PT to the normal range. PIVKA-II determinations can help to confirm the diagnosis retrospectively in confusing cases because this abnormal protein circulates with a halflife of 60 to 70 h even after therapy with vitamin K.[70] However, it has been determined that the subclinical state of vitamin K deficiency or estimation of vitamin K repletion produces conflicting results and makes it difficult to precisely assess effectiveness of neonatal prophylaxis. Recent studies which bear on this problem are summarized in Table 3.

The information summarized in Table 3 provides support for several impressions regarding vitamin K deficiency in the neonatal period.

1. The newborn infant is born with circulating levels of vitamin K which are less than half those found in normal adults and pregnant mothers. The equivocal results (Table 3) are probably due to methodological problems;[87] indeed the trend of recent results supports the concept of very low levels (<50 pg/ml) in cord plasma. This and the difficulty in raising cord levels substantially by maternal administration shortly before delivery[75,83] suggest that there is a significant placental barrier to the passage of the extremely lipophilic natural K vitamins.

2. A few infants are born with evidence of vitamin K deficiency as indicated by increased amounts of des-γ-carboxyprothrombin in their plasma; the deficiency in these babies, as noted by Shapiro et al.,[70] is not related to any particular risk group (preterm or maternal complications) and, therefore, cannot be predicted prenatally.

3. Most newborn infants display no clinical evidence of a vitamin K deficient state at birth.

TABLE 3
Studies of Nonbleeding Newborn Infants of Various Gestational Age

A. Studies for acarboxy prothrombin (PIVKA-II)

Year	Ref.	Method-subjects	No. positive/ no. studied	% positive
1977	Van Doorm et al.[37]	CIE-term, cord	0/43	0
1979	Muntean et al.[64]	CIE-term, cord	15/30	50
1980	Malia et al.[40]	CIEterm, cord	0/24	0
1982	Megura and Yamada[65]	Antibody coated beads-term, cord	2/12	16.6
1982	Atkinson et al.[66]	Chromogenic venom, S2238-term, cord	48/128	38.2
1984	Ekelund and Hedner[67]	CIE-term, cord	2/105	1.9
1985	Motohara et al.[68]	ELISA (monoclonal antibody)	21/99	21.2
		Term, cord, 5 d old	27/51	52.9
1985	von Kries et al.[69]	CIE-term, cord	0/40	0
1986	Shapiro et al.[70]	IE after BaCO$_3$ absorption-term, preterm, cord	27/934	2.9
1986	Motohara et al.[71]	ELISA (monoclonal antibody) 1 month old	21/171	12.2
1987	von Kries et al.[72]	CIE-term, 5 d old	93/183	50.8
1987	Motohara et al.[73]	ELISA (monoclonal antibody) 1 month old	26/50	51
1988	Ogata et al.[74]	ELISA (monoclonal antibody) pre-term, 7 d old	15/23	65.2

B. Vitamin K$_1$ assay studies.

Year	Ref.	Subjects	Levels (ng/ml)
1982	Shearer et al.[75]	30 Adults	0.10–0.66
		15 Infants (cord)	not detectable (<0.10)
1985	Pietersma-de Bruyn and van Haard[76]	22 Mothers	1.9–0.9
1985	Sann et al.[77]	103 Infants (cord)	0.9–0.3
1985	Sann et al.[78]	16 Prematures (age 1–6 h)	3–34; median = 9
		27 Mothers	9.03 ± 4.9
1985	McNinch et al.[61]	27 Cord	10.4 ± 5.3
		42 Infants	73
		4-h Postoral	
		1 mg/kl	
		20 Infants	178
		12-h post IM	
1987	McCarthy et al.[79]	1 mg K$_1$	
		20 Mothers	0.47(0.14–2.42)
		20 Cord	0.016(0.004–0.045)

TABLE 3 (continued)
Studies of Nonbleeding Newborn Infants of Various Gestational Age

B. Vitamin K_1 assay studies.

Year	Ref.	Subjects	Levels (ng/ml)
1987	Shirahata et al.[80]	Adults	3 ± 1.4
		19 Cord	n.d.(0.7,1.0,2.5)
1988	Greer et al.[81]	23 Mothers	1.7(0.4–4.4)
		23 Infants	1.1(0.5–2.9)
1988	Hiraike et al.[82]	13 Mothers	1.52(0.25–3.8)
		12 Cord	0.10(0.03–0.28)
1988	Mandelbrot et al.[83]	33 Mothers	0.38(0.07–1.1)
		13 Cord	0.02(0.005–0.98)
1989	Hathaway et al.[85]	20 Adults	0.5(0.18–1.2)
		15 Cord	0.22(0.05–0.82)
1988	Widdershoven et al.[84]	16 Cord	<0.07
1989	Yang et al.[86]	6 Mothers	0.33 (0.13–1.10)
		6 Cord	<0.02(n.d.–0.03)

Note: All samples were obtained prior to vitamin K except as noted.

4. Newborn infants absorb oral vitamin K_1 readily in almost all instances.
5. If vitamin K prophylaxis is not given at birth, a significant number of term and preterm infants develop vitamin K deficiency as evidenced by positive PIVKA by 5 to 7 d of age especially if they are breast fed or have poor oral intake.[68,72,74]
6. Vitamin K deficiency as judged by a positive PIVKA-II may be seen at 1 month of age in thriving breast fed infants not given neonatal prophylaxis.[71]

III. PREVENTION OF VITAMIN K DEFICIENCY IN INFANCY

As the previous discussion has indicated, the major reason for giving vitamin K to newborn infants is to prevent the bleeding tendency associated with the syndromes described in Table 2 (HDN, early, classical, and late). Administration of vitamin K to all infants in order to prevent HDN should no longer be considered controversial. However, the form of vitamin K (K_1, K_2, or K_3), the dose, the timing of dose(s), and the route of administration are still being actively discussed and investigated in many parts of the world. Current recommendations for preventing HDN should be based on recent studies using methods of detection which are indicative of a vitamin K deficiency state. Pertinent studies or lack thereof are discussed below.

The rare occurrence of early HDN, frequently associated with maternal drug therapy (anticonvulsants, etc.) is a special problem. As noted earlier, these infants may have a bleeding tendency which seems to be at least partly due to vitamin K deficiency. This coagulopathy can probably be prevented by giving relatively large doses of vitamin K to the mother prenatally. The Canadian Paediatric Society[88] recommends giving 20 mg of vitamin K_1 orally to the mother for 2 weeks prior to delivery. Further information regarding the placental transport of vitamin K is needed before it will be possible to give definitive recommendations on the dosage of vitamin K which should be given to pregnant mothers and to guarantee the efficacy and safety of the maternal route of vitamin K prophylaxis.

All newborn infants should receive vitamin K in order to prevent classical HDN. In line with previous recommendations which have been reviewed in this article and elsewhere,[52-54,56,88,89] vitamin K should be given to all newborn infants within a few hours of birth. Oral administration of vitamin K_1 appears to be as effective as parenteral prophylaxis in preventing the classical form of HDN in term infants.[90,91] Most recommendations agree, however, that the parenteral route should be used for preterm infants. Although the administration of vitamin K to the mother at term may provide effective neonatal prophylaxis in most instances, the details of timing and dosage have not been adequately worked out to allow a firm recommendation.

The most extensive experience with late HDN comes from Japan. Hanawa et al.[92] reviewed 543 cases of late HDN (January, 1981 to June, 1985) and determined that 427 cases were idiopathic occurring in mostly breast fed infants. Although most of these infants had received no vitamin K after birth, 11 had received oral prophylaxis with a vitamin K_2 (menaquinone-4) preparation one or two times before the onset of bleeding. Many of the idiopathic cases had associated transient mild abnormalities of liver function. Motohara et al.[73] using an enzyme-linked immunoabsorbent assay (ELISA) performed on dried blood spots, carried out an extensive screening program for PIVKA-II in infants at 1 month of age after one or two doses of oral menaquinone-4. The results suggested that such prophylaxis would not completely prevent vitamin K deficiency at 1 month. A third national survey on vitamin K deficiency in Japan[93] in 1988 revealed 129 cases of the idiopathic type of late HDN (4/100,000 incidence) of which 12 had received one to three doses of menaquinone-4 orally.

In contrast, a review of late HDN cases[94] indicated that, of 65 case reports in the literature, only 4 had been given vitamin K parenterally at birth; the rest had received no vitamin K. Of the four cases, three were reported in a letter by Verity et al.[95] one of infants had biliary atresia and the others were not extensively evaluated for secondary causes. The author is unaware of any documented cases of late HDN occurring in any infant given 1 mg parenteral K_1 at birth in the U.S. except for those with a secondary etiology.[96] A similar experience is reported from West Germany[97] where 2 of 16 cases of late HDN received oral prophylaxis, and from Switzerland,[98] where only one case of idiopathic late HDN after oral prophylaxis was seen (in 2 years).

While experience suggests that oral vitamin K_2 may not provide complete protection against late HDN the experience of pediatricians in U.S. and Europe

TABLE 4
Recommendations for Prevention of Hemorrhagic Disease of Newborn (HDN).

1. Early HDN (mother receiving anticonvulsants, etc.) Administer 10 mg vitamin K_1 orally per day for 2 weeks prior to delivery.
2. Classic HDN. Administer vitamin K_1 within 4 h of birth as follows: Term infant, 1 mg IM or 2 mg orally (Konakion drops, Hoffmann-LaRoche); preterm infant, 0.5–1 mg IM.
3. Late HDN (idiopathic acquired prothrombin complex deficiency). Best protection with parenteral vitamin K_1 at birth (2 above) but oral vitamin K_1, 2–5 mg, *may* also be effective. Breast-fed infants under 3 months of age who develop diarrhea or who are receiving oral antibiotics (for more than 5–7 d) should be given a repeat dose.
4. Infants with malabsorption syndromes. Administer vitamin K_1, 1 mg IM monthly while at risk.

suggests that the parenteral administration of vitamin K_1 to newborns gives excellent protection against both classical and late forms of HDN. Despite this observation, oral prophylaxis usually with vitamin K_1, is gaining in popularity. In Thailand, where oral prophylaxis is the most practical, an oral dose of 2 mg of vitamin K_1 was shown to be as effective as the intramuscular route in preventing the APCD syndrome (late HDN) as detected by the thrombotest[99] and plasma vitamin K levels.[85] Current recommendations in West Germany[97] include either 1 mg of vitamin K_1 given parenterally at birth or repeated oral doses (2 mg) given at each of the three checkup examinations (after delivery, then at 3 to 10 d, and 4 to 6 weeks of age). Based on recent recommendations[89] and the experiences reviewed here, our conclusions regarding prevention are summarized in Table 4.

REFERENCES

1. **Poncher, H. G.,** The role of vitamin K in hemorrhage in the newborn period, *Adv. Pediatr.,* 1, 151, 1942.
2. **Gelston, C. F.,** On the etiology of hemorrhagic disease of new-born, *Am. J. Dis. Child,* 22, 351, 1921.
3. **Townsend, C. W.,** The hemorrhagic disease of the new-born, *Arch. Pediatr.,* 11, 559, 1894.
4. **Schwarz, H. and Ottenberg, R.,** The hemorrhagic disease of the newborn, with special reference to blood coagulation and serum treatment, *Am. J. Med. Sci.,* 40, 17, 1910.
5. **Brinkhous, K. M., Smith, H. P., and Warner, E. D.,** Plasma prothrombin level in normal infancy and in hemorrhagic disease of the newborn, *Am. J. Med. Sci.,* 193, 475, 1937.
6. **Quick, A. J. and Grossman, A. M.,** Prothrombin concentration in the newborn, *Proc. Soc. Exper. Biol. Med.,* 4, 227, 1939.
7. **Nygaard, K. K.,** Prophylactic and curative effect of vitamin K in hemorrhagic disease of the newborn (hypothrombinemia hemorrhagica neonatorum), *Acta Obstet. Gynec. Scand.,* 19, 361, 1939.

8. **Waddell, W. W., Jr., Guerry, D., III, Bray, W. E., and Kelley, O. R.,** Possible effects of vitamin K on prothrombin and clotting time in newly-born infants, *Proc. Soc. Exp. Biol. Med.,* 40, 432, 1939.
9. **Dam, H., Tage-Hansen, E., and Plum, P.,** Vitamin-K lack in normal sick infants, *Lancet,* 2, 1157, 1939.
10. **Hellman, L. M. and Shettles, L. B.,** Factors influencing plasma prothrombin in the newborn infant, *Bull. Johns Hopkins Hosp.,* 65, 138, 1939.
11. **Salomonsen, L.,** On the prevention of hemorrhagic disease of the newborn by the administration of cow's milk during the first two days of life, *Acta Paediatr.,* 28, 1, 1940–41.
12. **Bohlender, G. P. and Rosenbaum, W. M., Sage, E. C.,** Antepartum use of vitamin K, *JAMA,* 116, 1763, 1941.
13. **Sells, R. L., Walker, S. A., and Owen, C. A.,** Vitamin K requirement of the newborn infant, *Proc. Soc. Exp. Biol. Med.,* 47, 441, 1941.
14. **Toohey, M.,** Vitamin K requirements of the newborn, *Arch. Dis. Child,* 17, 187, 1942.
15. **Parks, J. and Sweet, L. K.,** Does the antenatal use of vitamin K prevent hemorrhage in the newborn infant?, *Am. J. Obst. Gynec.,* 44, 432, 1942.
16. **Sanford, H. N., Shmigelsky, I., and Chapin, J. M.,** Is administration of vitamin K to the newborn of clinical value?, *JAMA,* 118, 697, 1942.
17. **Lehmann, J.,** Vitamin K as a prophylactic in 13,000 infants, *Lancet,* 1, 493, 1944.
18. **Potter, E. L.,** The effect on infant mortality of vitamin K administered during labor, *Am. J. Obstet. Gynecol.,* 50, 235, 1945.
19. American Academy Pediatrics Committee on Fetus and Newborn, Standards and recommendations for hospital care of newborn infants, November 18, 1948, 49.
20. **Dam, H., Dyggve, H., Larsen, H., and Plum, P.,** The relation of vitamin K deficiency to hemorrhagic disease of the newborn, *Adv. Pediatr.,* 5, 129, 1952.
21. American Academy Pediatrics, Standards and recommendations for hospital care of newborn infants, 1954, 92.
22. **Vest, M.,** Vitamin K in medical practice: pediatrics, *Vitam. Horm.,* 24, 649, 1966.
23. **Allison, A. C.,** Danger of vitamin K to newborn, *Lancet,* 1, 669, 1955.
24. **Aballi, A. J. and deLamerens, S.,** Coagulation changes in the neonatal period and in early infancy, *Pediatr. Clin. North Am.,* 9, 785, 1962.
25. **Aballi, A. J.,** The action of vitamin K in the neonatal period, *South Med. J.,* 58, 48, 1965.
26. **American Academy Pediatrics,** Committee on Nutrition, Vitamin K compounds and the water soluble analogs: use in therapy and prophylaxis in pediatrics, *Pediatrics,* 28, 501, 1961.
27. **Sutherland, J. M., Glueck, H. L., and Gleser, G.,** Hemorrhagic disease of the newborn, *Am. J. Dis. Child,* 113, 524, 1967.
28. **Kennan, W. J., Jewett, T., and Glueck, H. I.,** Role of feeding and vitamin K in hypoprothrombinemia of the newborn, *Am. J. Dis. Child,* 121, 271, 1971.
29. **Bhanchet, P., Bhamarapravati, N., Bukkavesa, S., and Tuchinda, S.,** A new bleeding syndrome in Thai infants. Acquired prothrombin complex deficiency, XIth *Congr. Int. Soc. Hematology,* 1966, 24 (abstract).
30. **Chan, M. C. K. and Wong, H. B.,** Late haemorrhagic disease of Singapore infants, *J. Singapore Pediatr. Soc.,* 9, 72, 1967.
31. **Lovric, V. A. and Jones, R. F.,** The haemorrhagic syndrome of early infancy, *Aust. Ann. Med.,* 16, 173, 1967.
32. **Goldman, H. I. and Deposito, F.,** Hypoprothrombinemic bleeding in young infants, *Am. J. Dis. Child,* 111, 430, 1966.
33. **Bhanchet, P., Tuchinda, S., and Hathirat, P. et al.,** A bleeding syndrome in infants due to acquired prothrombin complex deficiency, *Clin. Pediatr.,* 16, 992, 1977.

34. **Iizuka, A. and Nagao, T.,** Abnormal prothrombin in idiopathic and secondary vitamin K deficiency in young infants. Comparison with hemorrhagic disease of the newborn, *Blood Vessel,* 10, 649, 1979.

35. **Cooper, N. A. and Lynch, M. A.,** Delayed hemorrhagic disease of the newborn with extradural hematoma, *Br. Med. J.,* 1, 164, 1979.

36. **Minford, A. M. B. and Eden, O. B.,** Hemorrhagic responsive to vitamin K to a 6 weeks old infant, *Arch. Dis. Child,* 54, 310, 1979.

37. **Van Doorm, J. M., Muller, A. D., and Hemker, H. C.,** Heparinlike inhibitor, not vitamin K deficiency, in the newborn, *Lancet,* 1, 852, 1977.

38. **Göbel, U., Sonnenschein-Kosenow, S., Petrich, C., and Voss, H.,** Vitamin-K deficiency in newborn, *Lancet,* 2, 187, 1977.

39. **Mori, P. G., Bisogni, C., Odino, S., Tonini, G. P., Boeri, E., Serra, G., and Romano, C.,** Vitamin K deficiency in newborn, *Lancet,* 2, 188, 1977.

40. **Malia, R. G., Preston, F. E., and Mitchell, V. E.,** Evidence against vitamin K deficiency in normal neonates, *Thromb. Haemost.,* 44, 159, 1980.

41. **Aballi, A. J.,** Vitamin-K deficiency in the newborn, *Lancet,* 2, 559, 1977.

42. **Edson, J. R.,** Vitamin-K deficiency in the newborn, *Lancet,* 2, 187, 1977.

43. Editorial, *Lancet,* 1, 755, 1978.

44. **Corrigan, J. J., Jr. and Kryc, J. J.,** Factor II (prothrombin) levels in cord blood: correlation of coagulant activity with immunoreactive protein, *J. Pediatr.,* 97, 979, 1980.

45. **Lane, P. A., Hathaway, W. E., Githens, J. H., Krugman, R. D., and Rosenberg, D. A.,** Fatal intracranial hemorrhage in a normal infant secondary to vitamin K deficiency, *Pediatrics,* 72, 562, 1983.

46. **McNinch, A. W., Orme, R. L'E., and Tripp, J. H.,** Haemorrhagic disease of the newborn returns, *Lancet,* 1, 1089, 1983.

47. **O'Connor, M. E., Livingstone, D. S., Hannah, J., and Wilkens, D.,** Vitamin K deficiency and breastfeeding, *Am. J. Dis. Child,* 137, 601, 1983.

48. **Nagao, T. and Nakayama, K.,** Vitamin K deficiency in infancy in Japan, *Lett. Pediatr.,* 74, 315, 1984.

49. **Chaou, W. T., Chou, M. L., and Eitzman, D. V.,** Intracranial hemorrhage and vitamin K deficiency in early infancy, *J. Pediatr.,* 105, 880, 1984.

50. **Motohara, K., Matsukura, M., and Matsuda, I.,** Severe vitamin K deficiency in breast-fed infants, *J. Pediatr.,* 105, 943, 1984.

51. **Behrmann, B. A., Chan, W. K., and Finer, N. N.,** Resurgence of hemorrhagic disease of the newborn: a report of three cases, *Can. Med. Assoc. J.,* 133, 884, 1985.

52. **Lane, P. A. and Hathaway, W. E.,** Vitamin K in infancy, *J. Pediatr.,* 106, 351, 1985.

53. **Hathaway, W. E.,** ICTH subcommittee on neonatal hemostasis, *Thromb. Haemostas.,* 55, 145, 1986.

54. **Tripp, J. H., and McNinch, A. W.,** Haemorrhagic disease and vitamin K, *Arch. Dis. Child.,* 62, 436, 1987.

55. Hathaway, W. E. and Bonnar, J., *Hemostatic Disorders of the Pregnant Woman and Newborn Infant,* Elsevier, New York, 1987, 105.

56. **Hathaway, W. E.,** New insights on vitamin K, *Hem. Onc. Clin. N. Am.,* 1, 367, 1987.

57. **Argent, A. C., Rothberg, A. D., and Pienaar, N.,** Precursor prothrombin status in two mother-infant pairs following gestational anticonvulsant therapy, *Pediatr. Pharmacol.,* 4, 183, 1984.

58. **Bleyer, W. A. and Skinner, A. L.,** Fatal neonatal hemorrhage after maternal anticonvulsant therapy, *JAMA,* 235, 626, 1976.

59. **Mountain, K. R., Hirsh, J., and Gallus, A. S.,** Neonatal coagulation defect due to anticonvulsant drug treatment in pregnancy, *Lancet,* 1, 265, 1970.

60. **Hulac, P., Shapiro, A., Manco-Johnson, M., Jacobson, L. J., and Hathaway, W. E.,** Maternal anticonvulsants and neonatal vitamin K deficiency, *Pediatr. Res.,* 20, 390A, 1986.

61. **McNinch, A. W., Upton, C., Samuels, M., Shearer, M. J., McCarthy, P., Tripp, J. H., and Orme, R. L'E.,** Plasma concentrations after oral or intramuscular vitamin K in neonates, *Arch. Dis. Child.,* 60, 81, 1985.
62. **Motohara, K., Matsukura, M., Matsuda, I., Iribe, K., Ideda, T., Kondo, Y., Yonekubo, A., Yamamoto, Y., and Tsuchiya, F.,** Severe vitamin K deficiency in breast-fed infants, *J. Pediatr.,* 105, 943, 1984.
63. **Garrow, D., Chisholm, M., and Radford, M.,** Vitamin K and thrombotest values in full term infants, *Arch. Dis. Child.,* 61, 349, 1986.
64. **Muntean, W., Petek, W., Rosanelli, K., and Mutz, I. D.,** Immunologic studies of prothrombin in newborns. Pediatr. Res., 13, 1262, 1979.
65. **Meguro, M. and Yamada, K.,** A simple and rapid test for PIVKA-II in plasma. Thromb. Res., 25, 109, 1982.
66. **Atkinson, P. M., Bradlow, B. A., Moulineau, J. D., and Walker, N. P.,** Acarboxy prothrombin in cord plasma from normal neonates, *J. Pediatr. Gastroenterol. Nutr.,* 3, 450, 1984.
67. **Ekelund, H. and Hedner, U.,** Prothrombin and vitamin K deficiency in the newborn, *Eur. Paediatr. Haematol. Oncol.,* 1, 59, 1984.
68. **Motohara, K., Endo, F., and Matsuda, I.,** Effect of vitamin K administration on acarboxy prothrombin (PIVKA-II) levels in newborns, *Lancet* 2, 242, 1985.
69. **von Kries, R., Goebel, U., and Maase, B.,** Vitamin K deficiency in the newborn, *Lancet,* 2, 728, 1985.
70. **Shapiro, A. D., Jacobson, L. J., Armon, M. E., MancoJohnson, M. J., Hulac, P., Lane, P. A., and Hathaway, W. E.,** Vitamin K deficiency in the newborn infant: prevalence and perinatal risk factors, *J. Pediatr.,* 109, 675, 1986.
71. **Motohara, K., Endo, F., and Matsuda, I.,** Vitamin K deficiency in breast-fed infants at one month of age, *J. Pediatr. Gastroent. Nutr.,* 5, 931, 1986.
72. **von Kries, R., Becker, A., and Göbel, U.,** Vitamin K in the newborn: influence of nutritional factors on acarboxy-prothrombin detectability and factor II VII clotting activity, *Eur. J. Pediatr.,* 146, 123, 1987.
73. **Motohara, K., Endo, F., and Matsuda, I.,** Screening for late neonatal vitamin K deficiency by acarboxyprothrombin in dried blood spots, *Arch. Dis. Child.,* 62, 370, 1987.
74. **Ogata, T., Motohara, K., Endo, F., Kondo, Y., Ikeda, T., Kudo, Y., Iribe, K., and Matsuda, I.,** Vitamin K effect in low birth weight infants, *Pediatrics,* 81, 423, 1988.
75. **Shearer, M. J., Barkhan, P., Rahim, S., and Stimmler, L.,** Plasma vitamin K_1 in mothers and their newborn babies, *Lancet,* 2, 460, 1982.
76. **Pietersma-de Bruyn, A. L. J. M. and van Haard, P. M. M.** Vitamin K_1 in the newborn, *Clin. Chim. Acta,* 150, 95, 1985.
77. **Sann, L., Leclercq, M., Guillaumont, M., Trouyez, R., Bethenod, M., and Bourgeay-Causse, M.,** Serum vitamin K_1 concentrations after oral administration of vitamin K_1 in low birth weight infants, *J. Pediatr.,* 107, 608, 1985.
78. **Sann, L., Leclercq, M., Troncy, J., Guillaumont, M., Berland, M., and Coeur, P.,** Serum vitamin K_1 concentration and vitamin K-dependent clotting factor activity in maternal and fetal cord blood, *Am. J. Obstet. Gynecol.,* 153, 771, 1985.
79. **McCarthy, P., Gau, G., and Shearer, M.,** Plasma and liver levels of vitamin K in the newborn, *Thromb. Haemostas.,* 58, 218, 1987.
80. **Shirahata, A., Asakura, A., Nakamura, T., and Yamada, K.,** Contents of phylloquinone and menaquinone family in serum and feces from human newborn infants, *Thromb. Haemostas.,* 58, 217, 1987.
81. **Greer, F. R., Mummah-Schendel, L. L., Marshall, S., and Suttie, J. W.,** Vitamin K_1 (phylloquinone) and vitamin K_2 (menaquinone) status in newborns during the first week of life, *Pediatrics,* 81, 137, 1988.

82. **Hiraike, H., Kimura, M., and Itokawa, Y.,** Distribution of K vitamins (phylloquinone and menaquinones) in human placenta and maternal and umbilical cord plasma, *Am. J. Obstet. Gynecol.,* 158, 564, 1988.

83. **Mandelbrot, L., Guillaumont, M., Leclercq, M., Lefrere, J. J., Gozin, D., Daffos, F., and Forestier, F.,** Placental transfer of vitamin K_1 and its implications in fetal hemostasis, *Thromb. Haemost.* 60, 39, 1988.

84. **Widdershoven, J., Lambert, W., Motohara, K., Monnens, L., de Leenheer, A., Matsuda, I., and Endo, F.,** Plasma concentrations of vitamin K_1 and PIVKA-II in bottle-fed and breast-fed infants with and without vitamin K prophylaxis at birth, *Eur. J. Pediatr.,* 148, 139, 1988.

85. **Hathaway, W. E., Isarangkura, P. B., Mahasandana, C., Jacobson, L., Pintadit, P., Pung-Amritt, P., and Green, G. M.,** Comparison of oral parenteral vitamin K prophylaxis for prevention of late hemorrhagic disease of newborn (HDN), *Thromb. Haemostas.,* 62, 366, 1989.

86. **Yang, Y.-M., Simon, N., Maertens, P., Brigham, S., and Liu, P.,** Maternal-fetal transport of vitamin K_1 and its effects on coagulation in premature infants, *J. Pediatr.,* 115, 1009, 1989.

87. **Shearer, M. J.,** Absorption, metabolism, and storage of K vitamins in the newborn, in *Perinatal Thrombosis and Hemostasis,* Suzuki, S., Hathaway, W. E., Bonnar, J., and Sutor, A. H., Eds., Springer-Verlag, Tokyo, 1991, 203.

88. Canadian Paediatric Society, Fetus and Newborn Committee, The use of vitamin K in the perinatal period, *Can. Med. Assoc. J.,* 139, 127, 1988.

89. American Academy Pediatrics, Committee on Fetus and Newborn, Standards for hospital care of newborn infants, 1983, 85.

90. **O'Connor, M. E. and Addiego, J. E.,** Use of oral vitamin K_1 to prevent hemorrhagic disease of the newborn infant, *J. Pediatr.,* 108, 616, 1986.

91. **von Kries, R., Kreppel, S., Becker, A., Tangermann, R., and Göbel U.,** A carboxyprothrombin detectability after oral prophylactic vitamin K, *Arch. Dis. Child.,* 62, 938, 1987.

92. **Hanawa, Y., Maki, M., Murata, B., Matsuyama, E., Yamamoto, Y., Nagao, T., Yamada, K., Ikeda, I., Terao, T., Mikami, S., Shiraki, K., Komazawa, M., Shirahata, A., Tsuji, Y., Motohara, K., Tsukimoto, I., and Sawada, K.,** The second nation-wide survey in Japan of vitamin K deficiency in infancy, *Eur. J. Pediatr.,* 147, 472, 1988.

93. **Nagao, T. and Hanawa, Y.,** The third nationwide survey on vitamin K deficiency in infancy in Japan, in *Perinatal Thrombosis and Hemostasis,* Suzuki, S., Hathaway, W. E., Bonnar, J., and Sutor, A. H., Eds., SpringerVerlag, Tokyo, 1991, 249.

94. **von Kries, R., Shearer, M. J., and Göbel U.,** Vitamin K in infancy, *Eur. J. Pediatr.,* 147, 106, 1988.

95. **Verity, C. M., Carswell, F., and Scott, G. L.,** Vitamin K deficiency causing infantile intracranial haemorrhage after the neonatal period, *Lancet,* 1, 1439, 1983.

96. **Payne, D. R. and Hasegawa, D. K.,** Vitamin K deficiency in newborns: a case report in alpha 1 antitrypsin deficiency and a review of factors predisposing to hemorrhage, *Pediatrics,* 73, 712, 1984.

97. **Sutor, A. H., Kunzer, W., Gobel, U., Kries, R. V., and Landbeck, G.,** Vitamin-K-prophylaxe, *Pediat. Prax.,* 38, 625, 1989.

98. **Tonz, O. and Schubiger, G.,** Neonatale Vitamin-KProphylaxe und Vitamin-K-Mangelblutungen in der Schweiz 1986–1988, *Schweiz. Med. Wschr.,* 118, 1747, 1988.

99. **Isarangkura, P. B., Bintadish, P., Tejavej, A., Siripoonya, P., Chulajata, R., Green, G. M., and Chalermchandra, K.,** Vitamin K prophylaxis in the neonate by the oral route and its significance in reducing infant mortality and morbidity, *J. Med. Ass. Thailand.,* 69 (Suppl. 2), 56, 1986.

Chapter 12

VITAMIN K DEFICIENCY IN THE NEWBORN: ETIOLOGY AND INFLUENCE OF INFANT PHYSIOLOGY AND MATERNAL NUTRITION

Rüdiger von Kries and Martin J. Shearer

TABLE OF CONTENTS

0-8493-6423-X/93/$0.00 + $.50
© 1993 by CRC Press, Inc.

I. INTRODUCTION

It is now some 50 years since the pathogenic role of vitamin K deficiency in neonatal bleeding was first recognized. The fascinating history of the discovery of the association of a bleeding tendency in the newborn infant with vitamin K deficiency and how concepts of the incidence and nature of this deficiency syndrome have changed in the intervening years has been reviewed in depth by Hathaway elsewhere in this volume (see Chapter 11). Central to this topic, over the years, has been the issue of vitamin K prophylaxis and whether universal supplementation to the newborn represents a useful public health measure.[1] In this respect it is clearly important to establish, if possible, the etiology of the disease. This chapter addresses this problem both from the point of view of current knowledge of the normal physiology of vitamin K in the newborn period and how this may be influenced by other factors such as maternal nutrition.

The bleeding diathesis which results from vitamin K deficiency in the newborn is commonly called the "hemorrhagic disease of the newborn" (abbreviated to HDN), a phrase originally coined by Townsend[2] long before the association with vitamin K was known but which today is used synonymously with vitamin K deficiency bleeding of the newborn. This chapter will follow this convention. More recently,[3,4] the distinction has been made between different forms of HDN according to the time of presentation and, as also discussed in this chapter, their probable different etiologies. The first and longest known form of HDN refers to a temporary, vitamin K responsive bleeding tendency which presents in the first week of life and which is usually called "classic" or "classical" HDN.[3,4] Common bleeding sites in classical HDN are the gastrointestinal tract, skin, nose, and umbilicus. Bleeding may also occur after circumcision. Until the late 1960s the classical 'first week of life' syndrome was the only form of neonatal vitamin K deficiency that had been reported in the literature, even though there had been a period of intensive study of HDN in the 1940s and 1950s (For reviews see Dam et al.[5] and Chapter 11). A vitamin K responsive hemorrhagic syndrome of early infancy (as opposed to the first week of life) was first recognized in 1967.[6,7] Since then more than 1000 cases have been reported from Japan,[8,9] more than 100 cases from Southeast Asia,[10,11] significant numbers from Australasia,[12,13] and Europe[14-18] and a few cases from North America.[19] The peak incidence is from the fourth to sixth week of life. This hemorrhagic syndrome of early infancy has caused considerable clinical concern because of the site of bleeding with intracranial hemorrhage accounting for some 50% of the bleeding episodes at presentation. Despite this pathological difference vitamin K deficiency is central to both syndromes. To distinguish between them, however, the syndrome of early infancy is often called "late" or "late onset" hemorrhagic disease of the newborn. In this chapter the term late hemorrhagic disease of the newborn (abbreviated LHDN) will be used.

It should be emphasized that LHDN refers to a syndrome in which the presenting feature is bleeding whether or not the bleeding is subsequently shown to have been due to an identifiable disease. In fact, in most of the recent literature reports, the majority of cases of LHDN are "idiopathic" and the clotting defect in affected infants normalizes spontaneously after vitamin K and/or transfusion. On the other hand, vitamin K deficiency has long been recognized as a risk factor for bleeding in certain malabsorptive and cholestatic syndromes associated with disease states such as bile duct atresia[20] or cystic fibrosis.[21,22] Bleeding in these children may be seen at any time during the course of the underlying disease, unless sufficient vitamin K supplements are given.[23]

II. INFANT PHYSIOLOGY

Until recently, little was known about the physiology of vitamin K in the perinatal period. A major reason for this has been the lack of analytical techniques for measuring the low tissue concentrations of K vitamins. However, as reviewed in detail by Hart (Chapter 2) and Haroon (Chapter 3), the last decade or so has seen major advances in the development of chromatographic methodologies to resolve and detect the different molecular forms (phylloquinone and menaquinones) in small tissue samples. Although many analytical problems of tissue measurements still remain to be solved, it is now at least possible for the researcher to attempt to gain some insight into some of the major questions concerning the normal fetal and neonatal physiology and biochemistry of vitamin K. Some of these questions surrounding processes such as transplacental transfer, intestinal absorption, plasma transport, tissue distribution and turnover of the K vitamins have obvious relevance when trying to explain why the human newborn is at greater risk of developing vitamin K deficiency than the human adult. Under the broad physiological concepts outlined above it is also important to discover the way in which different molecular forms of vitamin K are handled; i.e., what relative contributions to fetal and neonatal requirements are made by phylloquinone (vitamin K_1), the plant synthesized form of vitamin K, and by the menaquinones (vitamins K_2) which are of bacterial origin? Recent progress made in our understanding of the normal physiology of vitamin K in the fetus and newborn infant is outlined below.

A. PLACENTAL TRANSPORT
The concentrations of fat-soluble vitamins tend to be lower in cord plasma than in the maternal circulation; this is often interpreted as providing evidence of a placental barrier. This interpretation is somewhat simplistic since the maternal/cord ratio alone at a single time point does not allow for other physiological possibilities that could account for a maternal/cord plasma gradient. For example, the capacity of plasma lipid transport may be lower in

the newborn; this apparently explains the lower (approximately halved) concentrations of vitamin E (α-tocopherol) in cord plasma.[24] On the other hand, there is now overwhelming evidence[25] that the concentrations of vitamin K in cord plasma are so low that they cannot be explained simply by the differential lipid concentrations between maternal and newborn circulations. Although there were initially serious methodological discrepancies there is now common agreement in the field that cord plasma levels of phylloquinone are below 50 pg/ml and that the average maternal/newborn concentration gradient of phylloquinone is within the range of 20:1 to 40:1.[26-29] This is by far the highest placental blood gradient of any of the fat-soluble vitamins.

Further evidence that phylloquinone does not readily cross the placenta is shown by the even higher maternal/newborn concentration gradients obtained when the vitamin is administered to mothers shortly before delivery.[27,29,30] The extent to which cord plasma concentrations can be raised depends on the dose, route and time interval between maternal administration and cord sampling. When single doses of 1–5 mg of phylloquinone were administered intravenously or intramuscularly, cord plasma levels were raised from 2 to 5-fold[29,30] whereas in mothers receiving 20 mg/day orally for at least 3 days cord levels were raised some 40-fold.[27] Such doses however represent massive doses compared to the average adult daily intake (normally in the range of 10–100 μg/day[31]; the comparatively mild increases in cord plasma levels in response to such high doses illustrates the inability of vitamin K to transfer *rapidly* across the placenta. Recent studies in a rat model support this concept and showed that after giving radiolabelled phylloquinone to pregnant rats the amount of vitamin reaching the fetal liver after 24 hours represented only about 2% of the amount in the maternal liver.[32]

B. FETAL AND NEONATAL LIVER RESERVES

In studies of the hepatic reserves of vitamin K in human fetal or neonatal samples obtained after abortion or at post-mortem it was shown by one of the authors[26] that phylloquinone is detectable in the liver as early as 10 weeks gestation at concentrations of 1–2 ng/g. Similar concentrations (median 1.3 ng/g) were measured in older fetuses with gestational ages ranging from 19–27 weeks, and at delivery in pre-term (1.4 ng/g) or term (1.0 ng/g) infants. These concentrations are about one-fifth the concentrations found in adult livers in the same study. Although significantly reduced, these fetal reserves are not as low as perhaps expected from the very low concentrations found in cord plasma.

A more surprising finding of the above analyses of fetal and neonatal liver tissue samples[26] has been the inability to detect significant concentrations of any of the menaquinone series of vitamin K at any stage of gestation or after birth until after the first week of life. These findings were in complete contrast to those in adults in whom a wide spectrum of menaquinones were detected and which represented some 75–97% (median 92%) of total hepatic stores of vitamin K. A similar inability to detect menaquinones in newborn livers has been reported by other investigators.[33,34]

III. MATERNAL NUTRITION

A striking similarity between classical and late HDN is that most of the affected babies reported in the literature have been exclusively breast fed.[3,4] The role of breastfeeding as a risk factor for classical HDN was recognized as early as 1940[35] and confirmed nearly 30 years later.[36] Following the more recent discovery of late HDN it has become equally evident that this syndrome too presents in exclusively breastfed babies.[3,4] This close association with breastfeeding has been observed in Japan,[9] Thailand,[10] Great Britain,[14] West Germany,[15,16] and North America.[3,19] Since human milk is usually considered to provide optimal concentrations of nutrients, including micronutrients such as vitamins, the apparent inability of human milk to meet the dietary requirements for vitamin K in some newborns is surprising and alarming. Several factors could account for this association between breast feeding and HDN, the most obvious being that breast milk may sometimes become deficient in vitamin K. The recent ability to make accurate and specific measurements of K vitamins in biological samples,[25] including milks,[37] is particularly pertinent to the questions surrounding HDN and breastfeeding, and is discussed below.

A. MEASUREMENTS OF VITAMIN K IN HUMAN MILK, COW'S MILK AND INFANT FORMULAS

1. Methodological Variability

In 1942, Dam et al.[38] reported the first measurements of vitamin K in human and cow's milk using a curative chick bioassay. Although the measurements provided by the bioassays of this time suffered from many disadvantages in terms of design and performance, they did allow relative estimations of the total vitamin K activity in different samples to be made. The most important basic information from these early analyses was that the concentrations of vitamin K in human milk were lower then in cow's milk; this has since been confirmed using modern physicochemical techniques mainly based on the technique of high-performance liquid chromatography (HPLC). With the availability of these highly specific and sensitive chromatographic assays some new insights have emerged on the vitamin K content of human milk and other infant foods.

The first measurements of vitamin K in milk samples using chromatographic methods were carried out by Haroon et al.[39] who were able to measure phylloquinone by a multi-stage procedure in which the final analytical stage was HPLC with UV absorbance detection. Although like Dam they found lower concentrations of phylloquinone in human milk compared to cow's milk, the concentrations measured by HPLC were considerably lower than the total vitamin K activity measured by the chick bioassay. The possibility

TABLE 1
Literature Values of Phylloquinone (Vitamin K$_1$)
Concentrations in Mature Human Milk

Year	Investigator and reference	Phylloquinone concentrations (µg/l)		
		Mean (±S.D.)	Median	Range
1982	Haroon et al.[39]	2.1	—	1.1–6.5
1983	Isarankura et al.[42]	8.8	—	4.0–16.0
1984	Motohara et al.[43]	3.8 (±0.9)	—	1.1–8.3
1987	Fournier et al.[44]	—	9.2	4.9–12.8
1987	von Kries et al.[45]	—	1.2	0.4–4.2
1988	Isshiki et al.[40]	2.1 (±0.9)	—	—
1989	Canfield et al.[37]	2.8 (±0.4)	—	—

that the higher levels measured by the bioassay are due to the presence of large concentrations of menaquinones has been largely discounted by newer, more specific detection methods which can detect both phylloquinone and menaquinones in milk and which suggest that phylloquinone is the predominant molecular form of vitamin K, especially in human milk[37,40,41] but also in cow's milk.[40,41] Instead, the methodological differences are probably mainly due to the problems of standardisation of the bioassay.

The advent of physicochemical methods for measuring vitamin K compounds has not seen the end of methodological controversies. Even though chromatographic methods all give lower values than bioassays there are considerable variations in values reported by different institutions. This is illustrated by the almost tenfold variation in reported values for the phylloquinone content of mature human milks[37,39,40,42-45] (Table 1). Several factors may account for these differences. From the methodological viewpoint the main problem areas would seem to be those associated with incomplete lipid extraction leading to underestimations or with chromatographic contamination leading to overestimations. Some of these methodological problems and a comparison between different procedures have been reviewed by Canfield.[37] Another important determinant of the phylloquinone concentration in milk is the way in which the breast milk is sampled; standardized milk collection techniques appear to be particularly important if reproducible and meaningful values are to be realised.[45] The lipid concentrations in human milk increases during the course of emptying of the breast[47,48] and as demonstrated recently there is a similar rise in the concentrations of phylloquinone.[45] The high phylloquinone concentrations reported by Fournier et al.[44] were measured in milk samples that had been collected after the mother had nursed the baby. This together with the lack of specificity of their particular chromatographic method may account for the abnormally high values obtained in their study.

2. Physiological Variations in Human Milk

Even when both sampling and assay techniques have been standardized, considerable variations in the phylloquinone content of human milk have been observed both within the same mother and between different mothers. One detailed study by the authors[45] followed the phylloquinone concentrations in nine individual mothers at regular intervals over the first 36 days of lactation. One finding from this study was that colostral milk (days 1–5) had significantly higher phylloquinone concentrations than mature milk (days 8–36), a finding generally in keeping with the higher concentrations in colostrum of other fat-soluble vitamins such as vitamins A and E.[48] For phylloquinone, the highest levels were in fact observed on the first day of lactation.

Within the same mothers, quite large variations were seen both within the same day and from day to day.[45,49] As would be expected, the maternal dietary intake of phylloquinone appears to be a major determinant of subsequent concentrations in mature human milk although there may be a lag phase of 12 hours or more between the increased dietary intake and the appearance of peak milk concentrations.[39,45] It is clear, however, that substantial increases in the phylloquinone concentration in human milk can be obtained either by giving supplements to the mother[39,45] or with a vitamin K-rich diet.[50]

3. Relative Concentrations in Human Milk, Cow's Milk, and Formula Feeds

Although the concentrations of phylloquinone in human milk may vary widely, they are almost always lower than those in cow's milk and cow's milk-based formulas.[39] As with human milk, however, variations also exist in the phylloquinone content of cow's milk. Seasonal variations have been observed with higher phylloquinone concentrations in summer and autumn as compared to winter and spring.[44] In addition, much higher phylloquinone concentrations were found in cow's milk from the Channel Islands (Jersey, Guernsey) as compared to milk from Friesian cows;[39] this may reflect the higher fat content of the former. Milk from the Channel Islands also contains higher concentrations of provitamin A carotenoids.[51]

The relevance of these measurements of vitamin K in cow's milk to infant nutrition is that many artificial feeds for young infants are derived from cow's milk and until recently were not supplemented with vitamin K. In 1982, analyses of formulas carried out in the laboratory of one of the authors using a newly developed HPLC method showed that the concentrations of phylloquinone in entirely or mainly milk-based formulas were generally lower than in unmodified cow's milk.[39] For this reason and because of possible losses during the manufacturing process it is now common commercial practice to supplement all artificial feeds with phylloquinone. Supplemented concentrations typically range from 30 to 70 μg/l compared to about 5 μg/l in cow's milk and about 2 μg/l in human milk.[39] In some countries, supplementation measures have been recommended by expert pediatric committees and the testing controlled by government legislation.[23,52]

Since most non-breast fed young infants in Europe and North America are fed artificial formulas which have been supplemented with phylloquinone, their dietary intake of vitamin K is much higher than in exclusively breastfed babies. For example, for a baby weighing 4 kg and drinking 750 ml per day of human milk containing 2 μg/l of phylloquinone, the daily phylloquinone intake would be 1.5 μg (0.37 μg/kg/day). With the same amount of commercial formula containing 40 μg/l, the baby would obtain 30 μg of phylloquinone per day (7.5 μg/kg/day). As yet, systematic studies of the impact of such different dietary intakes on the vitamin K status of breast or formula fed infants have not been performed. Preliminary data, however, have shown that the plasma levels of phylloquinone in formula fed infants are considerably higher than the levels in breast-fed infants.[28,54,55] (See also Section V. A)

IV. CLASSICAL HDN - CLUES TO ETIOLOGY

A. CLUES FROM VITAMIN K PHYSIOLOGY

As already outlined in Section II, current knowledge of the physiology of vitamin K in the perinatal period, although imperfect, does suggest that the newborn infant is born with precarious tissue reserves of vitamin K. This points to the need for a rapid and continuous vitamin K supply during the first week of life. For exclusively breastfed babies, the only secure source of vitamin K is the phylloquinone in breast milk, normally present in breast milk at concentrations around 1–2 μg/l. The role of menaquinones is less certain. There is now good evidence from more than one laboratory that the infant is born with virtually no liver stores of menaquinones;[26,33,34] in this respect the neonatal reserves are dramatically lower than adults in whom some 90% of the total vitamin K content in the liver consists of various menaquinones.[26,56,57] On the other hand, the nutritional significance of menaquinones and the degree to which they are able to participate in the gamma-carboxylation mechanism of clotting factors in the liver is questionable. Thus, biochemical abnormalities consistent with a very mild subclinical vitamin K deficiency can be detected in normal volunteers after a comparatively short period of avoidance of vitamin K-rich foods;[58] furthermore, in similarly deprived surgical patients, hepatic stores of phylloquinone become rapidly depleted whereas menaquinone stores remain relatively stable.[57] Recent experiments in rats[59] have confirmed the slower hepatic turnover of a long chain menaquinone such as menaquinone-9. On the other hand, even if the efficiency of utilization is low, the sheer size of the hepatic reserves of menaquinones compared to phylloquinone may act as a significant buffer in preventing the development of overt vitamin K deficiency. If this is true, newborn babies evidently do not possess this buffer and this may be a factor in their susceptibility to vitamin K deficiency. From the limited evidence available it seems that hepatic stores of menaquinones build up slowly and do not reach adult concentrations until several weeks after birth.[26] One implication of the above findings is that the needs of the human fetus and neonate (particularly in the first few days of life) are met largely by phylloquinone. On these grounds, the supply of this vitamen in breastmilk may be assumed to be of paramount importance in maintaining an adequate vitamin K status.

B. CLUES FROM EARLY COAGULATION STUDIES

As already mentioned, breastfeeding has been known to be a risk factor in the development of classical HDN since at least 1940. In this year Salomonsen[35] reported "on the prevention of hemorrhagic disease of the newborn by the administration of cow's milk during the first two days of life." Two years later, the classical studies by Dam and co-workers[38] gave a widely accepted explanation for these findings by demonstrating lower vitamin K concentrations in human milk than in cow's milk. Additionally, Dam[38] had suggested that a low milk intake during the first few days of life might be a further factor accounting for vitamin K deficiency in breastfed babies.

By the early 1950s some of the most important findings relating to the neonatal physiology of the prothrombin complex activity and the risk factors associated with classical HDN had already been elucidated by several groups of investigators of whom those of Salomonsen and Dam were notable. The main conclusions may be summarized:

1. Newborn babies exhibit a physiological hypoprothrombinemia with a nadir on about the third day of life.
2. The degree of hypoprothrombinemia is greatest in breast-fed infants and extreme depression of the prothrombin complex activity may be prevented by feeding supplements of cow's milk or cow's milk formulas or by the administration of vitamin K.
3. Human milk contains lower concentrations of vitamin K than cow's milk.

C. CLUES (REDISCOVERED) FROM LARGE CLINICAL STUDIES

This important pioneering work on the influence of breast feeding to the pathogenesis of HDN seems largely to have been forgotten until the late 1960s and early 1970s when it was confirmed in two extensive and equally conclusive studies from North America.[36,60]

The first study[36] showed that the incidence of moderate to severe bleeding among breastfed infants who were not given vitamin K was 15 to 20 fold higher than in infants who either received vitamin K or were fed with a cow's milk-based formula. A follow up study[60] confirmed the importance of breast feeding to the etiology of classical HDN by comparing the degree of hypoprothrombinemia in babies given different feeding regimes.

Among possible reasons for their findings the authors[60] cited the lower concentrations of vitamin K in human milk than in formula feeds, the lower volumes of milk a breastfed baby usually receives in the first few days of life and the possibilities of an inhibitor of vitamin K in human milk or that the intestinal flora of breastfed infants may be less active in producing vitamin K (i.e., menaquinones) than the microflora of formula-fed infants. Some of these suggestions have been substantiated. Thus, as discussed earlier in this article, (Section III.A) modern techniques of analysis have confirmed the lower concentrations of vitamin K in breast milk and as discussed later (Section IV.D) the volume of milk ingested is also now viewed as equally important. The question raised as to whether differences between the intestinal populations of bacteria in breast-fed versus formula-fed babies can influence the vitamin K status of neonates is also of interest but is more difficult to substantiate. Certainly, there are large differences in the bacterial spectrum of breast-fed and formula-fed neonates as judged from stool cultures[61] with breast-feeding promoting the luxuriant growth of bifidobacteria which do not synthesize menaquinones[62,63] and bottle-fed babies having significantly greater numbers of enterobacteria, enterococci, and *Bacteroides,* all of which synthesize menaquinones.[62-64] These differences would appear to be reflected in the concentrations of menaquinones in stools. One study[65] has shown that in the first week of life, the stools of formula-fed infants almost invariably contain readily detectable concentrations of menaquinones whereas these forms are rarely detected in the stools of breast-fed infants. However, since there is no direct evidence that the menaquinones synthesized in the large intestine are biologically available,[25] the relevance of these interesting differences between breast-fed and formula-fed neonates must remain open at the present time. As to whether there could be an inhibitor of vitamin K in breast milk, this also remains unanswered although with the increasing awareness of environmental pollution the possibility that polychlorinated biphenyls (PCBs), polychlorinated dibenzo-*p*-dioxins (PCDDs) and polychlorinated dibenzofurans (PCDFs) present in breast milk may be a cause of the recent resurgence of HDN, especially the late-onset form, has also been suggested.[66] This hypothesis, however, lacks any supportive biochemical evidence that such pollutants are inhibitors of vitamin K metabolism.

D. CLUES FROM PIVKA-II ANALYSES

With the recent availability of assays for the detection of low plasma concentrations of des-gamma-carboxyprothrombin (PIVKA-II) it has become possible to assess the effects of different infant feeding regimes using a more sensitive index of vitamin K deficiency than was previously possible with conventional coagulation assays. In such a study carried out by one of the authors and colleagues[67] the major findings in a group of infants who were not given vitamin K at birth and who were evaluated on the fifth day of life were as follows:

1.   The incidence of PIVKA-II in exclusively breastfed infants was significantly higher, and reduced factor II and VII activities were more

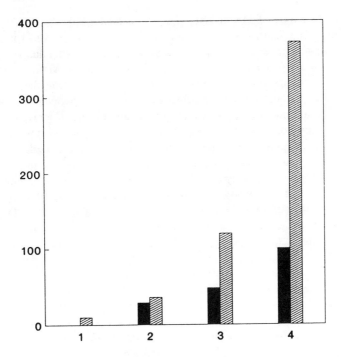

FIGURE 1. Average daily human milk intakes in PIVKA-II positive babies on days 1, 2, 3, and 4 after birth; intakes are shown for babies with factor II activities <25% (black columns) and for factor II activities ≥25% (hatched columns).

often observed, than in babies receiving supplementary or exclusive formula feeding.

2. Infants in whom PIVKA-II was detected had received significantly lower volumes of feed over the first 4 days of life than PIVKA-II negative babies regardless of whether they were breastfed or formula-fed.

3. All breastfed infants in whom PIVKA-II was detected on day 5 had received less than 100 ml per day of human milk during the first 2 days of life. Those with normal plasma factor II (prothrombin) activities had increased their milk intake on days 3 and 4 to more than 100 ml per day whereas those with lower than normal (<25%) factor II activities had not (Figure 1).

We concluded from this study that breastfed infants, in the first week of life, need a daily intake of 100 to 200 ml of milk per day to ensure an amount of vitamin K which is sufficient to prevent the appearance in plasma of des-gamma-carboxyprothrombin. Since lactation often needs some days to become fully established[68] the daily intake of human milk may be often less than 100 ml, a fact confirmed in our study.[67]

E. CLUES FROM CHANGING INFANT PRACTICES

Some of the confusion and disputation in the literature as to whether or not vitamin K deficiency in the newborn exists, is undoubtedly due to a failure to take into account changing infant feeding practices as well as different socio-economic and cultural factors. Thus a previous study from the institution of one of the authors showed no evidence of vitamin K deficiency as judged from the measurement of plasma prothrombin and factor VII activities on the third and fourth days of life.[69] Ten years later the same unit reported significantly reduced plasma activities of prothrombin in five day-old breastfed infants compared to infants receiving exclusive or supplementary formula feeds.[70] It now seems likely that the failure to detect evidence of vitamin K deficiency in the first study was due to the practice at that time of giving early supplementary formula feeds to many breastfed babies.[71] With the growing awareness that such early exposure to cow's milk based formulas may predispose the infant to the subsequent development of intolerance to cow's milk proteins,[72] the practice of giving supplementary feeds in the first few days of life has been abandoned in many nurseries.

In consequence, there is again today a greater proportion of exclusively breastfed infants and therefore a greater population at risk of developing classical HDN. Indeed, a recurrence of both classical and late HDN has been reported from units where vitamin K prophylaxis had been abandoned.[71,73]

V. LATE HDN - CLUES TO ETIOLOGY

Late HDN occurs at a time when lactation is fully established peaking at the fourth to sixth week of life. As with classical HDN, the disease is virtually confined to breastfed babies[3,4] which again points to the importance of maternal nutrition to the etiology. This and other aspects which may provide some clues to the etiology of late HDN are reviewed below.

A. CLUES FROM VITAMIN K PHYSIOLOGY

For obvious reasons, very little is known about the hepatic vitamin K reserves of infants after birth, neither to our knowledge is there any information about the extent of depletion of liver stores of vitamin K in babies who have had late HDN; such studies would only be possible in samples obtained at post-mortem. For these reasons, we have little idea as to the magnitude of hepatic reserves of vitamin K necessary to sustain clotting factor synthesis in the early weeks of life or how the relative concentrations of phylloquinone and menaquinones change post-delivery. It is suspected that liver menaquinone stores take some time to become established but, as already discussed (Section IV. A), their biological effectiveness in clotting factor biosynthesis remains as conjectural as their role in adult nutrition.[25]

Some information is now available on plasma levels of phylloquinone in infants. It has been confirmed that plasma levels of exclusively breastfed infants, while generally in the normal adult range, tend to be at the lower end of this range and are very much lower than the levels in infants fed on vitamin K supplemented formulas.[28,54,55] In the most recent of these studies,[55] plasma phylloquinone concentrations in breastfed infants were shown to remain low (mean < 0.25 ng/ml) throughout the first 6 months of life while concentrations in formula-fed infants ranged from 4–6 ng/ml and were several fold higher than the average adult concentration (0.5 ng/ml). This vast difference in plasma levels between breastfed and formula-fed infants can be attributed to the differential concentrations of phylloquinone in human milk which in this study averaged 0.6–0.9 μg/l at 4 time points over the 6-month period while the infant formula contained 55 μg/l. Thus, the exclusively formula-fed infants in this study received approximately 100 times the daily intake of the exclusively breast-fed infant. Although such differences between plasma levels and dietary intake are certainly impressive and give some quantitative expression to the protection against HDN afforded by modern infant formulas it should be reiterated that even the unsupplemented formulas of earlier times did provide substantial protection.[36] Many such formulas contained only slightly higher (often about double) concentrations of phylloquinone than those in breast milk.[39]

B. CLUES FROM COAGULATION STUDIES AND PIVKA-II DETECTION

Although a relative lengthening of prothrombin times in breast-fed babies compared to artificially-fed infants has often been demonstrated early after birth,[60,67,70] by the time of the peak incidence of HDN this difference disappears. Thus, in Germany, at the age of 4 to 6 weeks, identical distribution patterns of prothrombin activity were seen in a group of 78 exclusively breastfed infants and a group of 87 infants who had received infant formulas either exclusively or as supplemental feeds.[70] Similar results were obtained in Costa Rica for a smaller population sample of one-month-old infants who were either exclusively breast-fed or fed exclusively with cow's milk.[74] Conventional coagulation tests however will only detect babies with a more or less overt vitamin K deficiency. It seems likely, however, that subclinical vitamin K deficiency may be much more prevalent in breast-fed babies of this age than can be predicted from either the incidence of clinical bleeding or from conventional clotting factor assays. This diagnostic limitation of conventional coagulation tests for detecting biochemical vitamin K deficiency has been discussed by Widdershoven and co-workers.[75] Some investigators have therefore carried out studies in infants using the detection of des-gamma-carboxyprothrombin (PIVKA-II) as a more sensitive marker for vitamin K deficiency.

Studies designed to detect PIVKA-II in 4 to 8 week old infants, which is the age range of peak incidence of late HDN, have been carried out in Europe and Japan.[76-80] The proportion of the population in whom PIVKA-II was detected (i.e., PIVKA-II detection rates) in these studies has varied considerably (Table 2) and this is related to the sensitivity of the particular type of assay used to detect the des-gamma-carboxylated molecules of pro-thrombin.[81] As can be seen from Table 2, the highest detection rates for PIVKA-II were obtained for an enzyme-linked immunoabsorbent assay (ELISA) with a monoclonal antibody to PIVKA-II isolated by Motohara and co-workers.[82] This method allows the detection of very low concentrations of PIVKA-II. One problem however lies in the interpretation of values which lie only slightly above the cut-off levels for "normal" PIVKA-II and the fact that the cut-off level has often been applied in an arbitrary way.[83] For example, the most common cut-off level for the monoclonal assay and that which was originally applied by Motohara[84] is 0.13 arbitrary units (AU)/ml, 1 arbitrary unit corresponding to 1 μg of purified prothrombin. With this high sensitivity it is difficult to assess whether the detection of very low concentrations of PIVKA-II are truly specific for subclinical vitamin K deficiency. Indeed, some investigators have urged caution in the interpretation of studies which rely solely on the detection of PIVKA-II by sensitive immunoassays as a marker of subclinical vitamin K deficiency.[85,86] One of the present authors has suggested that only levels of PIVKA-II above 4 AU/ml assuredly reflect subclinical vitammin K deficiency.[87] Such levels may also be detected by crossed immunoelectrophoresis (CIE)[83,87] a long established method for PIVKA-II measurements.[88,89]

Reported detection rates of PIVKA-II in 4 to 8 week old infants in European and Japanese studies are shown in Table 2. In all studies, the incidence of "high" PIVKA-II concentrations (i.e., above 4 AU/ml) was low, such levels being detected in approximately 0.5% to 1% of exclusively breast-fed babies. In formula-fed babies (either given exclusively or as sup-plementary feeds) the incidence of "high" PIVKA-II levels is evidently even lower, being only 0.2% in Japan and so far indetermined in Europe.

These studies carry an important message: the "low" vitamin K intake from breast milk is a relevant risk factor for vitamin K deficiency in young infants. Latent vitamin K deficiency (i.e., PIVKA-II detectability without clinical bleeding) is more common than overt vitamin K deficiency (i.e., with bleeding) in breastfed infants. The reason why some of these babies with a "low" dietary vitamin K intake bleed is not well understood. The "low" dietary intakes might be insufficient to maintain normal hemostasis in some babies with an impaired vitamin K absorption, some babies may have a higher vitamin K requirement or some babies may be fed by mothers whose milk contains extremely low quantities of vitamin K.

C. MISCELLANEOUS CLUES

Of all the possible reasons as to why breast-fed babies should be at greater risk of developing late HDN, the concept of very low vitamin K concentrations in individual mother's milk is, at first sight, an appealing one because, as already discussed, concentrations of phylloquinone in milk from different mothers have been shown to vary considerably.[45,49] The maternal dietary

TABLE 2
PIVKA II Detection Rates in 4–8 Week-Old Infants

Study	Breast fed			Mixed feeding or formula only		
	PIVKA II (CIE)[a]	PIVKA II (monoclonal antibody)[b]		PIVKA II (CIE)	PIVKA II (monoclonal antibody)	
Country and author		>4 AU/ml[c]	>0,013 AU/ml		>4 AU/ml	>0,013 AU/ml
West Germany; v. Kries et al.[76]	1/113			0/89		
Holland; Büller et al.[77]	0/40			0/73		
Holland; Widdershoven et al.[78]		0/62 (day 30) 1/44 (day 60)	3/62 (day 30) 4/44 (day 60)			0/43 (day 30) 0/48 (day 60)
Japan; Motohara et al.[79]			21/171			
Japan; Motohara et al.[80]		26/5090			6/3256	

a   PIVKA II measured by crossed immunoelectrophoresis.
b   PIVKA II measured by enzyme-linked immunoabsorbent assay (ELISA) using a monoclonal antibody to des-gamma-carboxyprothrombin.
c   Arbitrary units/ml plasma.

vitamin K intake may vary widely[50] and extremely low phylloquinone concentrations in some mothers milk could be a consequence of such a low intake. Three studies reporting measurements of phylloquinone concentrations in milk samples from a total of 28 mothers of affected babies have now been published.[42,43,90] Two of the three studies found lower mean concentrations of phylloquinone in the samples from mothers whose children bled.[42,43] Phylloquinone concentrations below controls were reported in 5 of 9 cases in Thailand,[42] 3 of 10 cases from Japan[43] and none of 9 cases from West Germany.[90] These studies suggest that an extremely low vitamin K intake might account for late HDN in some of the affected babies, but certainly not in all.

Systematic studies on the absorption of vitamin K in babies with late HDN have not been performed as yet. There is, however, one well documented case report on the temporary malabsorption of vitamin K during the first months of life in a baby with late HDN.[91] The temporary malabsorption of vitamin K in this baby seems to have been related to a self-correcting episode of minor cholestasis. Bile acids are essential for the absorption of vitamin K[92] and subclinical cholestasis could be a relevant pathogenic factor for late HDN. In cases related to underlying disease such as alpha-1-antitrypsin deficiency, a pathogenic role for cholestasis is generally accepted, although in most reports the laboratory parameters of cholestasis in the affected patients have not been excessively high.[93-98] The same degree of cholestasis is frequently observed in infants with late HDN considered to be idiopathic and in whom underlying diseases such as alpha-1-antitrypsin deficiency, cystic fibrosis, bile duct atresia, hepatitis or a-beta-lipoproteinemia have been ruled out.[3,4] In a recent survey from Japan,[9] the direct bilirubin concentrations have been determined in 119 children with idiopathic late HDN: the mean bilirubin concentration (2.5 $\pm$ 1.6 mg/dl) was significantly higher than for healthy controls (0.37 $\pm$ 0.27 mg/dl). Malabsorption of vitamin K in children with minor cholestasis therefore might contribute to the pathogenesis of late HDN in a considerable proportion of cases.

A higher vitamin K requirement in babies with late HDN could also be a consequence of congenital or acquired defects of the vitamin K-dependent carboxylase or other enzymes of the vitamin K-epoxide cycle. As far as congenital defects are concerned, only seven cases of hereditary combined deficiency of vitamin K-dependent procoagulants have been reported in the literature.[99] Of these seven cases, the two most recent and best studied[99,100] suggest a hetereogeneous disorder resulting from distinct biochemical abnormalities possibly affecting the vitamin K carboxylase[99] or the vitamin K epoxide reductase[100] enzymes of the vitamin K-epoxide cycle.[25] The rarity of such hereditary disorders, however, suggests that they are not a significant cause of late HDN. The possibility that an acquired inhibition of the hepatic enzymes required to maintain vitamin K-dependent carboxylation could also cause late HDN also needs to be considered. Such a cause would be quite separate from other, well described, causes of acquired vitamin K deficiency resulting from an inherent, disease-related impairment of biological function (e.g., intestinal malabsorption or hepatic dysfunction). One example of an external factor causing vitamin K deficiency is the epidemic of late HDN reported from Vietnam in 1983 which was related to the use of talcum powder contaminated with warfarin.[101] Other compounds, such as certain cephalosporins, have a weak coumarin-like activity and have been shown to trigger vitamin K deficiency in patients with an impaired nutritional status (see Chapter 13). Finally, as already mentioned, a hypothesis has been forwarded that environmental pollutants may be a cause of late HDN.[66] Thus, although it is theoretically possible that drugs or some environmental pollutant may have the potential to cause hypothrombinemia and that this may affect the infant via the breast milk there is as yet little hard evidence to suggest that either of these possiblities is a major cause of late HDN.

REFERENCES

1. **von Kries, R.,** Vitamin K prophylaxis - a useful public health measure? *Paediatr., Perinatal Epidemiol.,* 6, 7, 1992.
2. **Townsend, C. W.,** The hemorrhagic disease of the newborn, *Arch. Pediatr.,* 11, 559, 1894.
3. **Lane, P. A. and Hathaway, W. E.,** Vitamin K in infancy, *J. Pediatr.,* 106, 351, 1985.
4. **von Kries, R., Shearer, M. J., and Göbel, U.,** Vitamin K in infancy, *Eur. J. Pediatr.,* 147, 106, 1988.
5. **Dam, H., Dyggve, H., Larsen, H., and Plum, P.,** The relation of vitamin K deficiency to hemorrhagic disease of the newborn, *Adv. Pediatr.,* 5, 129, 1952.
6. **Chan, M. C. K. and Boon, W. H.,** Late haemorrhagic disease of Singapore infants, *J. Singapore Paediatr. Soc.,* 9, 72, 1967.
7. **Lovric, V. A. and Jones, R. F.,** The haemorrhagic syndrome of early childhood, *Australasian Annals Med.,* 16, 173, 1967.
8. **Nakayama, K.,** The etiology of vitamin K deficiency in infants, *Perinat. Med.,* (Japanese), 12, 1029, 1982.
9. **Hanawa, Y., Maki, M., Murata, B., Matsuyama, E., Yamamoto, Y., Nagao, T., Yamada, K., Ikeda, I., Terao, T., Mikami, S., Shiraki, K., Komazawa, M., Shirahata, A., Tsuji, Y., Motohara, K., Tsukimoto, I., and Sawada, K.,** The second nation-wide survey in Japan of vitamin K-deficiency in infancy, *Eur. J. Pediatr.,* 147, 472, 1988.
10. **Bhanchet, P., Tuchinda, S., Hathirat, P., Visudhiphan, P., Bhamaraphavati, N., and Bukkavesa, S.,** A bleeding syndrome in infants due to acquired prothrombin complex deficiency. A survey of 93 affected infants, *Clin. Pediatr.,* 16, 992, 1977.
11. **Chuan, Y. T.,** Intracranial haemorrhage due to late haemorrhagic disease of infancy, *Med. J. Malaysia,* 42, 276, 1987.
12. **Forbes, K.,** Delayed presentation of haemorrhagic disease of the newborn, *Med. J. Australia,* 2, 136, 1983.
13. **Heron, P., Cull, A., Bourchier, D., and Lees, H.,** Avoidable hazard to New Zealand children: case reports of haemorrhagic disease of the newborn, *N. Z. Med. J.,* 101, 507, 1988.
14. **McNinch, A. W. and Tripp, J. H.,** Haemorrhagic disease of the newborn in the British Isles: two year prospective study, *Brit. Med. J.,* 303, 1105, 1991.

15. **Sutor, A. H. and Scharbau, O.,** Effect of vitamin K prophylaxis on the incidence of the late form of vitamin K deficiency bleeding, in *Perinatal Thrombosis and Hemostasis,* Suzuki, S., Hathaway, W. E., Bonnar, J., Sutor, A. H., Eds., Springer-Verlag, Tokyo, 1991, 263.

16. **von Kries, R. and Göbel, U.,** Vitamin K prophylaxis and vitamin K deficiency bleeding in early infancy, *Acta Paediatr. Scand.,* 81, 655, 1992.

17. **Tönz, O. and Schubiger, G.,** Neonatale Vitamin K Prophylaxe und Vitamin K-Mangel-blutungen in der Schweiz 1986–1988, *Schweiz. Med. Wschr.,* 118, 1747, 1988.

18. **Ekelund, H.,** Late haemorrhagic disease in Sweden 1987–89, *Acta Paediatr. Scand.,* 80, 966, 1991.

19. **Hathaway, W. E.,** New insights on vitamin K, *Hematol. Oncol. Clin. North Am.,* 1, 367, 1987.

20. **Fujimura, Y., Mimura, Y., Kinoshita, S., Yoshioka, A., Kitawaki, T., Yoshioka, K., and Takamiya, O.,** Studies on vitamin K-dependent factor deficiency during early childhood with special reference to prothrombin activity and antigen level, *Haemostasis,* 11, 90, 1982.

21. **Torstensen, O. L., Humphrey, G. B., Edson, J. R., and Warwick, W. J.,** Cystic fibrosis presenting with severe hemorrhage due to vitamin K malabsorption: A report of 3 cases, *Pediatrics,* 45, 857, 1970.

22. **Oppenheimer, E. H. and Schwartz, A.,** Easy bruisability and terminal coma in a "normal" 5-month-old infant, *J. Pediatr.,* 88, 1049, 1976.

23. American Academy of Pediatrics, Committee on Nutrition, Vitamin K supplementation for infants receiving milk substitute infant formulas and for those with fat malabsorption, *Pediatrics,* 48, 483, 1971.

24. **Martinez, F. E., Goncalves, A. L., Jorge, S. M., and Desai, I. D.,** Vitamin E in placental blood and its interrelationship to maternal and newborn levels of vitamin E, *J. Pediatr.,* 99, 298, 1981.

25. **Shearer, M. J.,** Vitamin K metabolism and nutriture, *Blood Reviews,* 6, 92, 1992.

26. **Shearer, M. J., McCarthy, P. T., Crampton, O. E., and Mattock, M. B.,** The assessment of human vitamin K status from tissue measurements, in *Current Advances in Vitamin K Research,* Suttie, J. W., Ed., Elsevier, New York, 1988, 437.

27. **Mandelbrot, L., Guillaumont, M., Leclercq, M., Lefrère, J. J., Gozin, D., Daffos, F., and Forestier, F.,** Placental transfer of vitamin K_1 and its implications in fetal hemostasis, *Thromb. Haemostas.,* 60, 39, 1988.

28. **Pietersma-de Bruyn, A. L. J. M., van Haard, P. M. M., Beunis, M. H., Hamalyák, K., and Kuijpers, J. C.,** Vitamin K_1 levels and coagulation factors in healthy term newborns till 4 weeks after birth, *Haemostasis,* 20, 8, 1990.

29. **Yang, Y.-M., Simon, N., Maertens, P., Brigham, S., and Liu, P.,** Maternal-fetal transport of vitamin K_1 and its effect on coagulation in premature infants, *J. Pediatr.,* 115, 1009, 1989.

30. **Shearer, M. J., Rahim, S., Barkhan, P., and Stimmler, L.,** Plasma vitamin K_1 in mothers and their newborn babies, *Lancet,* 2, 460, 1982.

31. Bolton-Smith, C. and Shearer M. J., unpublished data, 1992.

32. **Hamulyák, K, De Boer-van den Berg, M. A. G., Thijssen, H. H. W., Hemker, H. C., and Vermeer, C.,** The placental transport of [³H] vitamin K_1 in rats, *Brit. J. Haematol.,* 65, 335, 1987.

33. **Kayata, S., Kindberg, C., Greer, F. R., and Suttie, J. W.,** Vitamin K_1 and K_2 in infant human liver, *J. Pediatr. Gastroenterol. Nutr.,* 8, 304, 1989.

34. **Shirahata, A., Nakamura, T., and Ariyoshi, N.,** Vitamin K_1 and K_2 contents in blood, stool, and liver tissues of neonates and young infants, in *Perinatal Thrombosis and Hemostasis,* Suzuki, S., Hathaway W. E., Bonnar, J., Sutor, A. H., Eds., Springer-Verlag, Tokyo, 1991, 213.

35. **Salomonsen, L.,** On the prevention of hemorrhagic disease of the newborn by the administration of cow's milk during the first two days of life, *Acta Paediatr.,* 28, 1 1940.

36. **Sutherland, J. M., Glueck, H. I., and Gleser, G.,** Hemorrhagic disease of the newborn: Breast-feeding as a necessary factor in the pathogenesis, *Am. J. Dis. Child.,* 113, 524, 1967.

37. **Canfield, L. M. and Hopkinson, J. M.,** State of the art vitamin K in human milk, *J. Pediatr. Gastroenterol. Nutr.,* 8, 430, 1989.

38. **Dam, H., Glavind, J., Larsen, E. H., and Plum P.,** Investigations into the cause of the physiological hypoprothrombinemia in newborn children IV. The vitamin K content of woman's milk and cow's milk, *Acta Med. Scand.,* 112, 210, 1942.

39. **Haroon, Y., Shearer, M. J., Rahim, S., Gunn, W. G., McEnery, G., and Barkhan, P.,** The content of phylloquinone (vitamin K_1) in human milk, cow's milk and infant formula foods determined by high-performance liquid chromatography, *J. Nutr.,* 112, 1105, 1982.

40. **Isshiki, H., Suzuki, Y., Yonekubo, A., Hasegawa, H. and Yamamoto, Y.,** Determination of phylloquinone and menaquinone in human milk using high performance liquid chromatography, *J. Dairy Sci.,* 71, 627, 1988.

41. **Bach, A. and Shearer, M. J.,** unpublished data, 1990.

42. **Isarangkura, P. B., Mahadandana, C., Panstienkul, B., Nakayama, K., Tsijkimoto, I., Yamamoto, Y., and Yonekubo, A.,** Vitamin K level in maternal breast milk of infants with acquired prothrombin complex deficiency syndrome, *Southeast Asian J. Trop. Med. Pub. Hlth.,* 14, 275, 1983.

43. **Motohara, K., Matsukura, M., Matsuda, I., Iribe, K., Ikeda, T., Kondo, Y., Yonekubo, A., Yamamoto, Y., and Tsuchiya, F.,** Severe vitamin K deficiency in breast-fed infants, *J. Pediatr.,* 105, 943, 1984.

44. **Fournier, B., Sann, L., Guillaumont, M., and Leclercq, M.,** Variations of phylloquinone concentration in human milk at various stages of lactation and in cow's milk at various seasons, *Am. J. Clin. Nutr.,* 45, 551, 1987.

45. **von Kries, R., Shearer, M., McCarthy, P. T., Haug, M., Harzer, G., and Göbel, U.,** Vitamin K_1 content of maternal milk: influence of the stage of lactation, lipid composition, and vitamin K_1 supplements given to the mother, *Pediatr. Res.,* 22, 513, 1987.

46. **Ferris, A. M. and Jensen, R. G.,** Lipids in human milk: a review. 1. Sampling, determination and content, *J. Pediatr. Gastroenterol. Nutr.,* 3, 108, 1984.

47. **Harzer, G. and Haug, M.,** Abhängigkeit der Frauenmilchlipide von der Dauer der stillperiode, der Tageszeit, dem Stillvorgang und der mütterlichen Ernährung. *Z. Ernährungswiss,* 23, 113, 1984.

48. **Dostálová, L., Salmenperä, L., Václavinková, V., Heinz-Erian, P., and Schuep, W.** Vitamin concentration in term milk of European mothers, in *Vitamins and Minerals in Pregnancy and Lactation,* Berger, H., Ed., Nestlé Nutrition Workshop Series, Vol. 16, Vevey/Raven Press, New York, 1988, 275.

49. **von Kries, R., Gobel, U., Shearer, M. J., and McCarthy, P. T.,** Vitamin K deficiency in breast-fed infants (letter), *J. Pediatr.,* 107, 650, 1985.

50. **Sawada, K. and Hanawa, Y.,** Vitamin K_1 content of human milk in various maternal nutritional states, in *Vitamins and Minerals in Pregnancy and Lactation,* Berger H., Ed., Nestlé Nutrition Workshop Series, Vol. 16, Vevey/Raven Press, New York, 1988, 389.

51. **Porter, J. W. G.,** *Milk and Dairy Foods,* Oxford University Press, Oxford, 1975, 5.

52. American Academy of Pediatrics, Committee on Nutrition, Commentary on breast-feeding and infant formulas, *Pediatrics,* 57, 278, 1976.

53. Committee on Medical Aspects of Food Policy (U.K.), Artificial feeds for the young infant, *Department of Health and Social Security, Report on Health and Social Subjects No. 18,* HMSO, London, 1980, 38.

54. **Widdershoven, J., Lambert, W., Motohara, K., Monnens, L., de Leenheer, A., Matsuda, I., and Endo, F.,** Plasma concentrations of vitamin K_1 and PIVKA-II in bottle-fed and breast-fed infants, *Eur. J. Pediatr.,* 148, 139, 1988.

55. **Greer, F. R., Marshall, S., Cherry, J., and Suttie, J. W.,** Vitamin K status of lactating mothers, human milk, and breast-feeding infants, *Pediatrics,* 88, 751, 1991.

56. **Uchida, K., and Komeno, T.,** Relationships between dietary and intestinal vitamin K, clotting factor levels, plasma vitamin K, and urinary Gla, in *Current Advances in Vitamin K Research,* Suttie, J. W., Ed., Elsevier, New York, 1988, 477.

57. **Usui, Y., Tanimura, H., Nishimura, N., Kobayashi, N., Okanoue, T., and Ozawa, K.,** Vitamin K concentrations in the liver and plasma of surgical patients, *Am. J. Clin. Nutr.,* 51, 846, 1990.

58. **Suttie, J. W., Mummah-Schendel, L. L., Shah, D. V., Lyle, B. J., and Greger, J. L.,** Vitamin K deficiency from dietary vitamin K restriction in humans, *Am. J. Clin. Nutr.,* 47, 475, 1988.

59. **Will, B. H. and Suttie, J. W.,** Comparative metabolism of phylloquinone and mena-quinone-9 in rat liver, *J. Nutr.,* 122, 953, 1992.

60. **Keenan, W. J., Jewett, T., and Glueck, H.,** Role of feeding and vitamin K in hypo-prothrombinemia of the newborn, *Am. J. Dis. Child.,* 121, 271, 1971.

61. **Yoshioka, H., Iseki, K., and Fujita, K.,** Development and differences of intestinal flora in the neonatal period in breast-fed and bottle-fed infants, *Pediatrics,* 72, 317, 1983.

62. **Ramotar, K., Conly J. M., Chubb, H., and Louie, T. J.,** Production of menaquinones by intestinal anaerobes, *J. Infect. Dis.,* 150, 213, 1984.

63. **Mathers, J. C., Fernandez, F., Hill, M. J., McCarthy, P. T., Shearer, M. J., and Oxley, A.,** Dietary modification of potential vitamin K supply from enteric bacterial menaquinones in rats, *Br. J. Nutr.,* 63, 639, 1990.

64. **Collins, M. D. and Jones, D.,** Distribution of isoprenoid quinone structural types in bacteria and their taxonomic implications, *Microbiol. Rev.,* 45, 316, 1981.

65. **Greer, F. R., Mummah-Schendel, L. L., Marshall, S., and Suttie, J. W.,** Vitamin K_1 (phylloquinone) and vitamin K_2 (menaquinone) status in newborns during the first week of life, *Pediatrics,* 81, 137, 1988.

66. **Koppe, J. G., Pluim, E., and Olie, K.,** Breastmilk, PCBs, dioxins, and vitamin K deficiency: discussion paper, *J. Roy. Soc. Med.,* 82, 416, 1989.

67. **von Kries, R., Becker, A., and Göbel, U.,** Vitamin K in the newborn: influence of nutritional factors on acarboxyprothrombin detectability and factor II and VII clotting activity, *Eur. J. Pediatr.,* 146, 123, 1987.

68. **Rosegger, H. and Pürstner, P.,** Zufütterung von volladaptierter Kunstmilch oder ka-lorienlosem Tee in den ersten Lebenstagen, *Wien. Klin. Wochenschr.,* 97, 411, 1985.

69. **Gobel, U., Sonnenschein-Kosenow, S., Petrich, C., and von Voss, H.,** Vitamin K deficiency in the newborn (letter), *Lancet,* 2, 187, 1977.

70. **Gobel, U., von Kries, R., Bewersdorff, S., Henninghausen, B., and Schmidt, E.,** Erniedrigte Prothrombin – Gerinnungsaktivitäten bei gestillten Kindern? *Klin. Pädiatr.* 198, 13, 1986.

71. **McNinch, A. W., Orme, R., and Tripp, J. H.,** Haemorrhagic disease of the newborn returns, *Lancet,* 1, 1089, 1983.

72. **Stintzing, G. and Zetterström, R.,** Cow's milk allergy. Incidence and pathogenic role of early exposure to cow's milk formula, *Acta Paediatr. Scand.,* 68, 383, 1979.

73. **Behrmann, B. A., Chan, W. K., and Finer, N. N.,** Resurgence of hemorrhagic disease of the newborn: a report of three cases, *Can. Med. Assoc. J.,* 133, 884, 1985.

74. **Jimenéz, R., Navarrete, M., Jiménez, E., Mora, L. A., and Robles, G.,** Vitamin K-dependent clotting factors in normal breast-fed infants, *J. Pediatr.,* 100, 424, 1982.

75. **Widdershoven, J., Kollee, L., von Munster, P., Bosman, A. M., and Monnens, L.,** Biochemical vitamin K deficiency in early infancy: diagnostic limitation of conventional coagulation tests, *Helv. Paediatr. Acta,* 41, 195, 1986.

76. **von Kries, R., Maase, B., Becker, A., and Göbel, U.,** Latent vitamin K deficiency in healthy infants (Letter), *Lancet,* 2, 1421, 1985.

77. **Buller, H., Peters, M., Burger, B., Nagelkerke, N., Ten Cate, J. W., Breedervelt, C., and Heymans, H.,** Vitamin K status beyond the neonatal period: a prospective study in normal breast-fed and formula-fed infants, *Eur. J. Pediatr.,* 145, 496, 1986.

78. **Widdershoven, J., Motohara, K., Endo, F., Matsuda, I., and Monnens, L.,** Influence of the type of feeding on the presence of PIVKA-II in infants, *Helv. Paediatr. Acta,* 41, 25, 1986.

79. **Motohara, K., Endo, F., and Matsuda, I.,** Vitamin K deficiency in breast-fed infants at one month of age, *J.Pediatr. Gastroenterol.,* 5, 931, 1986.

80. **Motohara, K., Endo, F., and Matsuda, I.,** Screening for late neonatal vitamin K deficiency by acarboxyprothrombin in dried blood spots, *Arch. Dis. Child.,* 62, 370, 1987.

81. **Widdershoven, J., van Munster, P., De Abreu, R., Bosman, H., van Lith, T., van der Putten-van Meyel, M., Motohara, K., and Matsuda, I.,** Four methods compared for measuring des-carboxy-prothrombin (PIVKA-II), *Clin. Chem.,* 33, 2074, 1987.

82. **Motohara, K., Kuroki, Y., Kan, H., Endo, F., and Matsuda, I.,** Detection of vitamin K deficiency by use of an enzyme-linked immunoabsorbent assay for circulating abnormal prothrombin, *Pediatr. Res.,* 19, 354, 1985.

83. **von Kries, R., Shearer, M. J., Widdershoven, J., Motohara, K., Umbach, G., and Göbel, U.,** Des-gamma-carboxyprothrombin (PIVKA II) and plasma vitamin K_1 in newborns and their mothers, *Thromb. Haemostas.,* 68, 383, 1992.

84. **Motohara, K., Endo, F., and Matsuda, I.,** Effects of vitamin K administration on acarboxy prothrombin (PIVKA-II) levels in newborns, *Lancet,* 2, 242, 1985.

85. **von Kries, R., Göbel, U., and Maase, B.,** Vitamin K deficiency in the newborn (letter), *Lancet,* 2, 728, 1985.

86. **Shapiro, A. D., Jacobson, L. J., Armon, M. E., Manco-Johnson, M. J., Hulac, P., Lane, P. A., and Hathaway, W. E.,** Vitamin K deficiency in the newborn infant: prevalence and perinatal risk factors, *J. Pediatr.,* 109, 675, 1986.

87. **von Kries, R.,** Untersuchungen zur Bedeutung der Muttermilch-Ernährung für Vitamin K-Mangelblutungen bei Neugeborenen und Säuglingen. Thieme, New York, 1991.

88. **Nilehn, J. E., and Ganrot, P. O.,** Plasma prothrombin during treatment with dicumarol, *Scand. J. Clin. Lab. Invest.,* 22, 17, 1968.

89. **Ganrot, P. O., and Nilehn, J. E.,** Plasma prothrombin during treatment with dicumarol. II. Demonstration of an abnormal prothrombin fraction, *Scand. J. Clin. Lab. Invest.,* 22, 23, 1968.

90. **von Kries, R., Tangermann, R., Shearer, M. J., and Göbel, U.,** Vitamin K deficiency in breast-fed infants, in *Human Lactation. 3. The Effects of Human Milk on the Recipient Infant,* Goldman, A. S., Atkinson, S. A., and Hanson, L. A., Eds., Plenum Press, New York, 1987, 317.

91. **von Kries, R., Reifenhäuser, A., Göbel, U., McCarthy, P. T., Shearer, M. J., and Barkhan, P.,** Late onset haemorrhagic disease of newborn with temporary malabsorption of vitamin K_1 (letter), *Lancet,* 1, 1035, 1985.

92. **Shearer, M. J., McBurney, A., and Barkhan, P.,** Studies on the absorption and metabolism of phylloquinone (vitamin K_1) in man, *Vitam. Horm.,* 32, 513, 1974.

93. **Hope, P. L., Hall, M. A., Millward-Sadler, G. H., and Normand, I. C. S.,** Alpha-1-antitrypsin deficiency presenting as a bleeding diathesis in the newborn, *Arch. Dis. Child.,* 57, 68, 1982.

94. **Jenkins, H. R., Leonard, J. V., Kay, J. D. S., Pool, R. W., Sills, J. A., and Isherwood, D. M.,** Alpha-1-antitrypsin deficiency, bleeding diathesis, and intracranial haemorrhage, *Arch. Dis. Child.,* 57, 722, 1982.

95. **von Kries, R., Wahn, V., Koletzko, B., and Göbel, U.,** Späte Manifestation eines Vitamin-K-Mangels bei gestillten Säuglingen, *Monatsschr. Kinderheilkd.,* 132, 293, 1984.

96. **Mahdi, S., Bopp, E., Henke-Wolter, J. V., and Stockhausen, H. B.,** Zerebrale Blutung bei einem 4 Wochen alten Säugling mit homozytogem Alpha-1-Antitrypsinmangel, *Klin. Pädiatr.,* 196, 115, 1984.

97. **Payne, N. R. and Hasegawa, D. K.,** Vitamin K deficiency in newborns: a case report in α-1-antitrypsin deficiency and a review of factors predisposing to hemorrhage, *Pediatrics,* 73, 712, 1984.

98. **Radetti, G., Pittschieler, K., Dordi, B., and Mengarda, G.,** Neonatale Krampfe infolge einer Hirnblutung bei Alpha-1-Antitrypsin-Mangel, *Helv. Paediatr. Acta,* 40, 173, 1985.

99. **Brenner, B., Tavori, S., Zivelin, A., Keller, C. B., Suttie, J. W., Tatarsky, I., and Seligsohn, U.,** Hereditary deficiency of all vitamin K-dependent procoagulants and anticoagulants, *Brit. J. Haematol.,* 75, 537, 1990.

100. **Pauli, R. M., Lian, J. B., Mosher, D. F., and Suttie, J. W.,** Association of congenital deficiency of multiple vitamin K-dependent coagulation factors and the phenotype of the warfarin embryopathy: clues to the mechanism of teratogenicity of coumarin derivatives, *Am. J. Hum. Genet.,* 41, 566, 1987.

101. **Martin-Bouyer, G., Linh, P. D., Tuan, L. C., Barin, C., Khnah, N. B., Hoa, D. Q., Tourneau, J., Guerbois, H., and Binh, T. V.,** Epidemic of haemorrhagic disease in Vietnamese infants caused by warfarin-contaminated talcs, *Lancet,* 1, 230, 1983.

Chapter 13

ANTIBIOTIC-INDUCED HYPOPROTHROMBINEMIA: BIOCHEMICAL MECHANISM AND CLINICAL SIGNIFICANCE

John W. Suttie

TABLE OF CONTENTS

0-8493-6423-X/93/$0.00 + $.50

267

I. INTRODUCTION

Vitamin K deficiency in the adult, with associated hypoprothrombinemia, is a relatively rare but well documented condition. Because of the lipoidal nature of the vitamin, biliary obstruction, pancreatic insufficiency, sprue, bowel disease, and a number of miscellaneous intestinal disorders have been reported to be associated with a vitamin K responsive hypoprothrombinemia.[1] Most cases of adult vitamin K deficiency, however, have been associated with antibiotic administration. As early as the late 1940s and early 1950s, antibiotic therapy was recognized as a potential contributing factor in the development of a potentially serious hypoprothrombinemia.[2,3] The widely cited study of Frick et al.[4] clearly demonstrated the importance of antibiotic administration to the development of vitamin K deficiency in subjects given only parenteral glucose, electrolytes, and vitamins. Two more recent studies of hospital records[5,6] have adequately demonstrated that vitamin K deficiency in hospitalized patients can contribute to morbidity and mortality, and that these bleeding problems are almost always associated with antibiotic administration.

There are numerous case reports of antibiotic induced hypoprothrombinemia in the literature,[1,7] and a review of the available data indicates that these reactions are not limited to the use of a single antibiotic. In a retrospective study of 42 patients, Alperin[6] noted a predominant use of penicillin, semi-synthetic penicillins, and cephalosporins, but also reported the use of aminoglycosides, trimethoprim, chloramphenicol, amphotericin B, erythromycin, and clindamycin. As many patients received combination antibiotic treatment, it is difficult to assign relative risk, but it is clear that these adverse reactions were not limited to a single type of antibiotic.

II. HYPOPROTHROMBINEMIA AND THE CLINICAL USE OF NMTT-CONTAINING ANTIBIOTICS

Although antibiotic induced hypoprothrombinemia had been observed for nearly 40 years, an apparent increase in incidence in the early 1980s appeared to be associated with the use of a number of the newer β-lactam antibiotics.[8-12] These early reports were largely associated with the administration of the cephalosporin, cefamandole, or the related oxa-β-lactam, moxalactam, but subsequent studies[13] have implicated a number of other cephalosporins with a *N*-methylthiotetrazole (NMTT) side chain. Successful β-lactam antibiotics have a combination of high antibacterial properties, stability to β-lactamase action, and desirable pharmacokinetic characteristics. The NMTT group improves antibacterial action[14] and antibiotics with this functional group include cefoperazone, cefmetazole, cefotetan, and cefmenoxime (Figure 1). Cefazolin does not contain NMTT but does have a structurally related methyl-thiadiazole-thiol (MTD) side chain. Studies of antibiotic use by nearly 1500 patients in a single medical center[15] or reviews of a number of smaller studies[7]

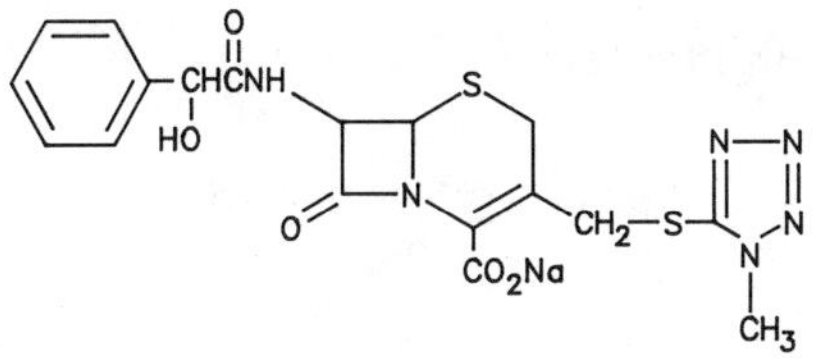

Cefamandole, Sodium

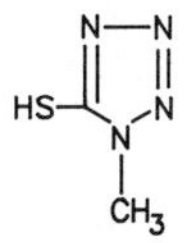

NMTT

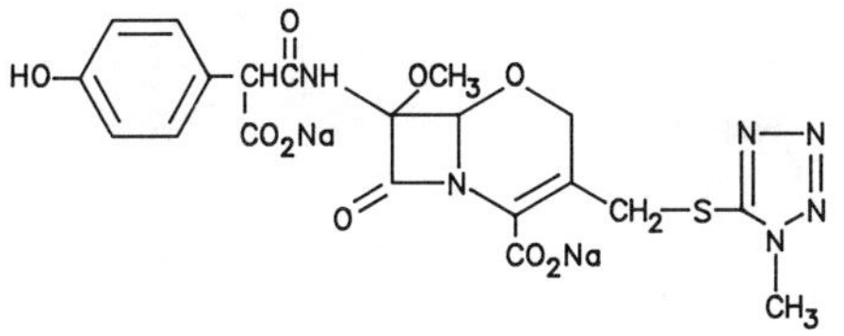

moxalactam, disodium

FIGURE 1. Structure of cefamandole and moxalactam. Both of these antibiotics contain a *N*-methyl-thiotetrazole side-chain linked to the dihydrothiazine ring of the cephalosporin cefamandole or to the dihydrooxazine ring of the analogous oxa-β-lactam, moxalactam. The other NMTT-containing antibiotics have different functional groups attached to the four-membered β-lactam ring.

clearly indicate that use of these antibiotics has increased the incidence of antibiotic related coagulopathies.

The early observations of adverse reactions prompted a series of investigations into the basis for the apparent increase in hypoprothrombinemic potential of this class of β-lactam antibiotics. Antibiotic-induced hypoprothrombinemia has historically been assumed to be due to a decrease in the synthesis of menaquinones by gut organisms and has been based on the premise that these menaquinones are important in satisfying at least a portion of the normal human requirement for vitamin K. Although this is a widely held position,[16] data to assess the relative contribution of dietary phylloquinone and gut menaquinones to the human requirement of vitamin K are nonexistent. It is also possible that an antibiotic could alter the absorption or metabolism of vitamin K, or that an antibiotic or a metabolite of an antibiotic could interfere with the action of the vitamin K-dependent carboxylase. This is the enzyme responsible for the formation of the γ-carboxyglutamyl (Gla) residues essential for the normal function of the vitamin K-dependent plasma clotting factors.[17] Interference with Gla formation could occur either by direct inhibition of the enzyme or by an interference with the generation of the active cofactor, reduced vitamin K from vitamin K-2,3epoxide. Inhibition of the vitamin K-epoxide reductase is the site of action of the commonly used coumarin anticoagulants.[18] These possibilities of a metabolic antagonism of vitamin K action by an antibiotic are summarized in Figure 2.

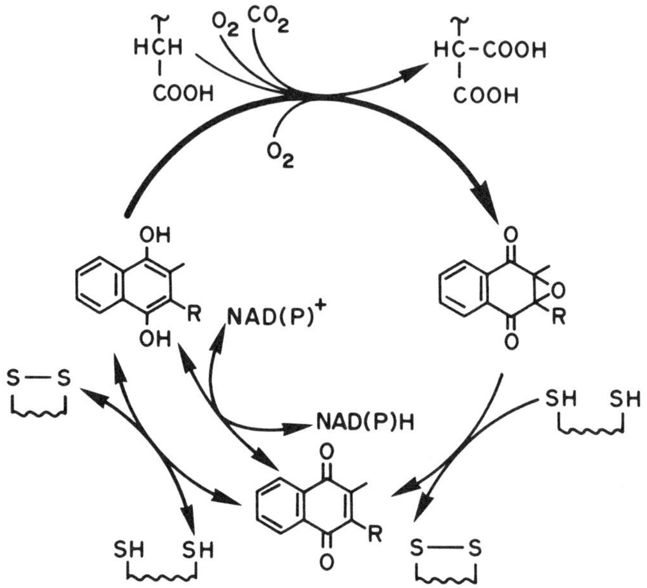

FIGURE 2. Vitamin K metabolism in liver. The vitamin K-dependent carboxylase catalyzes the O_2 and CO_2-dependent carboxylation of specific glutamyl residues of a limited number of proteins to γ-carboxyglutamyl residues. Vitamin K-2,3-epoxide is a second product of this reaction and is converted to the quinone form of the vitamin by a dithiol-dependent enzyme. A second dithiol-dependent activity, which may be catalyzed by the same enzyme, can reduce the quinone to the active cofactor for the carboxylase, hydroquinone form of the vitamin, vitamin KH_2. These two dithiol-dependent activities are effectively blocked by coumarin anticoagulants such as warfarin leading to an increase in vitamin K epoxide and a decrease in the concentration of vitamin KH_2.

A. EFFECT OF NMTT-CONTAINING ANTIBIOTICS ON MENAQUINONE PRODUCTION

The β-lactam and oxacepham antibiotics associated with bleeding problems are administered intravenously, but significant biliary excretion does occur,[19-21] and the potential for interference with the gut microflora does exist. *Escherichia coli* and *Bacterillum fragilis* organisms are the major producers of menaquinones in the gut,[22-24] and the population of these organisms in stool cultures has been shown to be decreased by moxalactam administration to healthy volunteers[25] or patients.[26] The influence of these antibiotics on menaquinone production is, however, not yet clearly defined. Ramotar et al.[27] found that moxalactam and ticarcillin or moxalactam and tobramycin significantly reduced fecal *E. coli* and *B. fragilis* numbers and fecal menaquinone concentrations in neutropenic patients. Suttie et al.[28] found that three of nine volunteers receiving NMTT-containing antibiotics (cefamandole, cefoperazone, and moxalactam) showed a decrease in total fecal menaquinones, while five of nine showed an increase. In a rat model, Ramotar et al.[29] demonstrated that moxalactam administration will decrease total cecum menaquinone concentrations, but no more than two other antibiotics, cefoxitin and gentamicin, that do not contain a NMTT side chain. The available data therefore, have demonstrated that those antibiotics whose clinical use has been most associated with a severe hypoprothrombinemia can influence both fecal flora distribution and menaquinone production. However, the effects appear variable and many non-NMTT containing antibiotics have similar effects.

B. EFFECTS OF NMTT-CONTAINING ANTIBIOTICS ON VITAMIN K-DEPENDENT γ-CARBOXYLATION

Most of the recent interest in the NMTT-containing antibiotics has centered on the possibility that they are directly or indirectly inhibiting the vitamin K-dependent γ-carboxylation of prothrombin and the other vitamin K-dependent plasma clotting factors. Uotila and Suttie[30] studied the effects of cefamandole and some of its structural analogs and found an I_{50} (50% inhibition level) for the carboxylase of 6 to 10 mM and reported that the epoxide reductase was less sensitive. These concentrations appeared to be much higher than tissue levels achievable with therapeutic doses of these antibiotics. Smith and Lipsky[31] first suggested that the NMTT side chain, which could be released from these antibiotics in the intestine or by metabolism,[32,33] could directly inhibit the vitamin K-dependent carboxylase. Lipsky[34] subsequently reported that NMTT could inhibit the vitamin K-dependent carboxylase with an I_{50} of 1.1 mM. These results were in an *in vitro* system where the active naphthoquinone cofactor, vitamin KH$_2$, was generated from NADH and vitamin K quinone by reductases present in the crude microsomal preparation. A similar degree of inhibition was not observed in the same system or in incubations where vitamin KH$_2$ was utilized as the active cofactor by other investigators.[35,36] In a more extensive study,[37] Lipsky demonstrated that the inhibition of the carboxylase by NMTT was time dependent and that the disulfide dimer of NMTT, with an I_{50} of about 0.1 mM, was a more potent inhibitor. These observations suggested that the dimer or some other metabolite whose formation was time dependent might be responsible for the inhibition, and other studies[38] suggested that thiol metabolism may have a significant effect on the inhibitory activity. The inhibition observed in the studies could have been caused by inhibition of the carboxylase or by the enzymes involved in generating vitamin KH$_2$. Suttie and co-workers[39] subsequently demonstrated that the microsomal quinone reductases are not inhibited by NMTT and that the presence of NADH in the incubation is required for the time-dependent inhibition. Similar observations have been reported by Uchida and Komeno[40] who have also shown that the enhancement of inhibition is specific for NADH and that NADPH is ineffective. These *in vitro* studies have shown that given the correct incubation conditions, the vitamin K-dependent carboxylase is inhibited by NMTT. Tissue levels of free NMTT in subjects administered cefamandole[41] do not reach those needed for *in vitro* inhibition, but metabolism to a more active compound cannot be ruled out. However, it is significant that in none of the *in vitro* studies was the inhibition by NMTT reversed by increasing the vitamin K concentration of the incubation, while most cases of hypoprothrombinemia induced by NMTT-containing antibiotics appear to be vitamin K responsive.

C. RELATIONSHIP OF HYPOPROTHROMBINEMIA TO ADMINISTRATION OF NMTT-CONTAINING ANTIBIOTICS

The ability of these antibiotics to produce a vitamin K deficiency in experimental subjects or animal models has also been studied. Bang et al.[42] administered moxalactam to normal male volunteers for 1 week with no influence on the plasma concentration of prothrombin or factors VII, IX, or X. There was also no evidence, by the use of a relatively sensitive assay, of an increase in the circulating levels of abnormal (des-γ-carboxy) prothrombin. Weitekamp et al.[43] administered latamoxef (moxalactam) or cefoperazone to healthy adult volunteers for 6 d with no change in prothrombin times or partial thromboplastin times, and Bowcock et al.[44] found no change in these he-mostatic parameters in six patients administered moxalactam. Allison et al.[45] fed male volunteers a low vitamin K diet (2 to 5 μg phylloquinone per day for 13 d and administered one of ten different antibiotics during the last 10 d of this regimen. Three of these antibiotics contained a NMTT side chain and seven did not. No changes in one-stage prothrombin times were observed, but 7 of 33 subjects exhibited a factor VII level below the normal range and 21 of the 33 showed an alteration in a specialized clotting assay designed to measure increases in circulating des-γ-carboxyprothrombin. The incidence of these apparent indices of vitamin K deficiency was not correlated to the administration of antibiotics containing a NMTT side chain.

The commonly used clinical one-stage prothrombin time is an extremely insensitive indication of vitamin K sufficiency, and immunochemical assay of circulating des-γ-carboxyprothrombin[46,47] provides a much more sensitive means of assessing what has been called a "subclinical" vitamin K deficiency. Barza et al.[48] have retrospectively studied the sera of neutropenic, febrile cancer patients receiving a course of treatment with tobramycin in combination with moxalactam, ticarcillin, or piperacillin. By the sensitive assay utilized in this study, 27 of 40 patients had an elevated level of abnormal prothrombin prior to a course of antibiotic treatment indicating a pre-existing subclinical deficiency. During the course of treatment, the level of abnormal prothrombin increased in only 2 of 31 patients receiving piperacillin or ticarcillin, but increased in 9 of 12 patients receiving moxalactam, including 6 of 9 who were also receiving supplemental vitamin K. These data confirm the hypoth-esis that large numbers of seriously ill patients, for whom antibiotic therapy is indicated, have borderline vitamin K status prior to treatment and that this is the population that develops problems following therapy with NMTT-containing antibiotics.

The ability of intact NMTT-containing antibiotics or NMTT to produce hypoprothrombinemia in an animal model also appears to depend on vitamin

K status. Wold et al.[49] reported that up to 500 mg/kg (s.c.) of NMTT in the rat or 100 mg/kg (i.v.) in the dog for 30 d did not influence prothrombin times. These levels were shown[50] to result in higher plasma NMTT concentrations than those resulting from the administration of moxalactam to patients. Lipsky et al.[51] subsequently demonstrated that either oral NMTT or intravenous moxalactam would enhance the degree of hypoprothrombinemia observed in rats fed a vitamin K-deficient diet for 10 d. The non-NMTT containing antibiotic, cefotaxime, did not have this effect. More extensive data were reported by Uchida et al.[52] who demonstrated that NMTT would increase prothrombin times in male rats fed a vitamin K-deficient diet, but not a normal diet. This increase was more pronounced in germ-free vitamin K-deficient rats.

D. INHIBITION OF THE VITAMIN K EPOXIDE REDUCTASE

A clearer understanding of the nature of the NMTT response was obtained by Bechtold et al.[53] who demonstrated the presence of significant amounts of circulating vitamin K 2,3-epoxide following vitamin K administration to hypoprothrombinemic patients receiving moxalactam. This response was identical to that observed following treatment with the oral anticoagulant phenprocoumon and is consistent with the known effect of coumarin anticoagulants in blocking the recycling of vitamin K epoxide to vitamin K.[18] The hypothesis that antibiotics containing NMTT are inhibitors of vitamin K epoxide reductase was confirmed in an animal model by Creedon and Suttie[54] who demonstrated that epoxide reductase activity was decreased in livers obtained from rats administered NMTT and that both plasma and liver vitamin K epoxide concentrations were increased by this treatment. The *in vitro* activity of the enzyme was not inhibited, suggesting that metabolism of NMTT is required to produce the effect.

The importance of a pre-existing marginal vitamin K status as a risk factor for antibiotic-induced hypoprothrombinemia has been recognized for some time.[55,56] The importance of vitamin K status to the development of a hypoprothrombinemic response to NMTT-containing antibiotics was pointed out by Shearer and his associates[57,58] who demonstrated that it was those patients with low circulating plasma phylloquinone concentrations and other indicators of low nutritional status who were susceptible to this response. Well-nourished patients with normal serum vitamin K levels were able to maintain normal prothrombin times and factor VII levels through a normal course of treatment with a NMTT-containing cephalosporin. In a subsequent study,[59] it was demonstrated that all patients receiving NMTT containing antibiotics showed an increase in circulating vitamin K epoxide following a test dose of vitamin K, but only those on parenteral nutrition with a pre-existing decreased concentration of circulating vitamin K developed a prolonged prothrombin time. Patients receiving non-NMTT containing antibiotics did not have prolonged prothrombin times, and did not respond by increasing circulating vitamin K epoxide when given a test dose of vitamin K.

The results of these recent studies appear to conclusively demonstrate that antibiotics containing a NMTT side chain or a MTD side chain (cefazolin) are capable of causing an inhibition of the hepatic epoxide reductase resulting in a coumarin-like response in the synthesis of vitamin K-dependent coagulation factors. However, these antibiotics are very weak anticoagulants and an adverse response is seen only in those patients with low vitamin K status. This response is similar to that previously observed in studies of the anticoagulant action of salicylate.[60-62] In most cases, the condition resulting from antibiotic administration appears to be readily reversible by vitamin K,[7] and prophylactic vitamin K is strongly recommended for all patients treated with these antibiotics who might have low vitamin K stores.

III. GENERALIZED ANTIBIOTIC EFFECTS ON HEMOSTASIS

The potential for bleeding episodes following antibiotic treatment is not restricted to effects on the synthesis of vitamin K-dependent clotting factors but may also involve platelet dysfunction. This dysfunction is measured clinically by a prolongation of the template bleeding time and biochemically by a suppression of ADP-induced platelet aggregation. This effect has been noted following the administration of a large number of different β-lactam antibiotics[13,42,63] and is not restricted to the NMTT-containing second generation cephalosporins. However, moxalactam appears to be more likely to interfere with platelet function than many other antibiotics,[43,44] and the high incidence of adverse reactions associated with this particular oxacephem may have been due to both its coumarin-like action and an induced platelet dysfunction.

The demonstration that NMTT containing antibiotics have a weak coumarin-like effect does not rule out the possibility that they also have an effect on the bacterial flora of the lower bowel and on menaquinone production. Cohen et al.[58] have reported on 11 patients with low vitamin K status that developed a hypoprothrombinemia following antibiotic treatment. Of these 11, 4 received a non-NMTT containing antibiotic that has no known coumarin-like effect. A review of the clinical literature clearly indicates that there have been numerous reports of antibiotic induced hypoprothrombinemia or bleeding episodes over the last 40 years[1,7] and that only recently have these involved NMTT-containing antibiotics. The early study of Frick et al.[4] indicated that parenterally fed patients receiving no oral vitamin K became hypoprothrombinemic only when an unspecified antibiotic was administered. Human liver has been shown to contain longchain bacterially synthesized menaquinones,[64-65] and recent data[40,66,67] suggest that the total amount of this form of vitamin K in human liver greatly exceeds that of phylloquinone. As most foods contain only small amounts of menaquinones, the assumption has been that the presence of liver menaquinones is evidence for the absorption of bacterially produced menaquinones from the large bowel. However, the ability to produce mild signs of vitamin K deficiency by dietary restriction of phylloquinone in subjects not receiving antibiotics[68] would suggest that menaquinones may not be an important factor in human nutrition. Clearly a great deal of additional information on menaquinone production, absorption, and turnover will be needed before inhibition of menaquinone production as a factor in antibiotic-induced hypoprothrombinemia can be accurately assessed.

REFERENCES

1. **Savage, D. and Lindenbaum, J.,** Clinical and experimental human vitamin K deficiency, in *Nutrition in Hematology,* Lindenbaum, J., Ed., Churchill Livingstone, New York, 1983, 271.
2. **Harris, H. J.,** Aureomycin and chloramphenicol in brucellosis: with special reference to side effects, *JAMA,* 142, 161, 1950.
3. **Haden, H. T.,** Vitamin K deficiency associated with prolonged antibiotic administration, *Arch. Intern. Med.,* 100, 986, 1957.
4. **Frick, P. G., Riedler, G., and Brögli, H.,** Dose response and minimal daily requirement for vitamin K in man, *J. Appl. Physiol.,* 23, 387, 1967.
5. **Ansell, J. E., Kumar, R., and Deykin, D.,** The spectrum of vitamin K deficiency, *JAMA,* 238, 40, 1977.
6. **Alperin, J. B.,** Coagulopathy caused by vitamin K deficiency in critically ill, hospitalized patients, *JAMA,* 258, 1916, 1987.
7. **Lipsky, J. J.,** Antibiotic-associated hypoprothrombinemia, *J. Antimicrob. Chemother.,* 21, 281, 1988.
8. **Reddy, J. and Bailey, R. R.,** Vitamin K deficiency developing in patients with renal failure treated with cephalosporin antibiotics, *N.Z. Med. J.,* 92, 378, 1980.
9. **Hooper, C. A., Haney, B. B., and Stone, H. H.,** Gastrointestinal bleeding due to vitamin K deficiency in patients on parenteral cefamandole, *Lancet,* i, 39, 1980.
10. **Weitekamp, M. R. and Aber, R. C.,** Prolonged bleeding times and bleeding diathesis associated with moxalactam administration, *JAMA,* 249, 69, 1983.
11. **Panwalker, A. P. and Rosenfeld, J.,** Hemorrhage, diarrhea, and superinfection associated with the use of moxalactam, *J. Infect. Dis.,* 147, 171, 1983.
12. **Fainstein, V., Bodey, G. P., McCredie, K. B., Keating, M. J., Estey, E. H., Bolivar, R., and Elting, L.,** Coagulation abnormalities induced by β-lactam antibiotics in cancer patients, *J. Infect. Dis.,* 148, 745, 1983.
13. **Sattler, F. R., Weitekamp, M. R., and Ballard, J. O.,** Potential for bleeding with the new beta-lactam antibiotics, *Ann. Int. Med.,* 105, 924, 1986.
14. **Webber, J. A. and Yoshida, T.,** Moxalactam: the first of a new class of β-lactam antibiotics, *Rev. Infect. Dis.,* 4, S496, 1982.
15. **Brown, R. B., Klar, J., Lemeshow, S., Teres, D., Pastides, H., and Sands, M.,** Enhanced bleeding with cefoxitin or moxalactam. Statistical analysis within a defined population of 1493 patients, *Arch. Intern. Med.,* 146, 2159, 1986.
16. **Olson, R. E.,** Vitamin K, in *Modern Nutrition in Health and Disease,* Goodhart, R. S. and Shils, M. E., Eds., Lea & Febiger, Philadelphia, 1980, 170.
17. **Suttie, J. W.,** Vitamin K-dependent carboxylase, *Annu. Rev. Biochem.,* 54, 459, 1985.
18. **Suttie, J. W.,** The biochemical basis of warfarin therapy, in *The New Dimensions of Warfarin Prophylaxis,* Wessler, S., Becker, C. G., and Nemerson, Y., Eds., Plenum Publishing, New York, 1987, 3.

19. **Quinn, E. L., Madhavan, T., Wixson, R., Guise, E., Levin, N., Block, M., Burch, K., Fisher, E., Suarez, A., and del Busto, R.,** Cefamandole: observations on its spectrum, concentration in bone and bile, excretion in renal failure, and clinical efficacy, in *Current Chemotherapy II,* Siegenthaler, W. and Luthy, R., Eds., American Society for Microbiology, Washington, D.C., 1978, 803.

20. **Shimada, J. and Ueda, Y.,** Moxalactam — absorption, excretion, distribution, and metabolism, *Rev. Infect. Dis.,* 4, S569, 1982.

21. **Uchida, K., Konishi, M., Akiyoshi, T., Igimi, H., and Asakawa, S.,** Biliary excretion of latamoxef and *N*-methyltetrazolethiol in humans and rats, *J. PharmacobioDyn.,* 8, 981, 1985.

22. **Collins, M. D. and Jones, D.,** Distribution of isoprenoid quinone structural types in bacteria and their taxonomic implications, *Microbiol. Rev.,* 45, 316, 1981.

23. **Ramotar, K., Conly, J. M., Chubb, H., and Louie, T. J.,** Production of menaquinones by intestinal anaerobes, *J. Infect. Dis.,* 150, 213, 1984.

24. **Fernandez, F. and Collins, M. D.,** Vitamin K composition of anaerobic gut bacteria, *FEMS Microbiol. Lett.,* 41, 175, 1987.

25. **Benno, Y., Shiragami, N., Uchida, K., Yoshida, T., and Mitsuoka, T.,** Effect of moxalactam on human fecal microflora, *Antimicrob. Agents Chemother.,* 29, 175, 1986.

26. **Conly, J. M., Ramotar, K., Chubb, H., Bow, E. J., and Louie, T. J.,** Hypoprothrombinemia in febrile, neutropenic patients with cancer: association with antimicrobial suppression of intestinal microflora, *J. Infect. Dis.,* 150, 202, 1984.

27. **Ramotar, K., Chubb, H., Rayner, E., Conley, J., Bow, E. J., and Louie, T. J.,** Effect of empiric antimicrobial regimens on fecal flora and menaquinone (MK) profiles in neutropenic patients, *Microecol. Ther.,* 15, 311, 1985.

28. **Suttie, J. W., Kindberg, C. G., Greger, J. L., and Bang, N. U.,** Effects of vitamin K (phylloquinone) restriction in the human, in *Current Advances in Vitamin K Research,* Suttie, J. W., Ed., Elsevier, New York, 1988, 465.

29. **Ramotar, K., Krulicki, W., Gray, G., and Louie, T. J.,** Studies on intestinal and hepatic concentrations of menaquinone and hypoprothrombinemia in vitamin K_1-deficient rats, in *Current Advances in Vitamin K Research,* Suttie, J. W., Ed., Elsevier, New York, 1988, 493.

30. **Uotila, L. and Suttie, J. W.,** Inhibition of vitamin K-dependent carboxylase in vitro by cefamandole and its structural analogs, *J. Infect. Dis.,* 148, 571, 1983.

31. **Smith, C. R. and Lipsky, J. J.,** Hypoprothrombinemia and platelet dysfunction caused by cephalosporin and oxalactam antibiotics, *J. Antimicrob. Chemother.,* 11, 496, 1983.

32. **Boyd, D. B. and Lunn, W. H. W.,** Electronic structures of cephalosporins and penicillins. IX. Departure of a leaving group in cephalosporins, *J. Med. Chem.,* 22, 778, 1979.

33. **Wise, R. and Dent, J.,** Stability of β-lactam antibiotics containing *N*-methylthiotetrazole side-chain, *Lancet,* ii, 624, 1983.

34. **Lipsky, J. J.,** *N*-methyl-thio-tetrazole inhibition of the gamma carboxylation of glutamic acid: possible mechanism for antibioticassociated hypoprothrombinaemia, *Lancet,* ii, 192, 1983.

35. **Uchida, K., Ishigami, T., and Komeno, T.,** Effects of latamoxef and methyltetrazolethiol on gamma-glutamylcarboxylase activity, *J. J. Pharmacol.,* 35, 330, 1984.

36. **Smith, G. F. and Sundboom, J. L.,** The effects of 1-methyl-5thiotetrazole in a rat liver vitamin K-dependent carboxylase assay, *Thromb. Res.,* 33, 633, 1984.

37. **Lipsky, J. J.,** Mechanism of the inhibition of the γ-carboxylation of glutamic acid by *N*methylthiotetrazole-containing antibiotics, *Proc. Natl. Acad. Sci. U.S.A.,* 81, 2893, 1984.

38. **Kerremans, A. L., Lipsky, J. J., Van Loon, J., Gallego, M. O., and Weinshilboum, R. M.,** Cephalosporin-induced hypoprothrombinemia: possible role for thiol methylation of 1-methyltetrazole-5-thiol and 2methyl-1,3,4-thiadiazole-5-thiol, *J. Pharmacol. Exp. Ther.,* 235, 382, 1985.

39. **Suttie, J. W., Engelke, J. A., and McTigue, J.,** Effect of *N*-methyl-thiotetrazole on rat liver microsomal vitamin K-dependent carboxylation, *Biochem. Pharmacol.,* 35, 2429, 1986.

40. **Uchida, K. and Komeno, T.,** Relationships between dietary and intestinal vitamin K, clotting factor levels, plasma vitamin K and urinary Gla, in *Current Advances in Vitamin K Research,* Suttie, J. W., Ed., Elsevier, New York, 1988, 477.

41. **Aronoff, G. R., Wolen, R. L., Obermeyer, B. D., and Black, H. R.,** Pharmacokinetics and protein binding of cefamandole and its 1-methyl-1 H-tetrazole-5-thiol side chain in subjects with normal and impaired renal function, *J. Infect. Dis.,* 153, 1069, 1986.

42. **Bang, N. U., Tessler, S. S., Heidenreich, R. O., Marks, C. A., and Mattler, L. E.,** Effects of moxalactam on blood coagulation and platelet function, *Rev. Infect. Dis.,* 4, S546, 1982.

43. **Weitekamp, M. R., Caputo, G. M., Al-Mondhiry, H. A. B., and Aber, R. C.,** The effects of latamoxef, cefotaxime, and cefoperazone on platelet function and coagulation in normal volunteers, *J. Antimicrob. Chemother.,* 16, 96, 1985.

44. **Bowcock, S., Mackie, E. J., Ho, D., Moulsdale, M., Billings, P., and Machin, S. J.,** Effects of various doses of latamoxef (moxalactam) on haemostasis, *J. Hosp. Infect.,* 8, 193, 1986.

45. **Allison, P. M., Mummah-Schendel, L. L., Kindberg, C. G., Harms, C. S., Bang, N. U., and Suttie, J. W.,** Effects of a vitamin K-deficient diet and antibiotics in normal human volunteers, *J. Lab. Clin. Med.,* 110, 180, 1987.

46. **Blanchard, R. A., Furie, B. C., Jorgensen, M., Kruger, S. F., and Furie, B.,** Acquired vitamin K-dependent carboxylation deficiency in liver disease, *N. Engl. J. Med.,* 305, 242, 1981.

47. **Blanchard, R. A., Furie, B. C., Kruger, S. F., Waneck, G., Jorgensen, M. J., and Furie, B.,** Immunoassays of human prothrombin species which correlate with functional coagulant activities, *J. Lab. Clin. Med.,* 101, 242, 1983.

48. **Barza, M., Furie, B., Brown, A. E., and Furie, B. C.,** Defects in vitamin Kdependent carboxylation associated with moxalactam treatment, *J. Infect. Dis.,* 153, 1166, 1986.

49. **Wold, J. S., Buening, M. K., and Hanasono, G. K.,** Latamoxef-associated hypo-prothrombinaemia, *Lancet,* ii, 408, 1983.

50. **Black, H. R., Buening, M. K., and Wolen, R. L.,** Latamoxef, its side chain, and coagulation, *Lancet,* ii, 1090, 1983.

51. **Lipsky, J. J., Lewis, J. C., and Novick, W. J., Jr.,** Production of hypoprothrombinemia by moxalactam and 1-methyl-5-thiotetrazole in rats, *Antimicrob. Agents Chemother.,* 25, 380, 1984.

52. **Uchida, K., Shike, T., Kakushi, H., Takase, H., Nomura, Y., Harauchi, T., and Yoshizaki, T.,** Effect of sex hormones on hypoprothrombinemia induced by *N*methyl-tetrazolethiol in rats, *Thromb. Res.,* 39, 741, 1985.

53. **Bechtold, H., Andrassy, K., Jahnchen, E., Koderisch, J., Koderisch, H., Weilemann, L. S., Sonntag, H.-G., and Ritz, E.,** Evidence for impaired hepatic vitamin K_1 metabolism in patients treated with *N*-methyl-thiotetrazole cephalosporins, *Thromb. Haemostas.,* 51, 358, 1984.

54. **Creedon, K. A. and Suttie, J. W.,** Effect of *N*-methyl-thiotetrazole on vitamin K epoxide reductase, *Thromb. Res.,* 44, 147, 153, 1986.

55. **Pineo, G. F., Gallus, A. S., and Hirsh, J.,** Unexpected vitamin K deficiency in hospitalized patients, *Can. Med. Assoc. J.,* 109, 880, 1973.

56. **Hands, L. J., Royle, G. T., and Kettlewell, M. G. W.,** Vitamin K requirements in patients receiving total parenteral nutrition, *Br. J. Surg.,* 72, 665, 1985.

57. **Mackie, I. J., Walshe, K., Cohen, H., McCarthy, P., Shearer, M., Scott, S. D., Karran, S. J., and Machin, S. J.,** Effects of *N*-methyl-thiotetrazole cephalosporin on haemostasis in patients with reduced serum vitamin K_1 concentrations, *J. Clin. Pathol.,* 39, 1245, 1986.

58. **Cohen, H., Scott, S. D., Mackie, I. J., Shearer, M., Bax, R., Karran, S. J., and Machin, S. J.,** The development of hypoprothrombinaemia following antibiotic therapy in malnourished patients with low serum vitamin K_1 levels, *Br. J. Haematol.,* 68, 63, 1988.

59. **Shearer, M. J., Bechtold, H., Andrassy, K., Koderisch, J., McCarthy, P. T., Trenk, D., Jahnchen, E., and Ritz, E.,** Mechanism of cephalosporin-induced hypoprothrombinemia: relation to cephalosporin side chain, vitamin K metabolism, and vitamin K status, *J. Clin. Pharmacol.,* 28, 88, 1988.

60. **Park, B. K. and Leck, J. B.,** On the mechanism of salicylate-induced hypoprothrombinaemia, *J. Pharm. Pharmacol.,* 33, 25, 1981.

61. **Hildebrandt, E. F. and Suttie, J. W.,** The effects of salicylate on enzymes of vitamin K metabolism, *J. Pharm. Pharmacol.,* 35, 421, 1983.

62. **Hildebrandt, E. and Suttie, J. W.,** Indirect inhibition of vitamin K epoxide reduction by salicylate, *J. Pharm. Pharmacol.,* 36, 586, 1984.

63. **Uchida, K., Kakushi, H., and Shike, T.,** Effect of latamoxef (moxalactam) and its related compounds on platelet aggregation in vitro — structure activity relationships, *Thromb. Res.,* 47, 215, 1987.

64. **Rietz, P., Gloor, U., and Wiss, O.,** Menachinone aus Menschlicher Leber und Faulschlamm, *Internat. Z. Vit. Forschung,* 40, 351, 1970.

65. **Duello, T. J. and Matschiner, J. T.,** Characterization of vitamin K from human liver, *J. Nutr.,* 102, 331, 1972.

66. **Shearer, M. J., McCarthy, P. T., Crampton, O. E., and Mattock, M. B.,** The assessment of human vitamin K status from tissue measurements, in *Current Advances in Vitamin K Research,* Suttie, J. W., Ed., Elsevier, New York, 1988, 437.

67. **Usui, Y., Tanimura, H., Nishimura, N., Kobayashi, N., Okanoue, T., and Ozawa, K.,** Vitamin K concentrations in the plasma and liver of surgical patients, *Am. J. Clin. Nutr.,* 51, 846, 1990.

68. **Suttie, J. W., Mummah-Schendel, L. L., Shah, D. V. Lyle, B. J., and Greger, J. L.,** Vitamin K deficiency from dietary vitamin K restriction in humans, *Am. J. Clin. Nutr.,* 47, 475, 1988.

Chapter 14

THE RELATIONSHIP BETWEEN THE DISPOSITION AND PHARMACOLOGICAL RESPONSE TO PHYLLOQUINONE (VITAMIN K₁) DURING COUMARIN ANTICOAGULATION

B. K. Park and M. J. Winn

TABLE OF CONTENTS

0-8493-6423-X/93/$0.00 + $.50
© 1993 by CRC Press, Inc.

I. INTRODUCTION

Recent cases of poisoning or overdose with coumarin anticoagulants have drawn our attention to the limited amount of information concerning the therapeutic administration of vitamin K_1 (phylloquinone). In particular, the development of novel long-acting coumarin rodenticides, such as difenacoum, brodifacoum, and chlorphacinone, has highlighted the need for a more fundamental understanding of the efficacy and mechanism of the antidotal action of the vitamin.[1-3] In patients poisoned with coumarins, the duration of the response to administration of phylloquinone, as measured by changes in prothrombin complex activity (PCA) may be unexpectedly short, and repeated administration of pharmacological doses (10 mg) of the vitamin may be required for several weeks to maintain normal clotting factor synthesis. In contrast, dietary requirements for the vitamin have been estimated to be of the order of 1 μg/kg/d.[4,5]

Coumarin anticoagulants (Table 1) are believed to block clotting factor synthesis by the inhibition of vitamin K epoxide reductase[6] and vitamin K quinone reductase,[7] in the physiologically important vitamin K-epoxide cycle[8] (Figure 1). This cycle seems to serve as a mechanism for maintaining a readily utilizable microsomal pool of vitamin K for vitamin K-dependent carboxylation; this active recycling may explain the very low dietary requirements for the vitamin. Inhibition of these enzymes prevents the regeneration of vitamin K and leads to anticoagulation. Warfarin is the coumarin most commonly used for therapeutic purposes, but several other 4-hydroxycoumarin compounds share the same mechanism of action. The pharmacokinetic properties, and therefore duration of action, of such compounds is determined largely by the nature of the substituent in the 3-position[9] (Table 1). Brodifacoum, which contains a large lipophilic side-chain has an extremely long duration of action, and has proved to be a useful model compound in both animal[10] and human studies.[11]

There are two important points which require consideration in any rationalization of the pharmacological response to phylloquinone. First, coumarin anticoagulants do not completely inhibit the response to a pharmacological dose of phylloquinone; this is in contrast to so-called direct inhibitors of vitamin K action such as 2-chlorophylloquinone.[12] Second, the duration of the response to administered phylloquinone is dependent on the dose and disposition of the vitamin, and the degree of exposure to the anticoagulant.

To address these points, we have carried out investigations in both man and in experimental animals. In the animal studies, we have attempted to determine the pharmacological relationships between clotting factor synthesis and tissue and subcellular disposition of phylloquinone and the coumarin anticoagulants. The development of a method based on the electrochemical detection of physiological and subphysiological concentrations of phylloquinone[13] (see Haroon, Chapter 11 of this book) has allowed us to determine the concentrations of phylloquinone in hepatic and subcellular

TABLE 1
Structure and Half-Lives of Coumarin Anticoagulants

Anticoagulant	Structure	$t_{1/2}$ (h)
Dicoumarol		80
Warfarin		42
Phenprocoumon		160
Acenocoumarol		9
Difenacoum		80
Brodifacoum		480

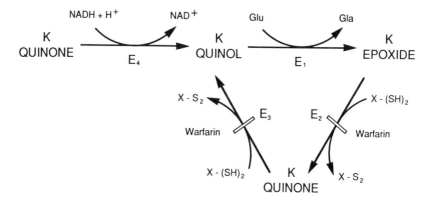

FIGURE 1. Scheme showing the vitamin K-epoxide cycle in relation to the conversion of glutamate residues (Glu) to gamma-carboxy glutamate (Gla) residues for the vitamin K-dependent coagulation proteins II, VII, IX, and X. Known enzyme activities are denoted by E_1, E_2, E_3, and E_4. The active form of vitamin K needed for carboxylation is the reduced form, vitamin K quinol. The carboxylation reaction is driven by a vitamin K-dependent carboxylase activity (E_1) coupled to a vitamin K-epoxidase activity (E_1) which simultaneously converts vitamin K quinol to vitamin K 2,3-epoxide. Vitamin K 2,3-epoxide is reduced back to quinone by vitamin K epoxide reductase (E_2). The cycle is completed by the reduction of recycled vitamin K quinone by a vitamin K reductase activity (E_3). Both vitamin K epoxide and vitamin K reductase activities E_2 and E_3 are dithiol-dependent [X-(SH)$_2$ and X-S$_2$ denote reduced and oxidized dithiols], and are inhibited by coumarin anticoagulants such as warfarin. Exogenous vitamin K may enter the cycle via an NAD(P)H-dependent vitamin K reductase activity (E_4) which is not inhibited by warfarin.

fractions of liver, and thereby assess the availability of the vitamin at its site of action. For the purpose of clinical studies we have used the measurement of plasma phylloquinone epoxide concentrations, after the administration of a pharmacological dose of phylloquinone, as an index of the amount of anticoagulant present at its site of action *in situ*.

II. THE PHARMACOLOGICAL RESPONSE TO PHYLLOQUINONE

In rats and rabbits previously dosed with a coumarin anticoagulant, the pharmacological response to phylloquinone may be studied by the measurement of changes in the PCA, or the activity of individual clotting factors. It is possible to calculate rates of clotting factor synthesis by mathematical transformation of the data obtained from the time-course of changes in clotting factor activity.[14] However, such calculations may now be limited by the recent discovery of other vitamin K-dependent proteins, since they do not take specific account of the changes in activity of the vitamin K-dependent anticoagulants, protein C, and protein S. The long-acting rodenticide, brodifacoum, has proved a useful pharmacological tool with which to assess the requirements for phylloquinone in the absence of a functional epoxide

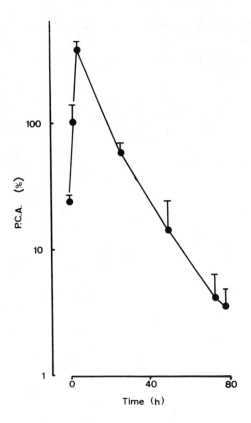

FIGURE 2.   Changes in prothrombin complex activity (PCA) against time following the administration of a pharmacological dose (10 mg/kg; i.v.) of phylloquinone in rabbits anticoagulated with the potent and long-acting coumarin, brodifacoum. PCA values are expressed as a percentage of normal (100%). Note logarithmic scale.

reductase enzyme.[15] Under these conditions the duration of the pharmacological response to phylloquinone is extremely short. After the intravenous administration of phylloquinone (10 mg/kg) to either rat or rabbits (dosed with brodifacoum 16 h previously), the PCA rose rapidly, reached a maximum at 3 h, and then declined at a rate that corresponded to complete inhibition of clotting factor synthesis (Figure 2). Further experiments showed that the duration of response to phylloquinone was directly proportional to dose.[10] The inability of coumarin anticoagulants to completely block the response to high doses of phylloquinone is consistent with the hypothesis that coumarins act indirectly by the inhibition of vitamin K epoxide reductase and vitamin K quinone reductase. 2-Chlorophylloquinone, in contrast, is a direct inhibitor of the epoxidase/carboxylase system and can, therefore, abolish the pharmacological response to phylloquinone.[16]

The structure of the side chain of vitamin K is an important determinant of pharmacological response in the presence of coumarin anticoagulants.

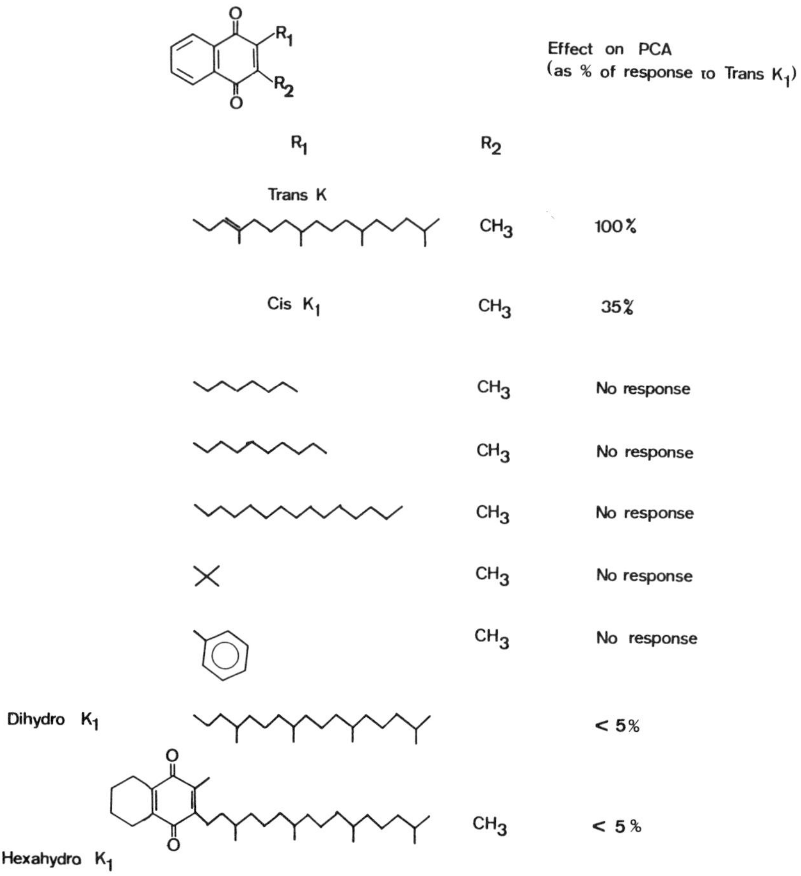

Effect on PCA
(as % of response to Trans K₁)

	R₁	R₂	
Trans K	(structure)	CH₃	100%
Cis K₁		CH₃	35%
	(structure)	CH₃	No response
	(structure)	CH₃	No response
	(structure)	CH₃	No response
	(structure)	CH₃	No response
	(structure)	CH₃	No response
Dihydro K₁	(structure)		< 5%
Hexahydro K₁	(structure)	CH₃	< 5%

FIGURE 3. The influence of changes in the side-chain of vitamin K on clotting factor synthesis in rabbits anticoagulated with brodifacoum (10 mg/kg; i.v.). The results are expressed as a percentage of the response in prothrombin complex activity (PCA) to *trans* phylloquinone (K₁).

Menaquinones (K₂ vitamins) were less effective than vitamin K₁ in promoting clotting factor synthesis, while menadione (2-methyl-1,4-naphthoquinone or vitamin K₃) and *cis*-phylloquinone had no effect. A higher dose of *cis*-phylloquinone (10 mg/kg) did produce a delayed increase in the PCA which coincided with the appearance of *trans*-phylloquinone in plasma, indicating that isomerization to the biologically active and naturally occurring *trans* isomer had occurred *in vivo*.

Further studies have been carried out with synthetic analogues of phylloquinone in which the side chain of each was selectively modified to determine the precise structural requirements for the vitamin (Figure 3). With the exception of *cis*-phylloquinone whose activity seems to be dependent on its conversion to the *trans* isomer, none of the analogues shown in Figure 3 proved to have significant procoagulant activity in the brodifacoum-anticoagulated rabbit. These results are similar to very early data of Fieser and co-workers, who used the curative chick bioassay to compare the activity of the analogues. These two models, however, differ in at least one important respect. Thus in our coumarin model the dithiol-dependent vitamin K epoxide reductase (Figure 1) is blocked and as suggested by recent results[17] (see also below) the production of the active hydroquinone can only proceed via a different NAD(P)H-dependent and coumarin insensitive pathway. In contrast, Fieser tested the biological activity in deficient animals with a functional vitamin K epoxide cycle. Although it is usually assumed that the specificity of vitamin K activity lies with the carboxylase our results would be also consistent with a specificity residing with the vitamin K reductase. Further work is required to resolve whether the specificity for the *trans*-phytyl side chain observed in our experiments is determined by the quinone reductase or by subsequent steps of the vitamin K-epoxide cycle.

III. THE DISPOSITION OF PHYLLOQUINONE

The short duration of action of phylloquinone during chronic coumarin poisoning may be explained, in part, by its rapid clearance. The plasma concentration of vitamin K_1 undergoes a triexponential decay following intravenous administration, with half-lives of 0.8 h, 1 to 2 h, and 20 h, for the α-, β-, and γ-phases, respectively.[16,18] Not only is clearance rapid, but the requirement for vitamin K increases significantly; clotting-factor synthesis is only observed when plasma concentrations of phylloquinone remain high (Figures 4 and 5). The need for very high plasma concentrations to drive clotting factor synthesis in situations of coumarin overdosage has been demonstrated in both rats and rabbits. Experiments indicate that the minimum plasma concentrations of vitamin K_1 required for clotting factor synthesis lies in the range 0.4 to 1.0 μg/ml.[16] This range is considerably higher than the normal physiological concentrations (between 10 to 20 ng/ml[18]).

The requirement for these high plasma concentrations of phylloquinone is not due to the inadequate uptake of the vitamin into either the liver or the endoplasmic reticulum of the liver because whole liver or microsomal concentrations of vitamin K_1 were not different in the presence or the absence of brodifacoum.[18] Moreover, the high plasma concentrations of phylloquinone are accompanied by liver concentrations which are at least 100-fold greater than normal, such that 24 h after the dose of phylloquinone the hepatic concentrations of the vitamin (2.67 $\pm$ 0.86 μg/g) remained in excess of the normal physiological levels (127 ng/g), but were insufficient to drive clotting factor synthesis. While these findings are difficult to reconcile with the apparent irreversibility of the inhibitions of vitamin K_1 epoxide reductase and quinone reductase by coumarin anticoagulants observed *in vitro*,[19] the data are consistent with the hypothesis proposed by Wallin and his co-workers.[17,20] These authors suggested that phylloquinone can be reduced to its hydroquinone derivative by a route independent of the coumarin sensitive quinone reductase.

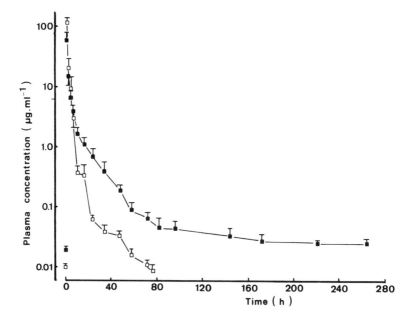

FIGURE 4.   Plasma concentrations of phylloquinone against time before and after the intravenous administration of a pharmacological dose (10 mg/kg) of phylloquinone to rabbits pretreated
with either brodifacoum (□) in polyethylene glycol vehicle (10 mg/kg; 0.5 ml/kg; i.v.) or the
vehicle (■) alone (0.5 ml/kg; i.v.). The results are the means of six rabbits in each group with
the SEM shown by vertical bars.

This NADPH-dependent pathway is less sensitive to vitamin K_1 than quinone
reductase, and therefore, requires considerably greater concentrations of vitamin K_1 to drive the reduction.[17]

IV. PLASMA PHYLLOQUINONE EPOXIDE AS AN INDEX OF COUMARIN OR INDANEDIONE ANTICOAGULATION

The metabolite phylloquinone 2,3-epoxide normally circulates in plasma
at very low concentrations (see Haroon, Chapter 11). After exposure to coumarins, however, the vitamin K epoxide cycle is inhibited and under these
conditions the administration of phylloquinone does result in readily measurable concentrations of the epoxide in plasma. Therefore, the presence of
higher than normal plasma concentrations of the epoxide provides a useful
screening test for the presence of coumarin (or indanedione) anticoagulants
or indeed other vitamin K antagonists which may inhibit the hepatic enzyme,
phylloquinone-epoxide reductase. In fact, this phylloquinone epoxide test has
proved to be a more sensitive test for the inhibition of phylloquinone-epoxide
reductase than either measurement of prothrombin time, or individual clotting
factors (see below).

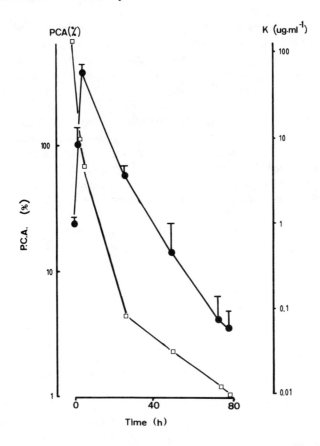

FIGURE 5. Decline in plasma concentrations of phylloquinone and the accompanying changes in prothrombin complex activity (PCA) in rabbits pretreated with brodifacoum (10 mg/kg; i.v.) showing the high concentrations of the vitamin needed to drive clotting factor synthesis.

In our laboratory the assessment of coumarin exposure by the phylloquinone epoxide test has been carried out by the intravenous administration of phylloquinone (Konakion; 10 mg) via the antecubital vein. While phylloquinone may also be given orally, its absorption is very erratic.[11,21] Therefore, intravenous dosing offers the most reliable route of administration. Until recently, one drawback of the phylloquinone epoxide test, which may have limited its acceptance, has been the reported incidences of cardiovascular toxicity which have been ascribed to the polyethoxylated oil-based preparation used to solubilize phylloquinone.[22,23] However, these problems seem largely to have been overcome by the recent development of a mixed-micelle based preparation of the vitamin, which appears much less toxic after intravenous administration than the polyethoxylated preparation, although oral uptake may be still variable.[24] After administration of the phylloquinone preparation, venous blood samples are obtained at predetermined timepoints over the next 24 h. In our laboratory, the measurement of phylloquinone epoxide is carried out using normal-phase high-performance liquid chromatography. The method[25] allows the rapid and reproducible separation of phylloquinone (including the resolution of the *cis-* and *trans-*isomers of phylloquinone) from phylloquinone epoxide. The ability of this method to detect the presence and duration of action of anticoagulants is illustrated by three cases of coumarin poisoning.

Cases 1 and 2 were both male caucasian factory employees who were exposed to coumarins at work. Both developed symptoms of anticoagulant effect: abnormal prothrombin times, hematuria, and spontaneous bruising. Both were treated for acute hypoprothrombinemia with fresh frozen plasma and phylloquinone after which the prothrombin times fell. There was then no subsequent exposure to coumarins. The patients were monitored over a period of 18 months, and on each of these occasions prothrombin times were normal.[26] Despite the normal prothrombin times, there was an apparent dissociation between pharmacodynamic half-life and kinetic effect because the phylloquinone epoxide test revealed the presence of the epoxide at each test session during this time, indicating the longterm inhibition of vitamin K epoxide reductase.[26] In case 1, who appeared to have been exposed to the very long-acting coumarin, brodifacoum, we have now been able to assess the long term residual presence of this anticoagulant over a period of years. While there has been a steady fall in the plasma concentrations, AUC and CP_{max} of phylloquinone epoxide when measured after administration of phylloquinone, the epoxide could still be detected 4 years after the original exposure (Figure 6). These data provided an apparent elimination half-life of brodifacoum of 6.1 months.

In case 3, chlorphacinone was thought to be the anticoagulant responsible for the alterations in clotting factor synthesis and for the disturbance in vitamin K metabolism. Chlorphacinone is an indanedione derivative used as a rodenticide.[27] A single case of chlorphacinone poisoning has been reported in which the anticoagulant action of the compound persisted for over 45 d.[28] In the patient reported here (case 3), clotting factor synthesis returned to normal within a week of chlorphacinone exposure, while abnormal vitamin K_1 metabolism persisted for over 7 weeks. Measurement of phylloquinone epoxide after periodic administration of phylloquinone during this time indicated a half-life for chlorphacinone of 9.4 d.

The apparent dissociation between the doses of coumarins required to prolong prothrombin times, and the doses of coumarins that lead to the appearance of vitamin K_1 epoxide in the plasma can also be seen with warfarin. Thus we have shown that the administration of a dose of 1 mg of warfarin daily to volunteers produced a very small, but significant (0.9 s) increase in mean prothrombin times,[29] whereas a dose of 0.2 mg daily had no effect on prothrombin times, nor on the activity of individual clotting factors II, VII, IX, and X, and protein C. However, all of the volunteers had detectable plasma concentrations of phylloquinone epoxide (after 10 mg of phylloquinone) at both doses of warfarin; and the CP_{max} and AUC for the epoxide could be seen to be dose dependent.

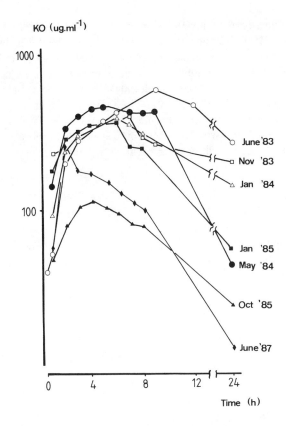

FIGURE 6. Plasma concentrations of phylloquinone 2,3-epoxide following the administration of phylloquinone (10 mg; i.v.) to a patient (case 1) who had been exposed to brodifacoum at work. The phylloquinone epoxide test was performed at each of the dates indicated.

Thus, the phylloquinone epoxide test provides a clear indication of the level of anticoagulation and inhibition of vitamin K epoxide reductase following coumarin exposure. Moreover, it can provide a highly accurate method for assessing the effective half-lives of the coumarins at their site of action in the liver.

The formation of phylloquinone epoxide independently of changes in prothrombin times or the activity of individual clotting factors also raises important questions about the available methods for testing anticoagulation, and about the relationship between γ-carboxylation, epoxidation, and functional activity of γ-carboxylated proteins. There are several possible explanations for the apparent dissociation between measurable epoxide formation and measurable changes in PCA or prothrombin times. First, the inability to measure small changes in either prothrombin times or the activities of individual clotting factors may be entirely due to the relative insensitivity of the techniques used. In this respect, resolution may be compromised because the prothrombin time bears an inverse relationship to the concentration of clotting factors in the plasma, so that when clotting factor synthesis falls between 100 and 70%, the prothrombin time changes only very slightly. Second, there may be a threshold for the inhibition of vitamin K epoxide reductase below which there is no further change in clotting factor synthesis. This is related to a third explanation, in that there may not be a stoichiometric relationship between formation of the epoxide and γ-carboxylation. This possibility is supported by evidence from *in vitro* sources which suggests that epoxide formation is not dependent on the presence of glutamic acid substrate in the incubation medium.[30]

V. ENANTIOMERS OF WARFARIN AND PHYLLOQUINONE METABOLISM

Warfarin has a single asymmetric center, and therefore exists as two separate enantiomers R(+)- and S(−)-warfarin. The S-enantiomer of warfarin has been reported to be 2.7 to 3.8 times more potent than the R-enantiomer.[31-33] Whether the difference in potency is due to a stereoselective interaction between R- or S-warfarin at the presumed vitamin K epoxide reductase receptor site is unclear. *In vitro* evidence would suggest that vitamin K epoxide reductase is inhibited equally by both enantiomers.[19] Yet the same authors found that S-warfarin inhibited vitamin K_1 epoxide reductase to a greater extent than R-warfarin in rat liver microsomes after the prior administration of the enantiomers *in vivo;* and others have found that the potency of racemic warfarin resides almost exclusively with the S-enantiomer.[34] In an attempt to investigate these differences in man, we have used the phylloquinone epoxide test. Previous studies in human volunteers using high doses of R- or S-warfarin failed to show any difference between the enantiomers and formation of the epoxide as judged from the accumulation of this metabolite in plasma.[35,36] This may have been due to the doses of warfarin exceeding those required for the maximum accumulation of the epoxide and therefore for any difference between the enantiomers to become apparent. In a more recent study, we have used smaller doses of the two enantiomers and found that CP_{max} and AUC of vitamin K_1 epoxide were significantly greater after S-warfarin than after R-warfarin,[37] suggesting a distinct functional difference between the two enantiomers in man. Nevertheless, the R-enantiomer of warfarin did produce significant inhibition of vitamin K epoxide reductase, as indicated by significant levels of phylloquinone epoxide in plasma.

The functional difference between the two enantiomers does not seem to be reflected in concentrations of R- or S-warfarin in liver microsomes. We have recently established a steadystate model of anticoagulation in rats, using either R- or S-warfarin.[38] The dose of S-warfarin needed to produce a consistent increase in the prothrombin time in this model (0.1 mg/kg/d was 4-times smaller than the concentration of R-warfarin required to cause a similar increase in prothrombin time. This difference in the pharmacodynamic effects was also reflected in differences between plasma, whole liver, and liver cytosolic concentrations of the two enantiomers (Table 2). However, microsomal concentrations were constant for both enantiomers, and remained constant for increasing doses of R-warfarin.[38] Thijssen et al.[39] have reported concentrations of warfarin in rat liver microsomes that were similar to ours, and concluded that this represented saturable binding of warfarin to epoxide reductase. But, our data showed that the pharmacodynamic index of warfarin action, the prothrombin time, was dose related, despite constant microsomal concentrations of warfarin. It would appear, therefore, that not all of the warfarin in microsomal tissue is bound to vitamin K epoxide reductase.

VI. CONCLUSIONS

The pharmacological relationships between the perturbation of vitamin K metabolism and clotting factor synthesis observed in man are consistent with the currently accepted mechanism of action of coumarin anticoagulants. Measurement of concentrations of anticoagulants in plasma, or at the site of action in the liver may not provide a clear indication of the degree of effect of these drugs. In contrast, the measurement of phylloquinone epoxide in plasma, after the administration of a single dose of vitamin K_1, provides a simple but very sensitive biochemical index of the pharmacological activity of coumarin anticoagulants. The phylloquinone epoxide test can detect concentrations of coumarins in liver which do not produce measurable changes in clotting factor activity, and may, therefore, be used to detect exposure to such compounds.

TABLE 2
Prothrombin Complex Activity and Concentrations of R(+) and S(−) Warfarin

Dose	Dose (mg/kg/d)	PCA (%)	Plasma (μg/ml)	Whole liver (μg/g · liver)	Cytosol (μg/g · protein)	Microsomes (μg/g · protein)
R-warfarin	0.1	16.3 ± 0.5	0.08 ± 0.00	0.8 ± 0.1	0.5 ± 0.0	2.8 ± 0.8
R-warfarin	0.4	21.6 ± 0.6	0.3 ± 0.04	1.3 ± 0.1	2.7 ± 0.6	3.9 ± 1.2
R-warfarin	0.8	55.1 ± 9.0	0.6 ± 0.05	2.3 ± 0.4	5.5 ± 1.2	4.0 ± 1.2
S-warfarin	0.1	19.7 ± 0.6	0.2 ± 0.02	0.9 ± 0.1	0.9 ± 0.6	3.9 ± 0.7

Note: The mean ± S.E.M. concentrations of either R- or S-warfarin in plasma, whole liver, and liver fractions (cytosol and microsomes) are shown in rats after steady-state anticoagulation had been established for at least 4 d. The pharmacodynamic effect of each regimen is shown by the prothrombin complex activity (PCA) expressed as a percentage of normal (100%).

REFERENCES

1. **Barlow, A. M., Gray, A. L., and Park, B. K.,** Difenacoum (neo-sorexa) poisoning, *Br. Med. J.,* 205, 541, 1982.
2. **Lipton, R. A. and Klass, E. M.,** Human ingestion of a "superwarfarin" rodenticide resulting in a prolonged anticoagulant effect, *J. Am. Med. Assoc.,* 252, 3004, 1984.
3. **Jones, E. L., Growe, G. H., and Naimann, S. C.,** Prolonged anticoagulation in rat poisoning, *JAMA,* 252, 3005, 1984.
4. **Frick, P. G., Riedler, G., Brogli, H.,** Dose response and minimal daily requirement for vitamin K in man, *J. Appl. Physiol.,* 23, 387, 1967.
5. **Barkhan, P. B. and Shearer, M. J.,** Metabolism of vitamin K (phylloquinone) in man, *Proc. Royal Soc. Med.,* 70, 83, 1977.
6. **Bell, R. G. and Matschiner, R. J.,** Warfarin and the inhibition of vitamin K activity by an oxide metabolite, *Nature,* 237, 32, 1977.
7. **Whitlon, D. S., Sadowski, J. A., and Suttie, J. W.,** Mechanism of coumarin action and significance of vitamin K epoxide reductase inhibition, *Biochemistry,* 17, 1371, 1978.
8. **Bell, R. G.,** Metabolism of vitamin K and prothrombin synthesis: anticoagulants and the vitamin K-epoxide cycle, *Fed. Proc.,* 37, 2599, 1978.
9. **Park, B. K.,** Warfarin: metabolism and mode of action, *Biochem. Pharmacol.,* 37, 19, 1988.
10. **Park, B. K. and Leck, J. B.,** A comparison of vitamin K antagonism by warfarin, difenacoum and brodifacoum in the rabbit, *Biochem. Pharmacol.,* 31, 3635, 1982.
11. **Park, B. K., Scott, A. K., Wilson, A. C., Haynes, B. P., and Breckenridge, A. M.,** Plasma disposition of vitamin K in relation to anticoagulant poisoning, *Br. J. Clin. Pharmac.,* 18, 655, 1984.
12. **Lowenthal, J. and McFarlane, J. A.,** The nature of the antagonism between vitamin K and indirect anticoagulants, *J. Pharmacol. Exp. Ther.,* 143, 273, 1964.
13. **Hart, J. P., Shearer, M. J., and McCarthy, P. J.,** Enhanced sensitivity for the determination of endogenous phylloquinone (vitamin K_1) in plasma using HPLC with dual-cell electrode electrochemical detection, *Analyst,* 110, 1181, 1985.
14. **Nagashima, R., O'Reilly, R. A., and Levy, G.,** Kinetics of pharmacologic effects in man: the anticoagulant action of warfarin, *Clin. Pharmacol. Ther.,* 10, 22, 1969.
15. **Park, B. K., Leck, J. B., Wilson, A. C., Serlin, M. J., and Breckenridge, A. M.,** A study of the effect of anticoagulants on [H]-vitamin K metabolism and prothrombin complex activity in the rabbit, *Biochem. Pharmac.,* 28, 1323, 1979.
16. **Hart, J. A. D., Haynes, B. P., and Park, B. K.,** A study of factors which determine the pharmacological response to vitamin K in coumarin anticoagulated rabbits, *Biochem. Pharmacol.,* 33, 3013, 1984.
17. **Wallin, R. and Martin, L. F.,** Warfarin poisoning and vitamin K antagonism in rat and human liver. Design of a system *in vitro* that mimics the situation *in vivo, Biochem. J.,* 241, 389, 1987.
18. **Winn, M. J., Cholerton, S., and Park, B. K.,** An investigation of the pharmacological response to vitamin K in the rabbit, *Br. J. Pharmacol.,* 94, 1077, 1988.
19. **Fasco, M. J. and Principe, L. M.,** R-warfarin and S-warfarin inhibition of vitamin K and vitamin K 2,3-epoxide reductase activities in the rat, *J. Biol. Chem.,* 257, 4894, 1982.
20. **Wallin, R.,** Vitamin K antagonism of coumarin anticoagulation. A dehydrogenase pathway in the rat liver is responsible for the antagonistic effect, *Biochem. J.,* 236, 685, 1986.
21. **Uchida, K. and Komeno, T.,** Relationships between dietary and intestinal vitamin K clotting factor levels, plasma vitamin K, and urinary Gla, in *Current Advances in Vitamin K Research,* Suttie, J. W., Ed., Elsevier, New York, 1988, 477.

22. **Barash, P., Kitahata, L. M., and Mandel, S.,** Acute cardiovascular collapse after intravenous phytonadione, *Anaesth. Analg.,* 55, 304, 1976.

23. **Rich, C. E. and Drage, C. N.,** Severe complication of intravenous phytadione therapy. Two cases with one fatality, *Postgrad. Med.,* 72, 303, 1982.

24. **Winn, M. J., White, P. M., Scott, A. K., Pratt, S. K., and Park, B. K.,** The bioavailability of a mixed-micellar preparation of vitamin K and its procoagulant effect, *J. Pharm. Pharmacol.,* 41, 257, 1989.

25. **Wilson, A. C. and Park, B. K.,** Quantitative analysis of pharmacological concentrations of vitamin K and vitamin K 2,3-epoxide in rabbit plasma by high-performance liquid chromatography, *J. Chromatogr.,* 277, 292, 1982.

26. **Park, B. K., Choonara, I. A., Haynes, B. P., Breckenridge, A. M., Malia, R. G., and Preston, F. E.,** Abnormal vitamin K metabolism in the presence of normal clotting factor activity in factory workers exposed to 4-hydroxycoumarins, *Br. J. Clin. Pharmacol.,* 21, 289, 1986.

27. **Lund, M.,** The toxicity of chlorophacinone and warfarin to house mice *(Mus musculus).,* J. Hygiene, 69, 69, 1971.

28. **Murdoch, D. A.,** Prolonged anticoagulation in chlorophacinone poisoning, *Lancet,* i, 355, 1983.

29. **Choonara, I. A., Malia, R. G., Haynes, B. P., Hay, C. R., Cholerton, S., Breckenridge, A. M., Preston, F. E., and Park, B. K.,** The relationship between inhibition of vitamin K_1 2,3-epoxide reductase and reduction of clotting factor activity with warfarin, *Br. J. Clin. Pharmacol.,* 25, 1, 1988.

30. **Cheung, A. Y., Wood, G. M., Funakawa, S., Grossman, C. P., and Suttie, J. W.,** Vitamin K-dependent carboxylase: substrates, products and inhibitors, in *Current Advances in vitamin K research,* Suttie, J. W., Ed., Elsevier, New York, 1988.

31. **Breckenridge, A. M., Orme, M. L. 'E. Wessling, H., Lewis, R. J., and Gibbons, R.,** Pharmacokinetics and pharmacodynamics of the enantiomers of warfarin in man, *Clin. Pharmacol. Ther.,* 15, 424, 1974.

32. **O'Reilly, R. A.,** Studies on the optical enantiomorphs of warfarin in man, *Clin. Pharmacol. Ther.,* 16, 348, 1974.

33. **Wingard, L. B., O'Reilly, R. A., and Levy, G.,** Pharmacokinetics of warfarin enantiomers: a search for intrasubject correlations, *Clin. Pharmacol. Ther.,* 23, 212, 1978.

34. **Chan, E., O'Reilly, R., and Rowland, M.,** Stereochemical aspects of warfarin in man: a combined pharmacokinetic-pharmacodynamic model, *Br. J. Clin. Pharmacol.,* 19, 545P, 1985.

35. **Shearer, M. J., McBurney, A., Breckenridge, A. M., and Barkhan, P.,** Effect of warfarin on the metabolism of phylloquinone (vitamin K_1): dose-response relationships in man, *Clin. Sci. Mol. Med.,* 52, 621, 1977.

36. **Choonara, I. A., Cholerton, S., Haynes, B. P., Breckenridge, A. M., and Park, B. K.,** Stereoselective interaction between the R-enantiomer of warfarin and cimetidine, *Br. J. Clin. Pharmacol.,* 21, 271, 1986.

37. **Choonara, I. A., Haynes, B. P., Cholerton, S., Breckenridge, A. M., and Park, B. K.,** Enantiomers of warfarin and vitamin K metabolism, *Br. J. Clin. Pharmacol.,* 22, 729, 1986.

38. **Pratt, S. K., Winn, M. J., and Park, B. K.,** The disposition of the enantiomers of warfarin following chronic administration to rats: relationship to anticoagulant response, *J. Pharm. Pharmacol.,* 44, 743, 1989.

39. **Thijssen, H. H. W. and Baars, L. G. M.,** Hepatic uptake and storage of warfarin. The relation with the target enzyme vitamin K 2,3-epoxide reductase, *J. Pharmacol. Exp. Ther.,* 243, 1082, 1987.

Chapter 15

METHODS FOR THE MEASUREMENT OF URINARY GAMMA-CARBOXYGLUTAMIC ACID AND SERUM OSTEOCALCIN AND THEIR USE IN THE CLINICAL SITUATION AS MARKERS OF BONE DISEASE

Caren M. Gundberg

TABLE OF CONTENTS

0-8493-6423-X/93/$0.00 + $.50
© 1993 by CRC Press, Inc.

I. INTRODUCTION

The skeleton provides for the mechanical support and protection of the body and for the maintenance of normal mineral metabolism. As such, bone is an active tissue constantly undergoing structural and metabolic changes. These events are controlled by several important cell types, of which two, the osteoblasts and osteoclasts, have been extensively studied. The osteoblasts, which are the bone forming cells, synthesize the matrix. The matrix is mineralized in the presence of normal concentrations of calcium and phosphate to form crystalline hydroxyapatite $[(Ca_{10}(PO_4)_6(OH)_2]$. The matrix consists of organic material, mainly collagen and a variety of sugars, lipids, and proteins. Among these proteins, osteocalcin and alkaline phosphatase, are found in the blood and their concentration in the circulation has been taken as an index of bone formation. The osteoclasts, the bone resorbing cells, degrade the mineralized matrix releasing mineral and matrix components. These components include hydroxyproline, γ-carboxyglutamic acid (Gla), and pyridinoline and deoxypyridinoline. These have been used as markers of bone resorption.

Although the cells account for only a minor fraction of the bone volume, they carry out two important functions. In concert with the calciotropic hormones, they regulate the content and distribution of mineral between bone and blood, thereby maintaining serum calcium and phosphorus within a narrow concentration range. Bone cells also control the modeling of bone during growth. After growth has stopped, existing bone is continually removed by resorption while new bone is being formed (termed bone turnover or remodeling). It is estimated that the skeleton is totally replaced every 8 to 10 years. This continuous remodeling of bone allows the skeletal system to respond to outside mechanical or hormonal forces. A number of systemic and local factors directly or indirectly influence growth and bone turnover. Parathyroid hormone (PTH) and the active form of vitamin D, $1,25(OH)_2D$ (dihydroxyvitamin D — calcitriol), stimulate bone resorption while calcitonin inhibits it. Bone resorption by osteoclasts and bone formation by osteoblasts are also linked in time and space by unknown factors. In the steady state, this "coupling" of bone formation and resorption maintains bone mass. Any disruption of this coupling can lead to debilitating bone disease.

The biochemical assessment of patients with metabolic disorders of bone is often difficult. Measurements of serum alkaline phosphatase activity and urinary total hydroxyproline excretion have been used routinely in the assessment of bone disease but both are strongly influenced by nonosseous metabolism and are subject to interference from systemic disorders. Alkaline phosphatase, the standard measure of bone formation is derived from several different sources and the quantitation of the bone isoenzyme is imprecise. Urinary hydroxyproline, a degradation product of collagen, reflects bone and nonbone collagen and requires careful urine collection.

Osteocalcin, the vitamin K-dependent protein of bone, is a specific product of the osteoblast. A fraction of that synthesized does not accumulate in bone but is secreted directly into the circulation. This protein is increasingly being used as a sensitive and specific marker for bone formation. Proteolytic degradation of osteocalcin contributes to the excretion of Gla. Urinary excretion of free Gla follows the catabolism of all vitamin K-dependent proteins. It can be used to measure the overall status of vitamin K-dependent processes, to directly monitor the actions of coumarin anticoagulants, and to indicate changes in bone turnover.

II. OSTEOCALCIN

A. ANALYTICAL METHODS AND CONSIDERATIONS

Because osteocalcin has no known function or bioassay, quantitation of the protein depends on standard chemical, physical, and immunological methods. The use of immunoassay for measurement of osteocalcin offers the advantages of specificity, sensitivity, and technical simplicity. The method can easily detect picogram quantities in bone extracts, cell cultures, and serum. Bovine osteocalcin, purified to homogeneity under non-denaturing conditions has been used as the antigen in establishing human osteocalcin RIA. Since antibody raised against cow osteocalcin cross-reacts identically with human osteocalcin. However, many current assays use mono- and polyclonal antibodies generated against human osteocalcin.[1-3, 151-153]

EDTA is used in all assay buffers in our laboratory. Removal of the chelator alters the binding curve. Since osteocalcin conformation depends upon calcium concentration antibody subpopulations are presumably present that are specific for the α-helical or random coil configurations. EDTA eliminates this binding heterogeneity for our antisera but the requirement for EDTA depends upon the antibody specificity. The epitope recognized by most characterized antibodies to osteocalcin resides in the carboxyl terminus,[2-5] the region that hydrophilicity calculations predict to be the most antigenic. However, two antisera, one raised against cow[6] and the other against human[1] osteocalcin, have atypical calcium requirements for antigen binding and may recognize the internal region of the molecule.

There are inconsistencies which appear in the literature regarding serum osteocalcin concentrations. First, there are wide variations in reported osteocalcin concentrations in control populations. There are also disagreements regarding the normal variation of osteocalcin with age (there are reports of increasing, decreasing, or unchanged osteocalcin concentrations with age). Although these discrepancies can be attributed to heterogeneous patient populations, some of the observed differences are due to analytical differences. Chemical reagents and methodology may contribute to the differences among assays, but antibodies and standards are the most likely source of variability. In the recent osteocalcin standardization report, in which an international osteocalcin standard and 10 unknown serum samples were provided to 8 different laboratories with their own assays, there were clear differences in absolute values of the samples from laboratory to laboratory.[154] These persisted even when the international standard was used to calibrate the individual assays, suggesting that the major variability resided in the various antibodies.

In another study, four different antibodies were used to measure osteocalcin in serum and bone extract. There were no differences in the amount of osteocalcin detected in the bone, but the amount of osteocalcin in the sera varied.[155] These data suggest that there are various forms of osteocalcin in the circulation but not in bone and that the individual antibodies recognized them differently. We have identified fragments of osteocalcin from the serum of patients with end-stage renal disease but not from normal individuals, and have suggested that limited proteolysis of osteocalcin occurs in extrarenal sites.[7] Other laboratories have since verified this circulating heterogeneity of osteocalcin in normal serum and in Paget's disease.[151,156,157] Furthermore, there may be some evidence that undercarboxylated forms of osteocalcin are present in serum.[158,159] It is clear that different antibodies detect different subforms or fragments of osteocalcin. The source of these various forms has not been established, but there is some evidence that they may be derivd not only from osteoclastic degradation but from extraosseous catabolism, such as the liver. Alternatively they may be nonspecific products of the osteoblast.[151,156,157]

All assays are sensitive to 0.5 μg/l with inter- and intra-assay variations of less than 15 and 10%, respectively. Nonspecific binding of tracer to serum proteins occurs when more than 200 μl of sample is used. Hemolysis and lipemia will interfere with the assay, resulting in reduced values, the extent of which is dependent upon the degree of hemolysis or lipemia. Freeze thawing considerably reduces values, and a decrease in concentration is often found by the second or third freeze-thaw cycle. Presumably, osteocalcin is degraded by serum proteinases, because purified osteocalcin is stable to repeated freeze-thaw cycles and to heating to 70°C for 15 min. All blood samples should be processed within 2 to 3 h and centrifuged at 4°C. Longterm storage of samples should be at −70°C.

B. ORIGIN OF OSTEOCALCIN IN THE CIRCULATION

Early studies showed that serum levels of osteocalcin were elevated in patients with diseases characterized by high bone turnover[8-14] and were normal in disorders not involving bone.[14] These were promising observations because, unlike conventional measures of alkaline phosphatase and hydroxyproline, serum osteocalcin could be used to assess bone disease in patients where other illnesses were also present. On the other hand, the precise aspect of bone metabolism reflected by these values is not known at this time. Although osteocalcin is synthesized and secreted by osteoblasts, the circulating form could result either from new osteoblastic synthesis or release of existing osteocalcin from the bone matrix. Furthermore, if circulating osteocalcin resulted from new synthesis, its synthesis might depend upon its function in bone. If osteocalcin serves as a structural protein, then its synthesis could reflect matrix deposition. If osteocalcin serves to regulate crystal growth, it might reflect mineralization. On the other hand, if osteocalcin signals or stimulates osteoclastic function, then its synthesis and appearance in serum could be linked to bone resorption.

The question of whether circulating osteocalcin originates from *de novo* synthesis or catabolism of bone has been answered by Price and co-workers in a series of experiments in which they exploited the well-known antagonism between vitamin K and warfarin in a rat model. Their studies were designed with the knowledge that (1) warfarin inhibits γ-carboxylation, resulting in osteocalcin containing little or no Gla, and (2) osteocalcin which contains Gla residues, has a greater binding affinity for hydroxyapatite than osteocalcin which is devoid of Gla.[18-23] In one experiment, the administration of warfarin as a bolus resulted in the complete turnover of rat serum osteocalcin in 4 to 6 h from a normal protein to an immunoreactive species with poor binding to hydroxyapatite;[24] this was long before any change was detectable in bone.[22,24] Similarly, rats chronically treated with warfarin had abnormal osteocalcin in their plasma which, upon vitamin K_1 injection, was fully replaced by normal hydroxyapatite-adsorbable osteocalcin within about 12 h, again before any increase in the Gla content of bulk bone could be identified.[24] In both experiments, the newly formed plasma osteocalcin could only have originated from bone cells and not from the breakdown of existing bone matrix.

Whether circulating osteocalcin reflects synthesis and secretion of the protein during bone formation or resorption has been addressed in human studies where dynamic histomorphometry has been performed. In this technique a bone biopsy (usually of the ilium) is taken. Quantitative measurements are made on the surfaces of the bone. These measurements include (among others) the total amount of bone relative to the marrow, the volume of trabecular bone, the degree of surface mineralization, and the numbers of osteoblasts and osteoclasts. Before the biopsy, tetracycline is given to the patient in two doses separated by a given time interval (usually 10 d). Since tetracycline is incorporated into the mineralizing front, a double line of fluorescence will be observed in the biopsy specimen. The rate of bone formation can be determined from the distance between the two fluorescent lines[25] (Figure 1). On the other hand, the rate of bone resorption cannot be measured directly but can be inferred from the osteoclast number, the amount of bone covered by the osteoclast, and the amount of eroded surface. Estimation of bone dynamics can also be done by isotopic calcium (^{47}Ca) kinetics in which calculations of the rate of transfer of calcium between the various pools of bone calcium and the bloodstream are made.[26]

Several studies have established that in normal individuals and in patients with bone disease (postmenopausal osteoporosis, thyroid disorders, and

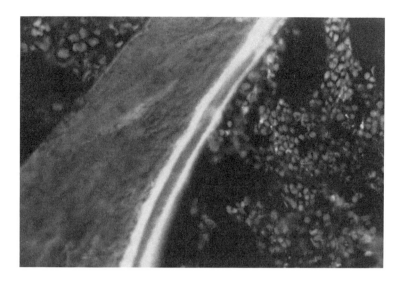

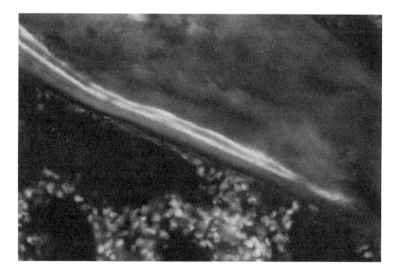

FIGURE 1. Transileal bone biopsy after administration of two time-spaced courses of oral tetracycline showing double fluorescent labels. (Top) Bone biopsy from a normal individual with a normal bone formation rate and clearly spaced lines of fluorescence. (Bottom) Bone biopsy from a patient with osteomalacia illustrating closely spaced lines of fluorescence and a reduced mineralization rate. (Kindly provided by Dr. Robert Weinstein, Department of Medicine, Medical College of Georgia, Augusta, Georgia.)

primary and secondary hyperparathyroidism) serum osteocalcin is highly correlated with histomorphometric measurements of bone formation ($r \geq 0.78$) but not resorption ($r < 0.30$).[29-32] Likewise, in calcium kinetic studies, there is a highly significant correlation between serum levels of osteocalcin and bone mineralization ($r = 0.89$) but not resorption.[33,34] Thus, the data clearly signify that osteocalcin does not reflect bone resorption but is associated with bone formation.

Early studies of the appearance of osteocalcin in embryonic bone tissue demonstrated that osteocalcin synthesis coincided with the onset of mineralization[35,37] and that osteocalcin increased in concert with hydroxyapatite deposition during the period of skeletal growth.[35] The constant osteocalcin to calcium ratio suggested an association of osteocalcin synthesis with mineralization. However, the interpretation of these data as well as the histomorphometric and calcium kinetic studies rely on the fact that mineral is deposited on a preformed matrix. It is difficult to make a distinction between matrix synthesis and mineralization because in a steady state and in the absence of osteomalacia (a defect in mineralization), formation of bone matrix and mineralization of that matrix occur at the same time and at identical rates.

In vitro and *in vivo* studies have addressed the question of whether osteocalcin synthesis is associated with matrix deposition or mineralization. First, in cultures of isolated chick or rat osteoblasts, low levels of alkaline phosphatase and osteocalcin are produced until cells reach confluence, at which time a dense collagenous extracellular matrix accumulates. Under certain conditions, this extracellular matrix can be stimulated to mineralize. When this occurs both alkaline phosphatate and osteocalcin synthesis increases. Alkaline phosphatase activity decreases after the cultures are mineralized but osteocalcin levels remain elevated for the lifespan of the cells.[38]

Other studies have utilized deer, in which antler growth and mineralization occur in two different stages making them a good model to distinguish between matrix synthesis and mineralization. We measured alkaline phosphatase, hydroxyproline, osteocalcin, and $1,25(OH)_2D$ in biweekly serum samples from six adult, four juvenile, and four fawn (<1 year old) white tailed deer for 1 year. Serum alkaline phosphatase, hydroxyproline, and osteocalcin were higher in fawns compared to juveniles and adults, reflecting increased bone growth in the younger deer. In adult deer, after bone growth had ceased, alkaline phosphatase and hydroxyproline levels were elevated during antler growth whereas serum osteocalcin and $1,25(OH)_2D$ were increased during antler mineralization. Finally, during fracture healing, osteocalcin message levels were found to coincide with endochondral ossification and remodelling but not during intramembranous bone formation or in the soft callus.[160] In all of these studies matrix synthesis and alkaline phosphatase expression preceded osteocalcin expression, suggesting that (1) osteocalcin is synthesized and secreated during matrix mineralization rather than matrix synthesis per se, and (2) osteocalcin is related to mineral maintenance and bone remodelling rather than initiation of bone formation or mineralization. In support of this, a recent immunolocalization study found osteocalcin to be unique among noncollagenous bone proteins in that its distribution in bone matrix is limited to mineralized areas only.[161]

These studies suggest that osteocalcin and alkaline phosphatase have related but separate functions in bone. It was initially thought that alkaline phosphatase acted by simply hydrolyzing organic phosphates, thereby providing phosphate as substrate for hydroxyapatite formation.[40] However, this is unnecessary since the bone extracellular fluid is supersaturated with respect to calcium and phosphate. On the other hand, in patients with hypophosphatasia, the bone isoenzyme is absent and there is a clinical and histological picture of defective bone calcification. These individuals excrete large amounts of pyrophosphate in their urine.[41] This has led to the theory that alkaline phosphatase acts by hydrolyzing pyrophosphate; pyrophosphate is an inhibitor of mineralization, and it is thus possible that alkaline phosphatase, by destroying local inhibitors, is involved in the initiation of mineralization.

The above discussion suggests that osteocalcin is synthesized and secreted during mineral deposition and maintenance rather than matrix synthesis per se, and that this may have important implications for the function of osteocalcin in bone. However, as noted above, matrix synthesis and mineralization are normally linked. When there is a dissociation between the two processes, the data are conflicting. A recent study showed that in human subjects with osteomalacia due to vitamin D deficiency, serum osteocalcin concentrations were better correlated with histomorphometric parameters of matrix synthesis than with mineralization. Therefore, it is more relevant to interpret osteocalcin data in terms of changes in bone formation *in toto*. Furthermore, in most clinical situations, bone formation and resorption are tightly coupled, i.e., when bone resorption is elevated bone formation is also elevated. Therefore, the assay of serum osteocalcin should be regarded as a measure of bone formation in particular, and bone turnover in general.

C. FACTORS AFFECTING CIRCULATING CONCENTRATIONS OF OSTEOCALCIN

The serum concentration of osteocalcin reflects that portion of newly synthesized protein that does not bind to the mineral phase of the bone but is released directly into the circulation. It is estimated that more than 90% of the newly synthesized osteocalcin is deposited in bone of 1 month-old rats, but as the animals mature, a greater proportion of protein is released directly into the serum.[24] In normal human adults, approximately one third of osteocalcin synthesis is destined for the circulation.[12,42] Deviations from normal concentrations of circulating osteocalcin are a consequence of changes in the synthesis or degradation of the protein. Such changes may result from physiological alterations in skeletal homeostasis that accompany normal development or may be associated with specific disease states. The rate of

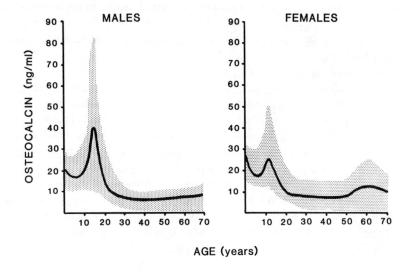

FIGURE 2. Serum osteocalcin concentrations in normal males and females as a function of age. The *solid line* is the mean value while the stippled area represents the 5 and 95% reference limits. Serum osteocalcin is higher in children than in adults. Peak values occur during the pubertal growth spurt. Elevations are also noted in women within the first ten to fifteen years after the menopause.

glomerular filtration or renal clearance of osteocalcin also influences circulating osteocalcin levels.

1. Normal Physiology
a. Age and Sex

Serum osteocalcin concentrations reflect osteoblastic activity. As a consequence, levels are elevated during bone growth and are higher in infants and children than in adults.[9,43] In neonates, levels range from 20 to 40 μg/l. Concentrations decline slightly thereafter (range: 10 to 25 μg/l) and remain relatively constant until the onset of puberty.[43-46] In boys a rapid increase in growth is seen around 15 years of age, while in girls this occurs earlier (12 years) but is of a smaller magnitude[43,44,46,47] (Figure 2). This growth spurt is mediated by the actions of sex steroids, growth hormone, and insulin-like growth factor (IGF-I, also called somatomedin C). Marked increases in serum osteocalcin at puberty show sex-related differences that are associated with the adolescent growth spurt. The changes in serum osteocalcin are strongly correlated with growth velocity rather than chronological age and parallel the related changes in alkaline phosphatase,[9] urinary hydroxyproline,[48] IGF-I,[47] as well as calcitonin, bone mineral content, and in boys, testosterone.[49]

Consistent with these observations is the finding that serum osteocalcin is lower in children with untreated growth hormone deficiency than in age-matched controls.[44] With treatment, serum osteocalcin increases slowly to normal levels[50] and decreases after therapy is discontinued.[44] Conversely, in children with accelerated growth associated with precocious puberty, osteocalcin levels were comparable to those in older pubertal adolescents and returned to the normal range with therapy.[47]

In young adults, serum osteocalcin varies between 2 and 12 μg/l, with a mean of about 7.2 μg/l.[13,51-53] Osteocalcin rises somewhat with aging in both men and women, although this effect has not been observed in all studies. Some authors report a continuous rise in serum osteocalcin in women over the age of 40.[51,53,55] However, in a cross-sectional study of 51 premenopausal and 114 postmenopausal normal women, we found osteocalcin increased only in the first 15 years following menopause and was normal thereafter.[56] This is consistent with the rapid bone loss that occurs in women in this perimenopausal period. In adult males 30 to 90 years old, serum osteocalcin concentrations are relatively constant.[53] Some variability in reported values may be due to decreasing renal function, a well-known concomitant of age,[57] and which has a significant effect on osteocalcin concentrations (see Section II.C.1.b below).

b. Circadian Rhythms

Serum osteocalcin concentrations show striking diurnal variations. In young adults on a normal light-dark cycle and meal schedule, levels decline in the morning, reach a nadir sometime after 12 noon, then rise again to reach a maximum around 4 a.m. This pattern is evident in males as well as females[58] (Figure 3). In a study of 10 adults, the osteocalcin levels varied almost twofold over the 24-h study period (range: 7 to 12 μg/l). In 2 adolescent males, the amplitude of the variation was similar (6 μg/l), but the mean 24-h value was 17 μg/l.[59] It is interesting to note that in children, there is an increased rate of skeletal mineralization and bone growth at night. One group has observed a nocturnal increase in the pulsatile release of growth hormone that paralleled the rise in serum osteocalcin.[60] However, subsequent studies have shown the nocturnal increase in these two proteins to not be causally related.[163,164] Rather, it appears that changes in endogenous cortisol are important for the changes that occur in serum osteocalcin during a 24 hour period.[165]

The large daytime variations (Figure 3) in osteocalcin concentrations may represent postprandial changes in metabolism. Unfortunately, there is little information regarding dietary influences on serum osteocalcin. Of the few observations which appear in the literature, osteocalcin changes are secondary to endocrine effects on calcium homeostasis. For example, phosphate loading will produce an increase in osteocalcin but this is also accompanied by hypocalcemia and hyperparathyroidism.[61] The diurnal pattern of serum osteocalcin is also not altered by age, sex, season, or smoking habits.[166] Clearly, these cyclical variations require the careful planning of blood collection times for any experimental protocol.

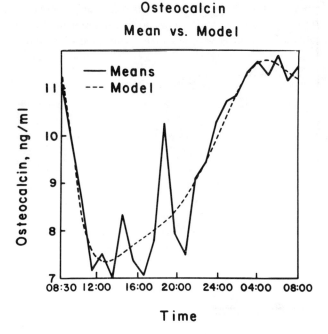

FIGURE 3. Osteocalcin circadian rhythm. Mean serum levels determined every 60 min in six normal 20- to 30-year-old men. *Solid line* indicates the mean values; the *dashed line* represents the mathematical model after all the data were smoothed. Serum osteocalcin was lowest around noon while the highest value occurred at 4 a.m. Consistent fluctuations were observed in all subjects in the afternoon and early evening. (From Gundberg et al., *J. Clin. Endocrinol. Metab.,* 60, 736, 1985. With permission.)

c. Clearance and Catabolism

Animal studies have shown that the chief route for the removal of circulating osteocalcin is through renal filtration and degradation. After administration of radiolabelled osteocalcin to rats the protein is taken up chiefly by the kidney with minor amounts of radioactivity being concentrated in bone, liver, and other soft tissues.[16,24,62] In fact, the best correlation between serum osteocalcin and bone formation is obtained when osteocalcin concentrations are normalized to creatinine clearance. Charles et al.,[33] noted that when serum levels were corrected for differences in renal function, osteocalcin was a significantly better predictor of bone formation than alkaline phosphatase.

When renal glomerular function is impaired, circulating osteocalcin concentrations are increased. In adults, this is not normally observed until the glomerular filtration rate (GFR) drops below 20 to 30 ml/min per 1.73 m² body surface area, or until the serum creatinine is greater than 160 μmol/l.[53,63] In children the increase in osteocalcin occurs when GFR drops below 40 ml/min per 1.73 m² (Figure 4). In patients with advanced renal

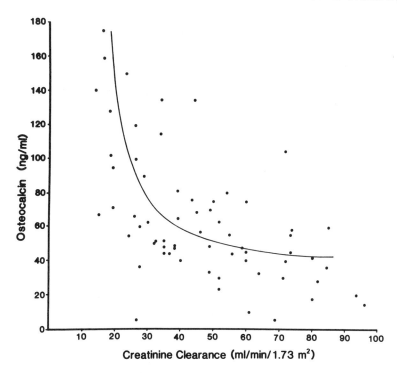

FIGURE 4. Serum osteocalcin as a function of creatinine clearance. Serum osteocalcin begins to rise above the normal range at a creatinine clearance of 40 ml/min.

failure, serum osteocalcin levels are invariably elevated. They range from 2 to 200 times higher than normal and are correlated to serum creatinine.[57,63-66]

In adults with end-stage renal disease, serum osteocalcin levels have been shown to reflect variations in histomorphometric parameters of both bone formation[64,66-68] and resorption.[7] This is in contrast to the findings that osteocalcin is related to bone formation but not resorption in individuals with normal renal function.[27-32] An explanation for this observation comes from our isolation of fragments of osteocalcin from the serum of patients with end-stage renal disease but not from normal individuals.[7] This suggests that limited proteolysis occurs in extrarenal sites and osteocalcin fragments produced by the osteoclast during bone resorption may accumulate in patients with impaired renal function. In normal individuals osteocalcin fragments are cleared from the circulation by the kidney.[7,69] Since antibodies raised against intact osteocalcin may be sensitive to peptide fragments when they are in high concentration, serum measurements will reflect both intact and epitope specific fragments. In the future, therefore, it will become increasingly important to establish the sensitivity of each particular assay to circulating osteocalcin fragments. Thus, the interpretation of osteocalcin levels in renal-failure patients requires consideration of at least two factors: decreased renal clearance and increased bone turnover (comprised of both bone formation *and* resorption).

2. Vitamin K

Osteocalcin production by osteoblasts is subject to transcriptional regulation by $1,25(OH)_2D$[70] and probable vitamin C-dependent hydroxylation of *Pro*$_9$ in most animals (but not humans).[71] In patients with pernicious anemia and vitamin B_{12} deficiency, osteocalcin levels are reduced and return to normal with replacement therapy, but the significance of this finding is not clear as there is no clinically significant bone disease known to be associated with this condition.[72] Vitamin K has the most profound influence on osteocalcin. It is essential for the production of Gla and the secretion and bone/plasma distribution of the protein.[18,20,72,74]

a. Effects on Synthesis and Hydroxyapatite Binding

In early pregnancy, the intake of coumarin anticoagulant drugs such as warfarin is associated with distinctive bony changes in the fetus producing a syndrome termed "chondrodysplasia punctata".[75-77] This fetal warfarin embryopathy is characterized by hypoplasia of the nasal bridge and distal phalanges, and punctate skeletal calcification which appears as radiographic stippling in the epiphyses and vertebrae. Animal models for warfarin teratogenicity in the developing chick embryo and rat fetus, show 50 to 80% reduction of total bone Gla content as a consequence of an exposure to 2 weeks of warfarin. Similar changes occur in growing chicks fed dicoumarol or vitamin K-deficient diets.[18] Chronic warfarin treatment of growing rats causes over 98% reduction of bone osteocalcin content[22] with premature growth plate closure.[78] These abnormalities could be caused by drug toxicity and/or hemorrhagic side effects, but more likely involve the presumptive skeletal vitamin K-dependent target proteins osteocalcin and matrix Gla protein. It has also been shown that the administration of vitamin K counteracts the effect of warfarin on the carboxylation of blood coagulation factors but does not overcome the effects of this drug on the carboxylation of osteocalcin.[79] A possible explanation for this disparity comes from a study[80] which suggested that the warfarin-insensitive and NADH-dependent vitamin K reductase, which is thought to mediate the antidotal effect of vitamin K on warfarin inhibition in the liver (i.e., by facilitating the reduction of the vitamin K quinone to the hydroquinone), is not present in an osteoblast-like, osteosarcoma cell line from rats. Wallin et al.[150] recently presented counter evidence that a human osteosarcoma cell line, which also has many similar characteristics to the human osteoblast, does possess this warfarin-insensitive reduction pathway suggesting that vitamin K can act as an antidote to warfarin in bone if enough vitamin K can accumulate in this tissue.

Prolonged administration of warfarin to rats results in a reduction in the overall rate of synthesis of osteocalcin. Importantly, the osteocalcin which is synthesized lacks its normal Gla complement and has a reduced affinity for hydroxyapatite. It might be expected, therefore, that warfarin treatment would result in a greater proportion of newly synthesized osteocalcin which is unable to bind to bone and finds its way into the circulation.

This is in fact observed when warfarin is given to young, rapidly growing rats (less than 4 weeks old). In such experiments the total concentration of osteocalcin antigen measurable in the serum is four to five times greater than that of control animals: if the animals are maintained on warfarin until maturity the osteocalcin concentrations decline to control levels although the protein remains undercarboxylated.[22,24] When mature rats are placed on a vitamin K-deficient diet their serum osteocalcin concentrations remain in the same range as vitamin K replete animals but once again the osteocalcin is undercarboxylated.[81] The difference in response between young and mature animals may be explained by the fact that periods of rapid bone growth are accompanied by an increased synthesis and accumulation of osteocalcin in bone. Therefore, in young rats, even if warfarin does reduce the normal rate of osteocalcin synthesis, this is more than outweighed by the lack of accretion of under-carboxylated osteocalcin to bone and hence the relative accumulation of the undercarboxylated species in blood. In the older rats, as bone growth declines (but never completely stops) osteocalcin synthesis stabilizes and declines to rates that are required for the maintenance of steady state levels in the bone. Under these circumstances the impact of warfarin on serum levels is minimal, with the decreased synthesis being countered by the decreased binding to bone. Likewise, in sheep, vitamin K is able to counteract the effect of the coumarin vitamin K antagonist, phenprocoumon, on the blood coagulation system, but not on osteocalcin synthesis or carboxylation.[82] In both adult sheep and humans, serum osteocalcin levels are actually lower in anticoagulated animals than in controls.[82] In these instances, in which bone growth stops at maturity, declining osteocalcin synthesis after the warfarin administration rather than increasing excretion into the circulation may be the greater factor in determining the concentrations of osteocalcin in serum.

Supportive evidence that vitamin K-dependent carboxylation of osteocalcin is essential for the normal development of embryonic bone has come recently from studies of a child with a multiple vitamin K-dependent factor deficiency.[83] In previous cases reported in the literature, this rare autosomal recessive disorder has presented solely as a severe bleeding disorder caused by the functional deficiency of the four vitamin K-dependent procoagulants.[84] In this most recent case,[83] in addition to the coagulopathy, the proband was born with the same phenotypic skeletal abnormalities which characterize the fetal warfarin syndrome. Biochemical studies of vitamin K metabolism pointed to an inborn deficiency of vitamin K epoxide reductase resulting in the undercarboxylation of all vitamin K-dependent proteins. Studies of the serum osteocalcin in this individual, revealed elevated levels and the presence of an abnormal osteocalcin species with properties consistent with a lack of Gla residues. This case has provided the first direct evidence that the teratogenic effect of warfarin on the skeleton is expressed through its known ability to inhibit vitamin K epoxide reductase and therefore to interfere with the carboxylation of the three specific glutamyl residues of osteocalcin to Gla residues in a posttranslational reaction.

b. Effects on Fracture Healing and Bone Density

Because of the possible role of osteocalcin in bone function, there is some concern that a deficit of vitamin K induced either nutritionally or by coumarin anticoagulants may have an adverse effect on bone metabolism. Plasma vitamin K_1 as well as MK-7 and MK-8 levels in elderly osteoporotic patients with fractures of the femoral neck were found to be reduced compared to aged matched controls.[85,167] Furthermore, in normal elderly individuals, there was reduced levels of MK-8 compared to younger individuals,[168] as well as an apperant undercarboxylation of osteocalcin in elderly women.[158,159] Whether these reflect a nutritional deficiency or are symptomatic of the disease process or normal aging is presently unclear. Since nearly 10% of the elderly population are on longterm anticoagulation therapy to prevent fatal pulmonary embolus, administration of vitamin K antagonists to hip-fracture patients may predispose them to disabling nonunions.

The effect of coumarin drugs on fracture healing has been studied in rats. In two such studies using dicoumarol, fracture healing was assessed histologically and impaired healing was observed.[22,86] However, high dose warfarin in combination with vitamin K, a situation that depletes the bone of osteocalcin, produced no radiologically discernible impairment of fracture repair.[22] To study the question of fracture healing in vitamin K deficiency, in a model that might resemble the condition observed in the osteoporotic crush-fracture patient, we produced vitamin K deficiency in rats by dietary deprivation. The fracture callus was tested by a biochemical as well as a mechanical method, a more accurate and quantifiable means of assessing callus strength. Nevertheless, the healing pattern and biomechanical properties of a standard closed fracture were still no different from controls and, although the degree of carboxylation of osteocalcin in the serum and the bone were reduced, the osteocalcin extracted from the fracture callus was normally carboxylated.[81] These findings can be explained in two ways. One explanation is that, in vitamin K deficiency, a small amount of osteocalcin becomes carboxylated and is thereby able to bind to the newly formed callus. (In the warfarin/ vitamin K rat model of Price,[22] approximately 2% of normal levels can be found in bone.) Alternatively callus osteoblasts may be influenced by different metabolic control mechanisms than those in the rest of the skeleton and may have a mechanism that ensures the gamma-carboxylation of glutamic acid residues at low tissue stores of vitamin K.

Although acute vitamin K deficiency may not affect fracture healing, the studies described above do not exclude the possibility that bone metabolism may be affected by protracted periods of vitamin K depletion or antagonism such as found in patients on long-term anticoagulant therapy. Although one study could find no statistically significant change in bone mass as assessed by single beam absorptiometry in seven patients who had been on coumadin (warfarin) therapy for 3 to 5 years, five of the seven patients showed a decrease in bone mass as compared to aged matched controls.[87] More recently, in a larger study of 57 patients (23 men, 34 women) maintained on phenprocoumon therapy, there was evidence of a decrease in bone mass compared to aged matched controls but interestingly only in women.[88]

3. Endocrine Effects

Hormonal status contributes to changes in circulating osteocalcin. Calcitriol thyroid and parathyroid hormone, cAMP, and estrogen directly affect osteocalcin gene transcription and mRNA levels.[89] Interpretation of osteocalcin data in clinical studies must be made with regard to endocrine status, as changes in osteoblastic function and activity are often secondary to shifting levels of calciotropic hormones.

a. 1,25 Dihydroxyvitamin D (Calcitriol)

The primary physiologic function of $1,25(OH)_2D$ is to increase intestinal absorption of calcium. It has a direct effect on bone metabolism by increasing bone resorption, perhaps by promoting the differentiation of progenitor cells to cells that are capable of bone resorption.[90] Calcitriol also modulates osteoblastic activity and its effect on osteocalcin synthesis and secretion is one of the best studied aspects of osteocalcin biology. The hormone will stimulate osteocalcin synthesis in osteoblasts by two-to tenfold depending upon the source of cells and culture medium.[70,91-93] Intravenous administration of a large dose of $1,25(OH)_2D_3$ to rats causes a fourfold rise in serum osteocalcin within 12 h.[72] These changes are consistent with changes in bone osteocalcin mRNA levels.[70] In adult humans, a single supraphysiological dose given at 7 a.m. increases serum osteocalcin within 6 and blunts or eliminates the normal morning fall that is characteristic of the circadian rhythm.[94] Treatment of vitamin D-dependent or hypophosphatemic rickets with daily doses of 1 μg/kg body weight increases serum osteocalcin within a week, while serum alkaline phosphatase activity remains unchanged.[95] Similar increases have also been observed in patients with postmenopausal osteoporosis and in controls.[96-98] On the other hand, lack of responsiveness to calcitriol has been demonstrated in vitamin D-dependent rickets type II, a disorder characterized by end organ resistance to vitamin D and its metabolites. Not only does serum osteocalcin remain the same after therapy in these patients,[9] but osteoblasts obtained from a 10 year old girl with this disorder also failed to respond to calcitriol stimulation.[99]

Although administration of calcitriol is associated with increases in circulating osteocalcin, endogenous levels of $1,25(OH)_2D$ do not always correlate with osteocalcin. Low to normal osteocalcin concentrations are observed in vitamin Ddeficiency,[19,43] a state which can be associated with low, normal, or elevated levels of circulating $1,25(OH)_2D$.[100] High concentrations of serum osteocalcin are observed in vitamin D-dependent rickets type I, but these patients have low circulating $1,25(OH)_2D$ due to reduced or absent renal 25-OH vitamin D 1-α-hydroxylase activity. In patients with hypophosphatemic rickets who have circulating $1,25(OH)_2D$ levels in the normal range, osteocalcin is elevated.[9,43,95] In fact, in most studies no sustained correlation between osteocalcin and $1,25(OH)_2D$ has been found,[45,94,101-104] although parallel increases in osteocalcin and $1,25(OH)_2D$ have been observed after diphosphonate[105] and glucocortinoid therapy.[106] Analysis of the osteocalcin gene indicates that several factors can modulate osteocalcin synthesis directly and in some cases may prevail over the influence of $1,25(OH)_2D$.

b. Parathyroid Hormone and Calcitonin

The action of PTH is to raise serum calcium by increasing renal calcium reabsorption and by increasing bone resorption. Its direct effect on bone is thought to be mediated through the osteoblast to produce a factor or factors which activate the osteoclast. It also indirectly affects bone resorption by stimulating the renal production of $1,25(OH)_2D$.[107] The precise relationship between parathyroid gland activity and serum osteocalcin concentrations has not been clearly established and may be subject to the interplay among the calciotropic hormones and circulating minerals. This is illustrated by the observations that patients with established hyperparathyroidism have osteocalcin levels that are elevated two- to fourfold above normal[10,13,32,108,109] while chronic hypoparathyroidism is associated with low osteocalcin concentrations.[13] This is consistent with the rates of bone turnover that are characteristic of these diseases. In individuals with normal levels of PTH, calcitriol stimulates osteocalcin synthesis two- to threefold.[78] In hypoparathyroidism, when PTH is absent and osteocalcin levels are diminished, calcitriol stimulates osteocalcin but it never reaches control levels.[110] In pseudohypoparathyroidism, a disorder in which PTH is elevated and in which bone is fully responsive to PTH but the renal response is diminished, osteocalcin levels are in the normal range. However, in this case, calcitriol therapy does not increase serum osteocalcin levels.[110] These observations suggest that PTH modulates the action of calcitriol on osteocalcin synthesis.

Attempts to clarify the direct action of PTH on osteocalcin synthesis have been made by studies of cultured osteoblasts or neonatal rat calvariae. In these cells bovine PTH alone has no effect on osteocalcin synthesis.[111] However, if the cells are first stimulated with $1,25(OH)_2D_3$ there is a suppression of osteocalcin secretion when physiologic amounts of bovine PTH (1–84) are added.[111,112] On the other hand, osteocalcin synthesis, secretion, and mRNA levels are increased when human PTH (1–34) is added to cultured rat osteoblast-like cells.[113] When bovine PTH (1–34) is infused into the rat hindlimb or intact animals, osteocalcin levels decline.[114] Conversely, rat PTH has no effect in these systems (unpublished observations). Patients with X-linked hypophosphatemia showed a significant decrease in osteocalcin concentrations within 15 min of a bPTH (1–84) infusion,[115] while a group of 18 healthy women showed a decrease in serum osteocalcin of 23% during a 24-h infusion of bPTH (1–34).[116] Bovine, rat, and human, 1–34 or 1–84, forms of the hormone have not been directly compared in the same system to determine if differences in the primary sequences affect the osteocalcin response.

Calcitonin has no apparent effect on osteocalcin synthesis *in vitro*,[112] and osteocalcin values have not been reported in isolated disorders of calcitonin metabolism. However, decreases in serum osteocalcin have been associated with calcitonin therapy of both Paget's disease[108] and osteoporosis.[117] Acute and chronic administration of calcitonin to rats also causes a rapid decrease in circulating osteocalcin.[118]

4. Alterations with Bone Disease
a. Correlations with Alkaline Phosphatase

The measurement of alkaline phosphatase is one of the most frequently performed assays in clinical medicine and its elevation in the circulation in various skeletal disorders has been recognized for 50 years. Bone alkaline phosphatase is expressed by the osteoblast and it is thought to have a function in bone formation. However, total alkaline phosphatase in the serum is comprised of several isoenzymes and an elevated value can be the result of increased activity of intestinal, spleen, kidney, placental, liver, or bone origin. The two most common sources of an elevated alkaline phosphatase, nevertheless, are liver and bone. Separation of the various enzymes by heat denaturation, electrophoresis, or wheat-germ agglutination may identify the source of the enzyme, but all methods have analytical problems and isoenzyme determinations are to be interpreted with caution.[119,120] It is for these reasons that a better marker for bone formation has long been sought.

Both circulating osteocalcin and alkaline phosphatase are elevated in patients with diseases characterized by high bone turnover. Unlike total alkaline phosphatase, serum osteocalcin levels are normal in disorders not involving bone. Many studies show correlations between serum osteocalcin and alkaline phosphatase in isolated bone diseases but there are often dissociations between the two (Table 1). Dissociations arise either because of contributions from nonosseous alkaline phosphatase or because the two parameters reflect differing aspects of osteoblastic activity.

Elevations of both osteocalcin and total alkaline phosphatase are observed in primary and secondary hyperparathyroidism, and in osteomalacia of various origins.[14,53] In nutritional or inherited rickets alkaline phosphatase is elevated while osteocalcin levels vary depending upon the type of disease.[53] In Paget's disease, both parameters are elevated. Alkaline phosphatase, however, correlates better with bone scintigraphy than does osteocalcin.[120] Alkaline

TABLE 1
Serum Alkaline Phosphatase (ALP) and Osteocalcin in
Various Disorders

Disorder	Total ALP	Bone ALP	Osteocalcin
Hyperparathyroidism	E	E	E
Paget's disease	E	E	E
Osteoporosis	N	E	D–E
Osteomalacia	E	ND	E
Rickets	E	ND	D–E
Fractures	N	ND	N,E
Osteogenesis imperfecta	N	ND	N,E
Renal failure	N	N	E
Osteolytic metastasis	E	E	E
Hypoparathyroidism	D	D	D
Hypothyroidism	D	D	D
Liver Disease	E	N	N

Note: N = normal; E = elevated; D = depressed; ND = not determined.

phosphatase activity is generally normal in osteogenesis imperfecta, but os-teocalcin can be normal or elevated.[121] This may be related to the incidence of fractures. Both bone and liver ALP are elevated in a high proportion of patients with malignancies. In primary tumors of bone, both osteocalcin and alkaline phosphatase are higher in patients with blastic lesions than with lytic lesions.[122] In patients with nonbone tumors that metastasize to bone, alkaline phosphatase is normal or elevated with high levels associated with hypocal-cemia. On the other hand, osteocalcin levels are decreased in patients with malignant hypercalcemia and correlate to histomorphometric parameters of bone formation.[32] Both alkaline phosphatase and osteocalcin are decreased in disorders characterized by low bone turnover, i.e., hypoparathyroidism[13,14] and hypothyroidism.[11]

There have been at least three reports of a direct comparison between the bone alkaline phosphatase isoenzyme activity and osteocalcin concentra-tion.[123-125] In two reports the correlation between the two parameters was greater for normal women than men.[123,124] In patients with metabolic bone disease concordant results were obtained in patients with hyper- and hypo-parathyroidism, hyperthyroidism, osteoporosis, and acromegaly. No associ-ation was found in patients with glucocorticoid excess, Paget's disease, chronic renal failure, or osteolytic metastasis[124] (Table 1). In the case of chronic renal failure, these differences are most likely due to differing clearances of the proteins.[125] (The clearance rate of osteocalcin is approximately 20 min, while that of alkaline phosphatase is 7 d.) In the other instances, the discordant results are most likely related to the differing roles of these two proteins in bone metabolism. Their simultaneous measurement in various diseases and under diverse experimental conditions may provide a better understanding of these functions.

The relevance of circulating osteocalcin in specific diseases has been extensively evaluated and the reader is directed toward recent reviews.[126,127,169]

b. Osteoporosis

Osteoporosis, by definition, is a state in which bone mass is so reduced that fractures occur after minimal or no trauma. Since osteoporosis is a very common debilitating disorder that lacks early diagnostic criteria, considerable attention has been focused on circulating osteocalcin as a possible biochemical marker. In women, bone mass is constant until the time of menopause, decreases rapidly in the first 5 to 10 years after menopause, and then stabilizes or declines slowly. Bone loss occurs due to an increase in bone resorption over formation. Normally, these processes are tightly coupled so that if one increases or decreases, the other changes in parallel, thereby maintaining normal bone mass. In osteoporosis, there is uncoupling of these two processes such that there is a net loss of bone.

Current methods for assessing skeletal density include quantitative computed tomography (CT), single and dual energy photon absorptiometry, dual energy X-ray absorptiometry and total body neutron activation. Quantitative CT measures the density of a small volume of trabecular bone within the vertebral body; absorptiometry is used primarily to measure bone density in the mid- or distal radius and in the spine or hip. Total body neutron activation which is primarily a research tool and not widely available, measures the amount of mineral in the entire skeleton. In normal postmenopausal women (that is, with no symptoms or documented fractures) increased serum osteocalcin is associated with decreased bone mineral density at the lumbar spine, midradius, and distal radius.[54,55,128] Likewise, in a study of 114 normal postmenopausal women, total body calcium and phosphorous determined by neutron activation analysis was significantly lower in a subset of women with elevated osteocalcin levels than in a similar group of women with normal osteocalcin levels.[56] High osteocalcin values were found only in those women who were within the first 15 years after the menopause (Table 2). These observations in normal women suggest that age-related bone loss resulting from increased bone turnover (with resorption increasing more than formation) leads to a negative calcium balance and progressive reduction in skeletal mass. It would be interesting to know which of these women develop frank osteoporosis and if the severity or timing is related to their ''pre-osteoporotic'' osteocalcin concentrations. In the same study, a group of women of the same age range but with proven osteoporosis had osteocalcin levels which were clearly elevated (Figure 5) while total body calcium was lower than any of the nonosteoporotic women (Table 2).

Osteocalcin levels have been reported to be low,[96,129] normal,[29,130] or high[55,56,128] in postmenopausal osteoporosis. This variability can be explained by the fact that in postmenopausal osteoporosis there is a wide variation in bone turnover rates (and therefore bone formation rates).[131] Serum osteocalcin

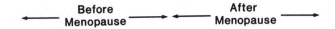

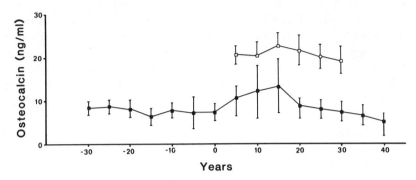

FIGURE 5.　Serum osteocalcin plotted against years (age minus 50) before or after the menopause. Serum osteocalcin was increased in some normal women in the decade following the menopause, but in those normal women who were more than 15 years postmenopausal, serum osteocalcin concentrations were in the normal premenopausal range. In postmenopausal osteoporotic women, mean serum osteocalcin levels were elevated.

TABLE 2
Serum Osteocalcin and Total Body Calcium in Normal and Osteoporotic Women

	Number	Total Body Calcium	Osteocalcin
Normal Women			
Premenopausal	51	898	8.8
Postmenopausal	114	807	10.1
		p <0.01[a]	p >0.1[a]
Osteoporotic Women			
	41	657	17.1
		p <.01[b]	p <.01[b]

[a]　Postmenopausal vs. premenopausal normal women.
[b]　Postmenopausal osteoporotic vs. postmenopausal normal women.

measurements have proven useful in osteoporosis in this regard. Concentrations are highly correlated to tetracycline-based indices of bone formation in affected postmenopausal women[29,30] and may predict those women most severely affected, i.e., those with high turnover rates and the most rapid bone loss.

It is thought that estrogen deficiency after the menopause is a major factor in postmenopausal bone loss. Estrogen administration to postmenopausal women may prevent bone loss by selectively reducing bone resorption. Unfortunately, there is also a secondary fall in bone formation and, after an initial period, a new steady state is reached in which formation is less than or equal to resorption. The skeleton remains osteoporotic although bone loss has been slowed. The effect of estrogen in suppressing bone turnover is supported by the observations that oophorectomy increases serum osteocalcin above normal levels,[132,133] while estrogen therapy decreases circulating osteocalcin in postmenopausal women.[104,134] When a sequential progestagen regimen is added, bone formation and osteocalcin levels increase.[135] Increased osteocalcin levels are also associated with administration of analogs of gonadotropin-releasing hormone which inhibit ovulation and lead to a reduction in circulating estrogen levels.[136,137]

The implication in the preceding discussion is that increased osteocalcin levels are detrimental to the maintenance of bone mass. This appears to be the case in those diseases in which bone formation and resorption are "negatively uncoupled". In osteoporosis there is an absolute increase in bone loss over bone formation, although both processes may be fast or normal. Obviously, those individuals with the fastest loss of bone are most at risk for debilitating fractures. An ideal therapeutic agent would be one which increases bone formation while maintaining or decreasing resorption. Many different factors contribute to the acceleration in bone loss. It is likely that optimal treatment will be dependent on accurate assessment of risk factors, early diagnosis of bone loss, and an individualized therapeutic strategy. It is in this context that osteocalcin measurements may be beneficial. If drugs that suppress or stimulate formation are indicated for a particular patient, the response to therapy may be individually monitored with serial osteocalcin measurements.

III. URINARY GLA EXCRETION

Since free Gla is not further metabolized,[138] its concentration in urine is an index of the turnover of all the Gla-containing proteins. The majority of urinary Gla results from the metabolism of liver-synthesized vitamin K-dependent clotting factors. Urinary Gla excretion has been quantitated by several procedures and is normally about 40 μmol/g creatinine in adults[52,139,140] but can reach 100 μmol/g creatinine in neonates and children[52,142](Figure 6). Day to day variation in Gla excretion for any one individual is small. However, Sadowski has reported that there are large differences in mean daily excretion among individuals and the differences are related to lean body mass.[142] Measurements of urinary Gla have been used as an indicator of vitamin K nutritional status in animals and humans[150] on vitamin K deficient diets and eliminates the need for repeated blood sampling to determine the extent of vitamin K depletion.

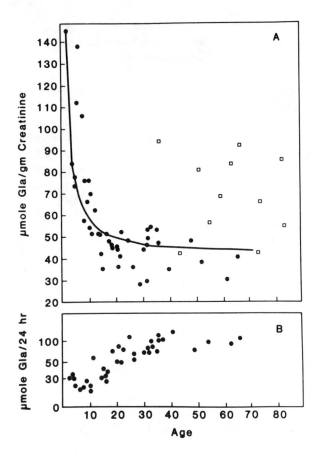

FIGURE 6. Urinary Gla excretion in relation to age when normalized to urine creatinine (A) or during a 24-h period (B) in normal subjects (●). In osteoporotic patients (□) urinary Gla is often elevated. (From Lian, J. B. and Grundberg, C. M., *Clin. Orthop. Rel. Res.*, 226, 267, 1988. With permission.)

An estimation of the contribution from osteocalcin to total Gla excretion is based on clinical data from warfarin-treated patients. At the limit of extreme anticoagulation, where the reduced Gla content of the vitamin K-dependent coagulation factors contributes minimally to urinary Gla, 20% of normal urinary Gla excretion persists.[143] Since less than 0.2% (50 nmol) of the total daily urinary output of Gla derives from circulating osteocalcin, the residual Gla may be presumed to come from degraded osteocalcin released by osteoclasts *in situ* during bone resorption. There should also be a contribution from the catabolism of matrix Gla protein in bone and slow-turnover nonosseous pools of Gla proteins (kidney, lung, spleen, etc.).

Urinary excretion of Gla has been quantitated in disorders of bone and calcium metabolism. Based on the presumed 20% contribution from

TABLE 3
Urinary Gla Excretion in
Various Disorders

Disorder	μmol Gla/gm Creatinine (Mean ± 5.0.)
Normal adults	44 ± 11
Chronic coumadin therapy	24 ± 8
Osteoporosis	69 ± 13
Paget's disease	45 ± 12
Dermatomyositis	109 ± 20
Scleroderma	81 ± 15

osteocalcin reserves in bone, a doubling of urinary Gla excretion would require a net fivefold increase in the rate of bone resorption in the absence of co-agulation factor changes. Urinary Gla excretion rates are elevated in some patients with osteoporosis, indicative of the enhanced bone resorption in that disease.[130] In disorders associated with ectopic calcification such as sclero-derma, dermatomyositis, and nephrocalcinosis, urinary Gla concentrations are altered[144-146] (Table 3). The origin of increased urine Gla in these patients is not clear but Gla proteins have been found to be associated with the calcific nodules and stones[147] (Table 3). In addition, free Gla has also been detected in the serum.[148] Because the major contribution to urinary Gla is from the catabolism of the vitamin K-dependent coagulation proteins, the measurement of serum or urine Gla in metabolic bone disease is of limited usefulness.

IV. SUMMARY AND CONCLUSIONS

Laboratory tests that are currently used for the diagnosis and treatment of metabolic bone disease are largely restricted to endocrine studies of bone mineral homeostasis, particularly those related to the calciotropic hormones — vitamin D and its metabolites, parathyroid hormone and calcitonin. In disorders that do not perturb hormonal status, the ability to monitor disease or judge the response to therapy is extremely limited. Bone status can be accurately assessed in biopsy specimens if dynamic histomorphometry is performed, but the technique is invasive, and results obtained with a single core biopsy may not apply to other areas of the skeleton. Quantitative bone absorptiometry may offer a very detailed and accurate assessment of the static structural changes and radioisotopic scintigraphy may provide a nonspecific measure of overall bone metabolism, but neither is very sensitive to the specific alterations in bone metabolism that lead to changes in general skeletal structure and integrity.

Studies monitoring serum osteocalcin in normal individuals and patients with metabolic bone disease indicate that serum osteocalcin can be a useful

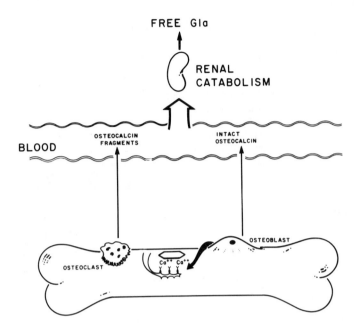

FIGURE 7. Proposed model for osteocalcin metabolism. Osteocalcin is synthesized by the osteoblast. The majority of newly synthesized osteocalcin accumulates in bone matrix where it interacts with Ca^{2+} in the hydroxyapatite crystal. A portion of the osteocalcin leaves the bone and is detectable in the circulation. During bone resorption, osteoclasts liberate osteocalcin fragments. With normal renal function, osteocalcin and these fragments are rapidly cleared by the kidney and contribute to the urine free Gla. In renal failure, these fragments accumulate and, with specific antisera, are detectable.

marker of bone formation. However, many factors contribute to osteocalcin concentrations in blood. Not only must sex, age, and circadian rhythms be considered, but other factors such as hormonal status, renal function, sensitivity of the assay to circulating fragments, and degree of carboxylation of the protein, must be assessed.

The physiological significance of serum osteocalcin and urine Gla measurements is outlined in Figure 7. Intact osteocalcin is a product of the osteoblast. The majority of the newly synthesized protein binds to the mineral and becomes a matrix component. A small portion, however, is released into the circulation during bone formation and is measurable in serum. The serum level is modulated by a variety of factors which affect osteoblast numbers and activity. Matrix osteocalcin may be released into the circulation during osteoclastic resorption, largely as nonimmune fragments. These are cleared efficiently and are not measurable when kidney function is normal. Renal filtration leads to the eventual excretion of unmetabolized free Gla.

REFERENCES

1. **Taylor, A. K., Linkhart, S. G., Mohon, S., and Baylink, D. J.,** Development of a new radioimmunoassay for human osteocalcin: evidence for a midmolecule epitope, *Metabolism,* 37, 872, 1988.
2. **Catherwood, B. D.,** Region-specific radioimmunoassay (RIA) for human gamma-carboxyglutamic acid-containing protein (BGP) in blood of normal subjects, *Calcif. Tissue Int.,* 3, 29, 1982.
3. **Juppner, H., Schettler, T., Giebel, G., Wenner, S., and Hesch, R.D.,** Radioimmunoassay for human osteocalcin using an antibody raised against the synthetic human (h37-49) sequence, *Calcif. Tissue Int.,* 39, 310, 1986.
4. **Gundberg, C. M., Hauschka, P. V., Lian, J. B., and Gallop, P. M.,** Osteocalcin: isolation, characterization and detection, in *Methods in Enzymology,* Moldave, K., Ed., Academic Press, 1984, 107.
5. **Price, P. A. and Nishimoto, S. K.,** Radioimmunoassay for the vitamin K-dependent protein of bone and its discovery in plasma, *Proc. Natl. Acad. Sci. U.S.A.,* 77, 2234, 1980.
6. **Delmas, P. D., Stenner, D. D., Romberg, R. W., Riggs, B. L., and Mann, K. G.,** Immunological studies of conformational alterations in bone gamma-carboxyglutamic acid containing protein, *Biochemistry,* 23, 4720, 1984.
7. **Gundberg, C. M. and Weinstein, R. S.,** Multiple immunoreactive forms of osteocalcin in uremic serum, *J. Clin. Invest.,* 77, 1762, 1986.
8. **Galli, M., Nuti, R., Franci, B., Righi, G., Martorelli, M. T., Turchetti, V., and Caniggia, M.,** Serum osteocalcin radioimmunoassay in bone diseases, *Ric. Clin. Lab.,* 15, 253, 1985.
9. **Kruse, D. and Kracht, U.,** Evaluation of serum osteocalcin as an index of altered bone metabolism, *Eur. J. Pediatr.,* 145, 27, 1986.
10. **Ljunghall, S., Hallgren, R., and Rastad, J.,** Serum osteocalcin levels in normal subjects and patients with primary hyperparathyroidism, *Exp. Clin. Endocrinol.,* 86, 218, 1985.
11. **Martinez, M. E., Herranz, L., de Pedro, C., and Pallardo, L. F.,** Osteocalcin levels in patients with hyper- and hypothyroidism, *Horm. Metab. Res.,* 18, 212, 1986.
12. **Melick, R. A., Farrugia, W., and Quelch, K. J.,** Plasma osteocalcin in man, *Aust. N.Z. J. Med.,* 15, 410, 1985.
13. **Price, P. A., Parthemore, J. B., and Deftos, L. J.,** New biochemical marker for bone metabolism: measurement by radioimmunoassay of bone Gla protein in the plasma of normal subjects and patients with bone disease, *J. Clin. Invest.,* 66, 878, 1980.
14. **Slovik, R. M., Gundberg, C. M., Neer, R. M., and Lian, J. B.,** Clinical evaluation of bone turnover by serum osteocalcin measurements, *J. Clin. Endocrinol. Metab.,* 59, 228, 1984.
15. **Hauschka, P. V. and Carr, S. A.,** Calcium-dependent alpha-helical structure in osteocalcin, *Biochemistry,* 21, 2538, 1982.
16. **Hauschka, P. V.,** Osteocalcin: the vitamin K-dependent calcium-binding protein of bone matrix, *in Heritable Disorders of Connective Tissue,* Akeson, W. H., Bornstein, P., Glimcher, M. J., Eds., Mosby, St. Louis, 1982, 195.
17. **Poser, J. W. and Price, P. A.,** A method for decarboxylation of gamma-carboxyglutamic acid in proteins: properties of the decarboxylated gamma-carboxyglutamic acid from calf bone, *J. Biol. Chem.,* 254, 431, 1979.
18. **Hauschka, P. V. and Reid, M. L.,** Vitamin K dependence of a calcium binding protein containing gamma-carboxyglutamic acid in chicken bone, *J. Biol. Chem.,* 253, 9063, 1978.
19. **Lian, J. B. and Friedman, P. A.,** The vitamin K-dependent synthesis of gamma-carboxyglutamic acid by bone microsomes, *J. Biol. Chem.,* 253, 6623, 1978.

20. **Nishimoto, S. K. and Price, P. A.**, The vitamin K-dependent bone protein is accumulated within cultured osteosarcoma cells in the presence of the vitamin K antagonist warfarin, *J. Biol. Chem.*, 260, 2832, 1985.
21. **Pan, L. C., Williamson, M. K., and Price, P. A.**, Sequence of the precursor to rat bone gamma-carboxyglutamic acid protein that accumulates in warfarin-treated osteosarcoma cells, *J. Biol. Chem.*, 260, 13,398, 1985.
22. **Price, P. A. and Williamson, M. K.**, Effects of warfarin on bone: studies on the vitamin K-dependent protein of rat bone, *J. Biol. Chem.*, 256, 12,754, 1981.
23. **Suttie, J. W.**, Vitamin K-dependent carboxylase, *Annu. Rev. Biochem.*, 54, 459, 1985.
24. **Price, P. A., Williamson, M. K., and Lothringer, J. W.**, Origin of the vitamin K-dependent bone protein found in plasma and its clearance by kidney and bone, *J. Biol. Chem.*, 256, 12,760, 1981.
25. **Melsen, F. and Mosekilde, L.**, Tetracycline double-labeling of iliac trabecular bone in 41 normal adults, *Calcif. Tiss. Res.*, 26, 99, 1978.
26. **Burkinshaw, L., Marshall, D. H., Oxby, C. B., Spiers, F. W., Nordin, B. E. C., and Young, M. M.**, Bone turnover model based on a continuously expanding exchangeable calcium pool, *Nature,* 222, 146, 1969.
27. **Eastell, R., Delmas, P. D., Hodgson, S. F., Eriksen, E. F., Mann, K. G., and Riggs, B. L.**, Bone formation rate in older women: concurrent assessment with bone histomorphometry, calcium kinetics, and biochemical markers, *J. Clin. Endocrinol. Metab.*, 67, 742, 1988.
28. **Garcia-Carrasco, M., Gruson, M., de Vernejovl, M. C., Denne, M. A., and Miravet, L.**, Osteocalcin and bone morphometric parameters in adults without bone disease, *Calcif. Tiss. Int.*, 42, 13, 1988.
29. **Brown, J. P., Delmas, P. D., Malaval, L., Eduoard, C., Chapuy, M. C., and Meunier, P. J.**, Serum bone Gla-protein: a specific marker for bone formation in postmenopausal osteoporosis, *Lancet,* i, 1091, 1984.
30. **Brown, J. P., Delmas, P. D., Arlot, M., and Meunier, P. J.**, Active bone turnover of the cortico-endosteal envelope in postmenopausal osteoporosis, *J. Clin. Endocrinol. Metab.*, 64, 954, 1987.
31. **Delmas, P. D., Malaval, L., Arlot, M. E., and Meunier, P. J.**, Serum bone Gla-protein compared to bone histomorphometry in endocrine diseases, *Bone,* 6, 339, 1985.
32. **Delmas, P. D., Demiaux, B., Malaval, L., Chapuy, M. C., Eduaord, C., and Meunier, P. J.**, Serum bone gamma carboxyglutamic acid-containing protein in primary hyperparathyroidism and in malignant hypercalcemia, *J. Clin. Invest.*, 77, 985, 1986.
33. **Charles, P., Poser, J. W., Mosekilde, L., and Jensen, F. T.**, Estimation of bone turnover evaluated by [47]Ca-kinetics. Efficiency of serum bone gammacarboxyglutamic acid-containing protein, serum alkaline phosphatase, and urinary hydroxyproline excretion, *J. Clin. Invest.*, 76, 2254, 1985.
34. **Charles, P., Mosekilde, L., and Taagehoj Jensen, F.**, Primary hyperparathyroidism: evaluated by [47]calcium kinetics, calcium balance and serum bone-Gla-protein, *Eur. J. Clin. Invest.*, 16, 277, 1986.
35. **Hauschka, P. V. and Reid, M. L.**, Timed appearance of calcium-binding protein containing gamma-carboxyglutamic acid in developing chick bone, *Dev. Biol.*, 65, 426, 1978.
36. **Hauschka, P. V., Frenkel, J., DeMuth, R., and Gundberg, C. M.**, Presence of osteocalcin and related higher molecular weight 4-carboxyglutamic acid-containing proteins in developing bone, *J. Biol. Chem.*, 258, 176, 1983.
37. **Yoon, K., Buenaga, R., and Rodan, G. A.**, Tissue specificity and developmental expression of osteopontin, *Biochem. Biophys. Res. Commun.*, 148, 1129, 1987.
38. **Gerstenfeld, L. C., Chipman, S. D., Glowacki, J., and Lian, J. B.**, Expression of differentiated function in mineralizing cultures of chicken osteoblasts, *Dev. Biol.*, 122, 49, 1987.

39. **Van Der Eems, K. L., Brown, R. D., and Gundberg, C. M.,** Circulating levels of 1,25 dihydroxyvitamin D, alkaline phosphatase, hydroxyproline, and osteocalcin associated with antler growth in white-tailed deer, *Acta Endocrinol.,* 118, 407, 1988.

40. **Robison, R.,** The possible significance of hexosephosphoric esters in ossification, *Biochem. J.,* 17, 286, 1923.

41. **Russell, R. G. G.,** Excretion of inorganic pyrophosphate in hypophosphatasia, *Lancet,* 2, 461, 1965.

42. **Melick, R., Farrugia, W., Heaton, C., and Scoggins, B.,** Plasma production rate of osteocalcin in sheep, *J. Bone Min. Res.,* (Suppl.) 1, 130A, 1986.

43. **Cole, D. E. C., Carpenter, T. O., and Gundberg, C. M.,** Serum osteocalcin levels in children with metabolic bone disease, *J. Pediatr.,* 106, 770, 1985.

44. **Delmas, P. D., Chatelain, P., Malaval, L., and Bonne, G.,** Serum bone Gla-protein in growth hormone deficient children, *J. Bone Min. Res.,* 1, 333, 1986.

45. **Delmas, P. D., Glorieux, F. H., Delvin, E. E., Salle, B. L., and Melki, I.,** Perinatal serum bone Gla-protein and vitamin D metabolites in preterm and fullterm neonates, *J. Clin. Endocrinol. Metab.,* 65, 588, 1987.

46. **Klein, G. L., Wadlington, E. L., Collins, E. D., Catherwood, B. D., and Deftos, L. J.,** Calcitonin levels in sera of infants and children: relations to age and periods of bone growth, *Calcif. Tiss. Int.,* 36, 635, 1987.

47. **Johansen, J. S., Giwercman, A., Hartwell, D., Nielsen, C. T., Price, P. A., Christiansen, C. and Skakkebaek, N. E.,** Serum Bone Gla-Protein as a marker of bone growth in children and adolescents: correlation with age, height, serum insulin-like growth factor I, and serum testosterone, *J. Clin. Endocrinol. Metab.,* 67, 273, 1988.

48. **Stepan, J. J., Tesarova, A., Havranek, T., Jodl, J., Formankova, J., and Pacovsky, V.,** Age and sex dependency of the biochemical indices of bone remodelling, *Clin. Chim. Acta,* 151, 273, 1985.

49. **Riis, B. J., Krabbe, S., Christiansen, C.., Catherwood, B. D., and Deftos, L. J.,** Bone turnover in male puberty: a longitudinal study, *Calcif. Tiss. Int.,* 37, 210, 1985.

50. **Lindstedt, G., Wejkum, L., and Lundberg, P. A.,** Increase in serum osteocalcin concentration is a slow indicator of therapeutic effect in children treated for somatotropin deficiency, *Clin. Chem.,* 32, 1589, 1986.

51. **Galli, M. and Caniggia, M.,** Osteocalcin in normal adult humans of different sex and age, *Horm. Metab. Res.,* 17, 165, 1985.

52. **Gundberg, C. M., Lian, J. B., and Gallop, P. M.,** Measurements of gamma-carboxyglutamate and circulating osteocalcin in normal adults and children, *Clin. Chim. Acta,* 128, 1, 1983.

53. **Johansen, J. S., Thomsen, K., and Christiansen, C.,** Plasma bone Gla protein in healthy adults. Dependence on sex, age, and glomerular filtration, *Scand. J. Clin. Lab. Invest.,* 47, 345, 1987.

54. **Delmas, P. D., Stenner, D., Wahner, H. W., Mann, K. G., and Riggs, B. L.,** Increase in serum bone gamma-carboxyglutamic acid protein with aging in women. Implications for the mechanism of age-related bone loss, *J. Clin. Invest.,* 71, 1316, 1983.

55. **Epstein, S., Poser, J. W., McClintock, R., Johnston, C. C., Jr., Bryce, G., and Hui, S.,** Differences in serum bone Gla protein with age and sex, *Lancet,* 1, 307, 1984.

56. **Yasumura, S., Aloia, J. F., Gundberg, C. M., Yeh, J., Vaswani, A. N., Yuen, K., LoMonte, A. F., Ellis, K. J., and Cohn, S. H.,** Serum osteocalcin and total body calcium in normal pre- and postmenopausal women and postmenopausal osteoporotic patients, *J. Clin. Endocrinol. Metab.,* 64, 681, 1987.

57. **Chung, A. K., Manolagas, S. C., Catherwood, B. D., Mosely, C. A., Jr., Mitas, J. A., Blantz, R. C., and Deftos, L. J.,** Determinants of serum 1,25(OH)$_2$D levels in renal disease, *Kidney Int.,* 24, 104, 1983.

58. **Gundberg, C. M., Markowitz, M. E., Mizruchi, M., and Rosen, J. F.,** Osteocalcin in human serum: a circadian rhythm, *J. Clin. Endocrinol. Metab.,* 60, 736, 1985.

59. **Markowitz, M. E., Gundberg, C. M., and Rosen, J. F.,** 24-hour variations in serum osteocalcin concentrations in teenage males, *Pediatr. Res.,* 18, 98A, 1984.

60. **Shima, M., Seino, Y., Tanaka, Y., Yabuuchi, H., Tsutsumi, C., and Moriuchi, S.,** Bone gamma-carboxyglutamic acid containing protein in the perinatal period, *Acta Paediatr. Scand.,* 74, 674, 1986.

61. **Silverberg, S. J., Shane, E., Clemens, T. S., Dempster, D. W., Segre, G. V., Lindsay, R., and Belezikian, J. P.,** Oral phosphate affects major indices of skeletal metabolism in normal human subjects, *J. Bone Min. Res.,* 1, 383, 1987.

62. **Farrugia, W. and Melick, R. A.,** Metabolism of osteocalcin, *Calcif. Tiss. Int.,* 39, 234, 1986.

63. **Delmas, P. D., Wilson, D. M., Mann, K. G., and Riggs, B. L.,** Effect of renal function on plasma levels of bone gla-protein, *J. Clin. Endocrinol. Metab.,* 57, 1028, 1983.

64. **Coen, G., Mazzaferro, S., Bonucci, E., Taggi, F., Ballanti, P., Bianchi, A. R., Donato, G., Massimetti, C., Smacchi, A., and Cinotti, G. A.,** Bone GLA protein in predialysis chronic renal failure. Effects of $1,25(OH)_2D_3$ administration in a long-term follow-up, *Kidney Int.,* 28, 783, 1985.

65. **Epstein, S., Traberg, H., Raja, R., and Poser, J.,** Serum and dialysate osteocalcin levels in hemodialysis and peritoneal dialysis patients after renal transplantation, *J. Clin. Endocrinol. Metab.,* 60, 253, 1985.

66. **Sebert, J. L., Ruiz, J. C., Fournier, A., Fardellone, P., Gueris, J., Marie, A., Moriniere, P. H., Codet, M. P., and Renaud, H.,** Plasma bone Gla-protein: assessment of its clinical value as an index of bone formation in hemodialyzed patients, *Bone Miner.,* 2, 21, 1987.

67. **Charhon, S. A., Delmas, P. D., Malaval, L., Chavassieux, P. M., Arlot, M., Chapuy, M. C., and Meunier, P. J.,** Serum bone Gla-protein in renal osteodystrophy: comparison with bone histomorphometry, *J. Clin. Endocrinol. Metab.,* 68, 892, 1986.

68. **Malluche, H. H., Faugere, M. C., Fanti, P., and Price, P.,** Plasma levels of bone Gla protein reflect bone formation in patients on chronic maintenance dialysis, *Kidney Int.,* 26, 869, 1984.

69. **Gundberg, C. M., Hanning, R. M., Liu, A., Zlotkin, A. H., Balfe, J. W., and Cole, D. E. C.,** Clearance of osteocalcin by peritoneal dialysis in children with end-stage renal disease, *Pediatr. Res.,* 21, 296, 1987.

70. **Pan, L. C. and Price, P. A.,** The effect of transcriptional inhibitors on the bone gamma-carboxyglutamic acid protein response to $1,25(OH)_2$-vitamin D_3 in osteosarcoma cells, *J. Biol. Chem.,* 259, 5844, 1984.

71. **Poser, J. W., Esch, F. S., Ling, N. C., and Price, P. A.,** Isolation and sequence of the vitamin K-dependent protein from human bone: undercarboxylation of the first glutamic acid residue, *J. Biol. Chem.,* 255, 8685, 1980.

72. **Carmel, R., Lau, K. H. W., Baylink, D. J., Saxena, S., and Singer, F. R.,** Cobalamin and osteoblast-specific proteins, *N. Engl. J. Med.,* 319, 70, 1988.

73. **Nishimoto, S. K. and Price, P. A.,** Secretion of the vitamin K-dependent protein of bone by rat osteosarcoma cells. Evidence for an intracellular precursor, *J. Biol. Chem.,* 255, 6579, 1980.

74. **Price, P. A.,** Vitamin K dependent formation of bone Gla protein (osteocalcin) and its function, *Vitam. Horm.,* 42, 65, 1985.

75. **Hall, J., Pauli, R. M., and Wilson, K. M.,** Maternal and fetal sequelae of anticoagulation during pregnancy, *Am. J. Med.,* 68, 1220, 1980.

76. **Hunter, A. G. W., Rimoin, D. L., Koch, U. M., MacConald, J., Cox, D. M., Lachman, R. S., and Adomian, G.,** Chondrodysplasia punctata in an infant with duplication 16p due to 7:16 translocation, *Am. J. Med. Genet.,* 21, 581, 1985.

77. **Spranger, J. W., Opitz, J. M., and Bidder, U.,** Heterogeneity of chondrodysplasia punctata, *Humangenetik,* 11, 190, 1971.

78. **Price, P. A., Williamson, M. K., Haba, T., Dell, R. B., and Jee, W. S.,** Excessive mineralization with growth plate closure in rats on chronic warfarin treatment, *Proc. Natl. Acad. Sci. U.S.A.,* 79, 7734, 1982.

79. **Price, P. A. and Kaneda, Y.,** Vitamin K counteracts the effect of warfarin in liver but not in bone, *Thromb. Res.,* 46, 121, 1987.

80. **Ulrich, M. W. W., Knapen, M. H. J., Herrmann-Erlee, M. P. M., and Vermeer, C.,** Vitamin K is no antagonist for the action of warfarin in rat osteosarcoma UMR 106, *Thromb. Res.,* 50, 27, 1988.

81. **Einhorn, T. A., Gundberg, C. M., Devlin, V. J., and Warman, J.,** Fracture Healing and osteocalcin metabolism in vitamin K deficiency, *Clin. Orthop. Rel. Res.,* 237, 219, 1988.

82. **Lian, J. B. and Gundberg, C. M.,** Osteocalcin: biochemical considerations and clinical applications, *Clin. Orthop. Rel. Res.,* 226, 267, 1988.

83. **Pauli, R. M., Lian, J. B., Mosher, D. F., and Suttie, J. W.,** Association of congenital deficiency of multiple vitamin K-dependent coagulation factors and the phenotype of the warfarin embryopathy: clues to the mechanism of teratogenicity of coumarin derivatives, *Am. J. Human Gen.,* 41, 566, 1987.

84. **McMillan, C. W. and Roberts, H. R.,** Congenital combined deficiency of coagulation factors II, VII, IX and X, *N. Engl. J. Med.,* 274, 1313, 1966.

85. **Hart, J. P., Shearer, M. J., Klenerman, L., Catterall, A., Reeve, J., Sambrook, P. N., Dodos, R. A., Bitensky, L., and Chayen, J.,** Electrochemical detection of depressed circulating levels of vitamin K in osteoporosis, *J. Clin. Endocrin. Metab.,* 60, 1268, 1985.

86. **Dodds, R. A., Catterall, A., Bitensky, L., and Chayen, J.,** Effects on fracture healing of an antagonist of the vitamin K cycle, *Calcif. Tiss. Int.,* 36, 233, 1984.

87. **Piro, L. D., Whyte, M. P., Murphy, W. A., and Birge, S. J.,** Normal cortical bone mass in patients after long term coumadin therapy, *J. Clin. Endocrinol. Metab.,* 54, 470, 1982.

88. **Resch, H., Pietschmann, P., Krexner, E., Willvonseder, R., and Brüder, K. H. B.,** Reduced peripheral bone density in patients under anticoagulant therapy, *Calcif. Tiss. Int.,* 44S, I23, 1989.

89. **Lian, J., Stewart, C., Puchacz, E., Mackowiak, S., Shaloub, V., Collart, D., Zambetti, G., and Stein, G.,** Structure of the rat osteocalcin gene and regulation of vitamin D-dependent expression, *Proc. Natl. Acad. Sci. U.S.A.,* 86, 1143, 1989.

90. **Tanaka, H., Abe, E., Mijaura, C., Kuribayaski, T., Konna, K., Nishi, Y., and Suda, T.,** 1α,25-Dihydroxycholecalciferol and a human myeloid leukaemia cell line (HL-60): the presence of a cytosol receptor and induction of differentiation, *Biochem. J.,* 204, 713, 1981.

91. **Chen, T. L., Hauschka, P. V., and Feldman, D.,** The effects of $1,25(OH)_2$-vitamin D_3 and dexamethasone on rat osteoblastlike primary cell cultures: receptor occupancy and functional expression patterns for three different bioresponses, *Endocrinology,* 118, 250, 1986.

92. **Canalis, E. and Lian, J. B.,** Effects of bone associated growth factors on DNA, collagen, and osteocalcin synthesis in cultured fetal rat calvariae, *Bone,* 9, 243, 1988.

93. **Price, P. A. and Baukol, S. A.,** $1,25(OH)_2D_3$ increases synthesis of the vitamin K dependent protein by osteosarcoma cells, *J. Biol. Chem.,* 255, 11,660, 1980.

94. **Markowitz, M. E., Gundberg, C. M., and Rosen, J. F.,** The circadian rhythm of serum osteocalcin concentrations: effects of 1,25-dihydroxyvitamin D administration, *Calcif. Tiss. Int.,* 40, 179, 1987.

95. **Gundberg, C. M., Cole, D. E. C., Lian, J. B., Reade, T. M., and Gallop, P. M.,** Serum osteocalcin in the treatment of inherited rickets with 1,25-dihydroxyvitamin D_3, *J. Clin. Endocrinol. Metab.,* 56, 1063, 1983.

96. **Caniggia, A., Nuti, R., Galli, M., Lore, F., Turchetti, V., and Righi, G. A.,** Effect of a long-term treatment with 1,25-dihydroxyvitamin D_3 on osteocalcin in postmenopausal osteoporosis, *Calcif. Tiss. Int.,* 38, 328, 1986.

97. **Duda, R. J., Kumar, R., Nelson, K. I., Zinsmeister, A. R., Mann, K. G., and Riggs, B. L.**, 1,25 dihydroxyvitamin D stimulation test for osteoblast function in normal and osteoporotic postmenopausal women, *J. Clin. Invest.*, 79, 1249, 1987.

98. **Zerwekh, J. E., Sakhaee, K., and Pak, C. Y. C.**, Short-term 1,25-dihydroxyvitamin D_3 administration raises serum osteocalcin in patients with postmenopausal osteoporosis, *J. Clin. Endocrinol. Metab.*, 60, 615, 1985.

99. **Silve, C., Grosse, B., Tau, C., Garabedian, M., Fritsche, J., Delmas, P., Cournot-Witmer, G., and Balsan, S.**, Response to parathyroid hormone and 1,25 dihydroxy-vitamin D_3 of bone-derived cells isolated from normal children and children with abnormalities in skeletal development, *J. Clin. Endocrinol. Metab.*, 62, 583, 1986.

100. **Garabedian, M., Vainsel, M., Mallet, E., Guillozo, H., Toppet, M., Grimberg, R., Nguyen, T. M., and Balsan, S.**, Circulating vitamin D metabolite concentrations in children with nutritional rickets, *J. Pediatr.*, 103, 381, 1983.

101. **Dandona, P., Menon, R. K., Shenoy, R., Houlder, S., Thomas, M., and Mallinson, W. J.**, Low 1,25-dihydroxyvitamin D, secondary hyperparathyroidism, and normal osteocalcin in elderly subjects, *J. Clin. Endocrinol. Metab.*, 63, 459, 1986.

102. **Dandona, P., Menon, R. K., Houlder, S., Thomas, M., Hoffbrand, A. V., and Flynn, D. M.**, Serum 1,25 dihydroxyvitamin D and osteocalcin concentrations in thalassaemia major, *Arch. Dis. Child*, 62, 474, 1987.

103. **Epstein, S., Bell, N. H., Shary, J., Shaw, S., Greene, A., and Oexmann, M. J.**, Evidence that obesity does not influence the vitamin D-endocrine system in blacks, *J. Bone Min. Res.*, 1, 181, 1986.

104. **Stock, J. L., Coderre, J. A., and Mallette, L. E.**, Effects of a short course of estrogen on mineral metabolism in postmenopausal women, *J. Clin. Endocrinol. Metab.*, 61, 595, 1985.

105. **Papapoulos, S. E., Frolich, M., Mudde, A. H., Harinck, H. I., van Den Berg, H., and Bijvoet, O. L.**, Serum osteocalcin in Paget's disease of bone: basal concentrations and response to bisphosphonate treatment, *J. Clin. Endocrinol. Metab.*, 65, 89, 1987.

106. **Reid, I. R., Chapman, G. E., Fraser, T. R., Davies, A. D., Surus, A. S., Meyer, J., Huq, N. L., and Ibbertson, H. K.**, Low serum osteocalcin levels in glucocorticoid-treated asthmatics, *J. Clin. Endocrinol. Med.*, 62, 379, 1986.

107. **Garabedian, M., Holick, M. F., DeLuca, H. F., and Boyle, I. T.**, Control of 25-hydroxycholecalciferol metabolism by parathyroid glands, *Proc. Natl. Acad. Sci. U.S.A.*, 69, 1673, 1971.

108. **Deftos, L. J., Parthemore, J. G., and Price, P. A.**, Changes in plasma bone Gla protein during treatment of bone disease, *Calcif. Tiss. Int.*, 34, 121, 1982.

109. **Rico, H. and Hernandez, E. R.**, Serum levels of osteocalcin in hypercalcemia of primary hyperparathyroidism and tumor-related hypercalcemia, *Rev. Clin. Esp.*, 178, 358, 1986.

110. **Mizunashi, K., Furukawa, U., Miura, R., Yumita, S., Sohn, H. E., Yoshinaga, K.**, Effects of active vitamin D_3 and parathyroid hormone on the serum osteocalcin in idiopathic hypoparathyroidism and pseudohypoparathyroidism, *J. Clin. Invest.*, 82, 861, 1988.

111. **Lian, J. B., Couttes, M. C., and Canalis, E.**, Studies of hormonal regulation of osteocalcin synthesis in cultured fetal rat calvaria, *J. Biol. Chem.*, 260, 8706, 1985.

112. **Beresford, J. N., Gallagher, J. A., Poser, J. W., and Russell, R. G. G.**, Production of osteocalcin by human bone cells in vitro. Effects of $1,25(OH)_2D_3$, $24,25(OH)_2D_3$, parathyroid hormone, and glucocorticoids, *Metab. Bone Dis. Rel. Res.*, 5, 229, 1984.

113. **Noda, M., Yoon, K., and Rodan, G. A.**, Cyclic AMP-mediated stabilization of osteocalcin mRNA in rat osteoblast-like cells treated with parathyroid hormone, *J. Biol. Chem.*, 263, 18,574, 1988.

114. **Calvo, M. S., Freyer, M. J., Laakso, K. J., Nissenson, R. A., Price, P. A., Murray, T. M., and Heath, H.**, Structural requirements for parathyroid hormone action in mature bone. Effects on release of cyclic adenosine monophosphate and bone gamma-carboxyglutamic acid-containing protein from perfused rat hindquarters, *J. Clin. Invest.*, 26, 2348, 1985.

115. **Cole, D. E. C. and Gundberg, C. M.,** Changes in serum osteocalcin associated with parathyroid hormone infusion in X-linked hypophosphatemic rickets, *Clin. Chem. Acta,* 151, 1, 1985.

116. **Riggs, B. L., Tsai, K. S., and Mann, K. G.,** Effect of acute increases in bone matrix degradation on circulating levels of bone-Gla protein, *J. Bone Min. Res.,* 1, 539, 1986.

117. **Rico, H., Cabranes, J. A., Nunez-Torron, M., Higueras, J. C., and Hernandez, E. R.,** Osteocalcin, (BGP) values in postmenopausal osteoporosis before and after treatment with calcitonin, *Med. Clin.,* 86, 791, 1986.

118. **Gundberg, C. M. and Fawzi, M.,** Effects of chronic and acute administration of parathyroid hormone and calcitonin on serum osteocalcin in vivo, *J. Bone Min. Res.,* 2, (Suppl.)1, 59A, 1987.

119. **Moss, D. W.,** Alkaline phosphatase isoenzymes, *Clin. Chem.,* 28, 2007, 1982.

120. **Delmas, P. D., Demiaux, B., Malaval, L., Chapuy, M. C., and Meunier, P. J.,** Serum Bone Gla-protein is not a sensitive marker of bone turnover in Paget's disease of bone, *Calcif. Tiss. Int.,* 38, 60, 1986.

121. **Castells, S., Yasumura, S., Fusi, M. A., Colbert, C., Bachtell, R. S., and Smith, S.,** Plasma osteocalcin levels in osteogenesis imperfecta, *J. Pediatr.,* 109, 88, 1986.

122. **Bataille, R., Delmas, P., and Sany, J.,** Serum BGP in multiple myeloma, *Cancer,* 59, 329, 1987.

123. **Steinberg, K. K. and Rogers, T. N.,** Alkaline phosphatase isoenzymes and osteocalcin in serum of normal subjects, *Ann. Clin. Lab. Med.,* 17, 241, 1987.

124. **Duda, R. J., O'Brien, J. F., Katzmann, J. A., Peterson, J. M., Mann, K. G., and Riggs, B. L.,** Concurrent assays of circulating bone Gla-protein and bone alkaline phosphatase: effects of sex, age, and metabolic bone disease, *J. Clin. Endocrinol. Metab.,* 66, 951, 1988.

125. **Stephan, J. J., Lackmanova, J., Strakova, M., and Pacovsky, V.,** Serum osteocalcin, bone alkaline phosphatase isoenzyme and plasma tartrate resistant acid phosphatase in patients on chronic maintenance hemodialysis, *Bone Min.,* 3, 177, 1987.

126. **Lian, J. B. and Gundberg, C. M.,** Osteocalcin: biochemical considerations and clinical applications, *Clin. Orthop. Rel. Res.,* 226, 267, 1988.

127. **Hauschka, P. V., Lian, J. B., Cole, D. E. C., and Gundberg, C. M.,** Osteocalcin and matrix Gla protein: vitamin K-dependent proteins in bone, *Physiol. Rev.,* 69, 990, 1989.

128. **Delmas, P. D., Wahner, H. W., Mann, K. G., and Riggs, B. L.,** Assessment of bone turnover in postmenopausal osteoporosis by measurement of serum bone Gla-protein, *J. Lab. Clin. Med.,* 102, 470, 1983.

129. **Ismail, F., Epstein, S., Pacifici, R., Drake, D., Thomas, S. B., and Avioli, L. V.,** Serum bone Gla protein (BGP) and other markers of bone mineral metabolism in postmenopausal osteoporosis, *Calcif. Tiss. Int.,* 39, 230, 1986.

130. **Gundberg, C. M., Lian, J. B., Gallop, P. M., and Steinberg, J. J.,** Urinary gamma-carboxyglutamic acid and serum osteocalcin as bone markers: studies in osteoporosis and Paget's disease, *J. Clin. Endocrinol. Metab.,* 57, 1221, 1983.

131. **Whyte, M. P., Bergfeld, M. A., Murphy, W. A., Avioli, L. V., and Teitelbaum, S. L.,** Postmenopausal osteoporosis — a heterogeneous disorder as assessed by histometric analysis of iliac bone from untreated patients, *Am. J. Med.,* 82, 193, 1982.

132. **Stepan, J. J., Presl, J., Broulik, P., and Pacovsky, V.,** Serum osteocalcin levels and bone alkaline phosphatase isoenzyme after oophorectomy and in primary hyperparathyroidism, *J. Clin. Endocrinol. Metab.,* 64, 1079, 1987.

133. **Ismail, F., Epstein, S., Fallon, M. D., Thomas, S. B., and Reinhardt, T. A.,** Serum bone Gla protein and the vitamin D endocrine system in the oophorectomized rat, *Endocrinology,* 122, 624, 1988.

134. **Podenphant, J., Christiansen, C., Catherwood, B. D., and Deftos, L. J.,** Serum bone Gla protein variations during prophylaxis of postmenopausal women with estrogen and calcium, *Calcif. Tiss. Int.,* 36, 536, 1984.

135. **Christiansen, C., Riis, B. J., Nilas, L., Rodero, P., and Deftos, L.,** Uncoupling of bone formation and resorption by combined estrogen and progestagen therapy in post-menopausal osteoporosis, *Lancet,* 1, 800, 1985.

136. **Gudmundsson, J. A., Ljunghall, S., Bergquist, C., Wide, L., and Nillius, S. J.,** Increased bone turnover during gonadotropin-releasing hormone superagonist-induced ovulation inhibition, *J. Clin. Endocrinol. Metab.,* 65, 159, 1987.

137. **Johansen, J. S., Riis, B. J., Hassager, C., Moen, M., Jacobson, J., and Christiansen, C.,** The effect of a gonadotropin-releasing hormone agonist analog (Nafarelin) on bone metabolism, *J. Clin. Endocrinol. Metab.,* 67, 701, 1988.

138. **Shah, D. V., Tews, J. K., Harper, A. E., and Suttie, J. W.,** Metabolism and transport of gamma-carboxyglutamic acid, *Biochem. Biophys. Acta,* 539, 209, 1978.

139. **Fernlund, P.,** Gamma-carboxyglutamic acid in human urine, *Clin. Chim. Acta,* 72, 147, 1976.

140. **Gundberg, C. M., Lian, J. B., and Gallop, P. M.,** Gamma-carboxyglutamate analysis by selective anion exchange elution and fluorescent detection, *Anal. Biochem.,* 98, 219, 1979.

141. **Sann, L., Leclercq, M., Fouillit, M., Chapuis, M. C., and Bruyere, A.,** Gamma-carboxyglutamic acid in urine of newborn infants, *Clin. Chim. Acta.,* 142, 31, 1984.

142. **Sadowski, J. A., Bacon, D. S., Hood, S., Davidson, K. W., Ganter, C. M., Haroon, Y., and Shepard, D. C.,** The application of methods used for the evaluation of vitamin K nutritional status in human and animal studies, in *Current Advances in Vitamin K Research,* Suttie, J. W., Ed., Elsevier, New York, 1988, 459.

143. **Levy, R. J. and Lian, J. B.,** Gamma-carboxyglutamate excretion and warfarin therapy, *Clin. Pharmacol. Ther.,* 25, 562, 1979.

144. **Lian, J. B., Pachman, L. M., Gundberg, C. M., Partridge, M., and Maryjowski, M. C.,** Gamma-carboxyglutamate excretion and calcinosis in juvenile dermatomyositis, *Arth. Rheum.,* 25, 1094, 1982.

145. **Lubinsky, M., Angle, C., Marsh, P. W., and Witkop, C. J., Jr.,** Syndrome of amelogenesis imperfecta, nephrocalcinosis, impaired renal concentration, and possible abnormality of calcium metabolism, *Am. J. Med. Genet.,* 20, 233, 1985.

146. **Nakagawa, Y., Abram, V., Kezdy, F. J., Kaiser, E. T., and Coe, F. L.,** Purification and characterization of the principal inhibitor of calcium oxalate monohydrate crystal growth in human urine, *J. Biol. Chem.,* 258, 12,594, 1983.

147. **Lian, J. B., Skinner, M., Glimcher, M. J., and Gallop, P. M.,** The presence of gamma-carboxyglutamic acid in the proteins associated with ectopic calcification, *Biochem. Biophys. Res. Commun.,* 73, 349, 1976.

148. **Wallin, R., Rossi, F., Loeser, R., and Key, L., Jr.,** The vitamin K-dependent carboxylation system in human osteosarcoma U2-OS cells, *Biochem. J.,* 269, 459, 1990.

149. **Suttie, J. W., Mummah-Schendel, L. L., Shah, D. V., Lyle, B. J., Greger, J. L.,** Vitamin K deficiency from dietary restriction in humans, *Am. J. Clin. Nutr.,* 47, 475, 1987.

150. **Garnero, P., Grimaux, M., Preaudat, C., Seguin, P., and Delmas, P. D.,** Measurement of serum osteocalcin with a human-specific two-site immunoradiometric assay, *J. Bone Min. Res.,* 7, 1389, 1992.

151. **Jaouhari, J., Scheile, F., Dragacci, S., Tarallo, P., Siest, J., Henney, J., and Siest G.,** Avidin-Biotin enzyme immunoassay of osteocalcin in serum or plasma, *Clin. Chem.,* 38, 1968, 1992.

152. **Hosoda, K., Eguchi, H., Nakamoto, T., Kubota, T., Honda, H., Jindai, S., Hasegawa, R., Kiyoki, M., Yamaji, T., and Shiraki, M.,** Sandwich immunoassay for intact human osteocalcin, *Clin. Chem.,* 38, 2233, 1992.

153. **Delmas, P. D., Christiansen, C., Mann, K. G., and Price, P. A.,** Bone gla protein (osteocalcin) assay standardization report, *J. Bone Min. Res.,* 5, 5, 1990.

154. **Power, M. J., Gosling, J. P., and Fottrell, P. F.,** Radioimmunoassay of osteocalcin with polyclonal and monoclonal antibodies, *Clin. Chem.,* 35, 1408, 1989.

155. **Tracy, R. P., Andrianorivo, A., Riggs, B. L., and Mann, K. G.,** Comparison of monoclonal and polyclonal antibody-based immunoassays for osteocalcin: a study of sources of variation in assay results, *J. Bone Min. Res.,* 5, 451, 1990.

156. **Taylor, A. K., Linkhart, S., Mohan, S., Christenson, R. A., Singer F. R., and Baylink, D. J.,** Multiple osteocalcin fragments in human urine and serum as detected by a midmolecule osteocalcin radioimmunoassay, *J. Clin. Endocrinol. Metab.,* 70, 467, 1990.

157. **Plantalech, L., Guillaumont, M., Vergnaud, P., Leclercq, M., and Delmas, P. D.,** Impairment of gamma carboxylation of circulating osteocalcin (bone gla protein) in elderly women, *J. Bone Min. Res.,* 6, 1211, 1991.

158. **Knappen, M. H. J., Hamulyak, K., and Vermeer, C.,** The effect of vitamin K supplementation on circulating osteocalcin (bone gla protein) and urinary calcium excretion, *Ann. Int. Med.,* 111, 1001, 1989.

159. **Jinguishi, S., Joyce, M. E., and Blander, M. E.,** Genetic expression of extracellular matrix proteins correlates with histologic changes during fracture repair, *J. Bone Min. Res.,* 7, 1045, 1992.

160. **Carlson, C. S., Tulli, H. M., Jayo, M. J., Loeser, R. F., Tracy, R. P., Mann, K. G., and Adams, M. R.,** Immunolocalization of noncollagenous bone matrix proteins in lumbar vertebrae from intact and surgically menopausal cynomologus monkeys, *J. Bone Min. Res.,* 8, 71, 1993.

161. **Demiaux, B., Arlot, M. E., Chapuy, M. C., Meunier, P. J., and Delmas, P. D.,** Serum osteocalcin is increased in patients with osteomalacia: correlations with biochemical and histomorphometric findings, *J. Clin. Endocrinol. Metab.,* 74, 1146, 1992.

162. **Ebling, P. R., Butler, P. C., Eastell, R., Rizza, R. A., and Riggs, B. L.,** The nocturnal increase in growth hormone is not the cause of the nocturnal increase in serum osteocalcin, *J. Clin. Endocrinol. Metab.,* 73, 368, 1991.

163. **Nielsen, H. K., Brixen, K., Kassem, M., Christensen, E., and Mosekilde, L.,** Diurnal rhythm in serum osteocalcin: relation with sleep, growth hormone, and PTH (1-84), *Calc. Tiss. Int.,* 49, 373, 1991.

164. **Nielsen, H. K., Brixen, K., Kassem, M., Charles, P., and Mosekilde, L.,** Inhibition of the morning cortisol peak abolishes the expected morning decrease in serum osteocalcin in normal males: evidence of a controlling effect of serum cortisol on the circadian rhythm in serum osteocalcin, *J. Clin. Endocrinol. Metab.,* 74, 1410, 1992.

165. **Nielsen, H. K., Brixen, K., and Mosekilde, L.,** Diurnal rhythm and 24-hour integrated concentrations of serum osteocalcin in normals: influence of age, sex, season, and smoking habits, *Calc. Tissue Int.,* 47, 284, 1990.

166. **Hodges, S. J., Pilkington, M. J., Stamp, T. C. B., Catterall, A., Shearer, M. J., Bitenshky, L., and Chayen, J.,** Depressed levels of circulating menaquinones in patients with osteoporotic fractures of the spine and femoral neck, *Bone,* 12, 387, 1991.

167. **Hodges, S. J., Pilkington, M. J., Shearer, M. J., Bitenshky, L., and Chayen, J.,** Age-related changes in the circulating levels of congeners of vitamin K_2, menaquinone-7 and menaquinone-8, *Clin. Sci.,* 78, 63, 1990.

168. **Power, M. J., and Fottrell, P. F.,** Osteocalcin: diagnostic methods and clinical applications, *Crit. Rev. Clin. Lab. Sci.,* 28, 287, 1991.

Chapter 16

EXTRA-HEPATIC GLA-CONTAINING PROTEINS IN THE HUMAN

Cees Vermeer and Marjo H. J. Knapen

TABLE OF CONTENTS

0-8493-6423-X/93/$0.00 + $.50

I. ENZYMES INVOLVED IN THE VITAMIN K CYCLE

Vitamin K functions as a coenzyme in a post-translational carboxylation reaction in which protein-bound glutamic acid (Glu) residues are converted into γ-carboxyglutamic acid (Gla) residues. The energy required for this reaction is provided by the oxidation of vitamin K hydroquinone (KH_2) into its epoxide (KO). On the basis of the daily requirement of vitamin K and the urinary Gla excretion it may be calculated that the vitamin must be re-used several thousand times before it is metabolized to inactive degradation products. Hence KO is not an end-product, but it is re-converted into KH_2 by the action of several reductases. It is not our aim here to elaborate on the details of the various reactions known to play a role in the vitamin K cycle (for more complete reviews see References 1 through 3), but we want to summarize briefly some basic knowledge, which is pertinent to this chapter.

The carboxylase and KO reductase enzymes are mainly located in the rough endoplasmic reticulum and behave like typical integral membrane proteins. Assay systems have been developed for both enzymes,[4,5] but because of their hydrophobic nature, the purification of the active enzymes has raised serious problems. Only recently has the complete purification of the carboxylase been reported.[6] Oral anticoagulants of the 4-hydroxycoumarin type block the vitamin K cycle because they inhibit the reductase rather than carboxylase activity. However, because of this blockade, vitamin K is no longer recycled and the reserves of KH_2 rapidly become exhausted. This prevents almost all new Gla-formation, so that the production of normal blood coagulation factors is effectively inhibited.

II. HUMAN TISSUES CONTAINING CARBOXYLASE/ REDUCTASE

Until the late 1970s it was generally thought that the carboxylase was exclusively involved in the production of the Gla-containing proteins already known to play a central role in blood coagulation and to be synthesized in the liver. Consequently the first *in vitro* carboxylating systems were developed using liver homogenates as a source of enzyme.[7,8] A few years later, however, it was shown that vitamin K-dependent carboxylase was present in many different types of tissue.[9] The relative concentrations of carboxylase and reductase in human tissues are given in Table 1.

The enzymes of the vitamin K cycle are also present in such varied cells as hepatocytes, endothelial cells, renal tubular cells, and osteoblasts.[11] With the knowledge that many tissues and cell types containing vitamin K-dependent carboxylase activity were not involved in the production of blood coagulation factors many investigators, in the early 1980s, turned their attention to the nature and possible function of this new class of vitamin K-dependent proteins. To date, the most extensively characterized extrahepatic Gla proteins are the bone proteins osteocalcin and matrix Gla protein.[12] Other Gla proteins

TABLE 1
Carboxylase and KO Reductase in
Human Tissues

Tissue	Carboxylase (%)	KO reductase (%)
Liver	100 ± 24	100 ± 21
Kidney	29 ± 4	46 ± 15
Lung	15 ± 4	41 ± 14
Spleen	9 ± 3	26 ± 11
Testis	37 ± 12	64 ± 25
Artery	18 ± 3	27 ± 7
Muscle	8 ± 2	28 ± 4
Epidermis	20 ± 3	32 ± 6

Note: The enzyme concentrations were calculated per milligram of microsomal proteins. In both cases, the hepatic enzymes are arbitrarily defined as 100%. Carboxylase was quantified by the rate of $^{14}CO_2$ incorporation into a pentapeptide substrate,[4] KO reductase by direct HPLC analysis.[10] The data represent the means of 5 different donors ± SD.

have been found in spermatozoa,[13] urine,[14] and calcified atherosclerotic plaques.[15] The function(s) of these extrahepatic Gla proteins, however, remains to be elucidated.

III. INFLUENCE OF VITAMIN K-ANTAGONISTS ON LIVER AND ON EXTRAHEPATIC TISSUES

During the last 40 years 4-hydroxycoumarin anticoagulant drugs (e.g., warfarin, acenocoumarol, and phenprocoumon) have been used extensively for the control of thrombogenic episodes after surgery or thromboembolic events. In fact, it is by no means unusual for these drugs to be administered for periods of 10 years or longer. In anticoagulant treatment, the therapeutic aim is to inhibit the enzymes of the vitamin K cycle to such an extent that the plasma concentration of each of the Gla-containing blood coagulation factors is below 30% of normal. In the content of potential long term management, it is clearly important to find out whether anticoagulant therapy also affects the enzymes of the vitamin K cycle in extrahepatic tissues. Such studies which have been carried out in experimental animals and *in vitro* clearly indicate that oral anticoagulants inhibit the hepatic and the extrahepatic carboxylase/reductase systems to a similar extent.[16] To demonstrate that this was also the case in humans, tissue donors had to be found who had been taking oral anticoagulants up to the time of death. After a 2-year survey we succeeded in obtaining tissue samples (liver, kidney, lung, spleen, testis, artery, and muscle) from five anticoagulated patients.[10] Preliminary results seemed to indicate that only the hepatic enzyme systems had been blocked, but later it became clear that, if measured at low reducing cofactor concentrations, the hepatic and extrahepatic KO reductase were affected to a similar extent.

Considering that vitamin K-dependent carboxylase occurs in nearly all tissues and cell types investigated, and that several extrahepatic Gla-proteins have been identified, it is remarkable that so few side-effects of coumarin derivatives have been noticed — other than the self evident risk of bleeding due to over-anticoagulation. The first reports of nonhemorrhagic side-effects of oral anticoagulants were published in 1975, describing a high frequency of bone malformations in newborns from mothers who had been anticoagulated during the first trimester of pregnancy.[17] Similar effects were reported in young rats that had been treated with warfarin during the first nine 9 months after birth.[18] Hence it was clear that Gla proteins play a vital role in bone formation, especially in rapidly growing bone. In a number of subsequent experiments, we have tried to establish whether vitamin K and vitamin K antagonists may also effect calcium metabolism in adult bone; some of our results are presented below.

IV. SERUM OSTEOCALCIN DURING ORAL ANTICOAGULANT TREATMENT

Osteocalcin (bone Gla protein) is exclusively synthesized in the osteoblasts of bone tissue. After its secretion the majority of the newly produced osteocalcin remains bound to the hydroxyapatite matrix, but a small fraction is set free into the blood stream, where it may be detected using a radioimmunoassay (RIA).[19] The direct quantitation of the Gla content of serum osteocalcin includes the extraction of osteocalcin from the serum with monospecific antibodies followed by Gla analysis.[20] The procedure, which was developed in bovine plasma, is laborious and its sensitivity does not permit the application of the same procedure in human plasma or serum. Therefore, the Gla content of human serum osteocalcin is usually estimated from its hydroxyapatite-binding (HAB) capacity.[21]

In our first study we compared a group of 74 male patients (mean age: 62 years) on stable, longterm (>3 years) anticoagulant treatment with an age-matched control group of healthy volunteers. In both groups we measured the serum concentration of immunoreactive osteocalcin (irOC) as well as its HAB capacity. As is shown in Figure 1, both parameters were significantly ($p < 0.001$) reduced in the coumarin-treated group. These data were confirmed in short-term studies in human subjects and in experimental animals (sheep), showing that both the serum irOC and the HAB capacity decrease in parallel at the onset of anticoagulant treatment.[22] The observation that vitamin K antagonists induce a decrease of the osteocalcin Gla content is consistent with their effect on blood coagulation factor synthesis. The fact that these drugs

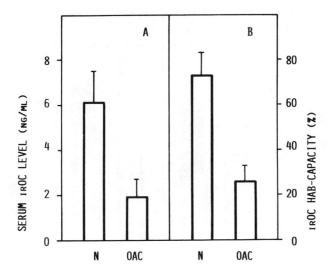

FIGURE 1.   Serum osteocalcin during oral anticoagulant treatment. Two groups of subjects were compared. The first one consisted of patients on stable longterm anticoagulant treatment (OAC) with Thrombotest® values between 5 and 15% of normal. The second group consisted of nontreated individuals (N), whose blood coagulation characteristics were well within the normal range. Blood was taken by venipuncture for the preparation of citrated plasma and serum. (A) The concentration of circulating immunoreactive osteocalcin (irOC) was measured with a radioimmunoassay (INCSTAR, Stillwater, Minnesota). The lines on top of each bar indicate the standard deviation. (B) The hydroxyapatite binding (HAB) capacity of serum osteocalcin was measured by extracting 300 μl of serum with 30 mg of hydroxyapatite and measuring the concentration of irOC before and after the extraction. The amount of irOC bound is expressed as a percentage of the total irOC present in the starting serum.

also reduce the serum irOC level is surprising, because on theoretical grounds one would expect that the low Gla content would lead to a decreased affinity of the partially carboxylated osteocalcin for the inorganic bone matrix and hence to an increased excretion of irOC into the blood stream. Mechanisms explaining this phenomenon may be either a poor cellular excretion of descarboxyosteocalcin by the osteoblasts or an increased catabolism of irOC in serum.

V. SERUM OSTEOCALCIN IN POSTMENOPAUSAL WOMEN

Having found that vitamin K-antagonists strongly interfere with osteocalcin biosynthesis, it seemed of interest to investigate whether low serum irOC levels and/or Gla deficient osteocalcin also occur in untreated subjects and whether vitamin K normalizes these variables. Because it had been shown by Hart et al.[23] that serum vitamin K_1 (phylloquinone) levels were about 30% of normal in a group of 16 osteoporotic subjects (1 male, 15 females with

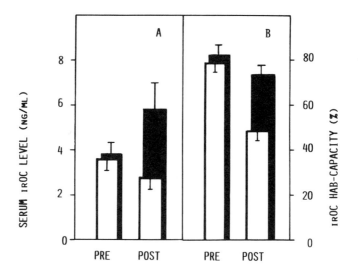

FIGURE 2.   Effect of vitamin K administration on serum osteocalcin. The two groups compared consisted of pre- and post-menopausal women, respectively. (Open bars) before treatment; (solid bars) the same variables after 2 weeks of vitamin K-administration. All data are ± SD. (A) The concentration of serum irOC. (B) The HAB-capacity of serum irOC.

ages ranging from 63 to 68 years) with femoral neck fractures, we compared a group of 50 post-menopausal women (55 to 75 years old) with a similar group of pre-menopausal women (25 to 40 years old). Using a number of blood coagulation tests, including the Thrombotest® and the plasma prothrombin concentration, no indication of vitamin K deficiency was obtained in any of these subjects. Both groups received vitamin K (1 mg/d) for 2 weeks and blood was taken by venipuncture before and after this period. As is shown in Figure 2A the serum irOC levels before treatment were comparable in both groups, but only in the post-menopausal group was this marker increased by vitamin K administration. Before treatment, the osteocalcin HAB capacity was low in the post-menopausal group (Figure 2B) but after vitamin K administration it had increased to the pre-menopausal level. These results were statistically significant ($p < 0.0001$) and indicate that, although the vitamin K supply in post-menopausal women is adequate for normal blood coagulation, it may be too low for the production of fully carboxylated osteocalcin. Whether this situation should be regarded as a state of vitamin K deficiency is presently unclear.

It is remarkable that before the start of the experiment the serum irOC levels in the post-menopausal women were comparable to those in the pre-menopausal ones. This is in contrast to data from the literature, where it is claimed that the serum irOC concentration increases with age.[24] Only after all participants had been treated with vitamin K were our data consistent with this tendency. From these results we conclude that, without taking into account

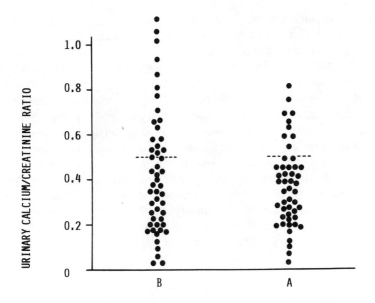

FIGURE 3.   Effect of vitamin K on urinary calcium excretion. The urine was collected during the last 2 h of a 16-h fasting period, and calcium concentrations were established with an atomic absorption spectrophotometer (Perkin-Elmer, Norwalk, Connecticut). Creatinine concentrations were assayed with a commercial kit (Hoffmann-La Roche, Basle, Switzerland) using a Cobas® centrifugal analyzer. The urinary calcium excretion was expressed as the calcium/creatinine ratio and was determined before (B) and after (A) vitamin K administration (14 d, 1 mg daily). All subjects were post-menopausal women.

the subject's vitamin K status, the reliability of serum irOC as a marker for bone diseases may be seriously questioned.

VI. EFFECT OF VITAMIN K ON URINARY CALCIUM EXCRETION

Gla-containing proteins other than osteocalcin have been identified in bone (matrix Gla protein),[12] kidney,[25] and in urine.[14] It seems likely that at least some of these proteins are involved in calcium metabolism. If so, one could expect that the urinary calcium excretion is affected during periods of vitamin K deficiency or during oral anticoagulant therapy. Second, in the former group the calcium excretion should be normalized by vitamin K administration. To test this hypothesis we have started a number of studies in which the HAB capacity of serum osteocalcin was taken as a marker for the vitamin K status of our subjects. In the experiment, which is reported here, the effect of vitamin K-administration on urinary calcium excretion was measured in a group of 50 post-menopausal women (mean age: 68 years). Before the start of the experiment their urinary calcium/creatinine ratio varied between 0.1 and 1.1 (Figure 3). Among the 50 participants we found 18 subjects with a calcium/creatinine ratio >0.5. The measurements were repeated after a 14-d period in which the women received an oral dose of 1 mg of vitamin K (phylloquinone) daily. In the group of the 18 "fast losers" of calcium this treatment resulted in a decrease of the calcium/creatinine ratio from 0.73 to 0.52 (mean values). This decrease was significant at $p < 0.001$ and showed a strong positive correlation with the urinary hydroxyproline excretion.[21]

At this stage it is too early to speculate about a possible contribution of vitamin K administration to the prevention of post-menopausal osteoporosis. First, because the subjects were recruited from a religious community, living in a convent, they may not be representative of the general population. Second, the undercarboxylation of circulating irOC was found in almost all participants, whereas only about 30% had a degree of urinary calcium loss which could be regarded as high. This demonstrates that there was no strict correlation between the degree of undercarboxylation of osteocalcin and the urinary calcium/creatinine ratio. Finally, it may be questioned whether the urinary calcium excretion over a relatively short time-span (as in this experiment) may be taken as a marker of the chronic bone loss of post-menopausal osteoporosis. Accordingly, more elaborate longterm investigations, with several hundred subjects, are presently in progress with the aim of gaining further insight into the possible extrahepatic role of vitamin K in calcium homeostasis.

VII. GLA-CONTAINING PROTEINS IN ATHEROSCLEROTIC PLAQUES

Another interesting vitamin K-dependent protein is known as plaque Gla protein (PGP). This protein was discovered only recently,[15] and as yet has been characterized less extensively than osteocalcin. PGP was isolated from the calcified lesions in the atherosclerotic vessel wall from which it could be extracted by dissolving the calcified material in EDTA. With the aid of polyacrylamide gel electrophoresis in SDS it was shown that PGP is a single chain molecule with an M_r of 23 kDa.

As yet the origin of PGP is unknown. One possibility is that it is synthesized by the vessel wall, either constitutively or only during the calcification process. Alternatively the protein might be produced elsewhere and subsequently be transported to the calcifying vessel wall via the blood stream. In both cases the occurrence of PGP in plasma may be expected. After a suitable assay had been developed,[26] PGP was indeed discovered in normal plasma and in serum. The concentration ranged from 0.5 to 1.5 mg/l. With the aid of the PGP test it was also shown that the plasma-PGP levels were relatively low in 37 patients suffering from severe atherosclerosis. It is not clear whether this phenomenon is due to decreased biosynthesis of PGP or due to the adsorption of PGP from the blood stream to the calcifying plaques.

A serious drawback of the PGP assay in its present form is that the sensitivity is not sufficient to accurately quantitate the plasma-PGP levels in the subnormal range. For this reason the question of whether plasma-PGP levels may be used as a marker for atherosclerosis cannot be answered as yet.

ACKNOWLEDGMENTS

The authors wish to thank Dr. K. Hamulyák for helpful discussions and advice and Mrs. T. Camphuisen-Engel for typing the manuscript. Our research is supported by grants 28–2140 (Prevention Fund) and 88–200 (Netherlands Heart Foundation).

REFERENCES

1. **Olson, R. E.**, The function and metabolism of vitamin K, *Annu. Rev. Nutr.*, 4, 281, 1984.
2. **Suttie, J. W.**, Vitamin K-dependent carboxylase, *Annu. Rev. Biochem.*, 54, 459, 1985.
3. **Vermeer, C.**, γ-Carboxyglutamate-containing proteins and the vitamin K-dependent carboxylase, *Biochem. J.*, 266, 625, 1990.
4. **Soute, B. A. M., Ulrich, M. M. W., and Vermeer, C.**, Vitamin K-dependent carboxylase: increased efficiency of the carboxylation reaction, *Thrombos. Haemostas.*, 57, 77, 1987.
5. **Fasco, M. J. and Principe, L. M.**, R- and S-warfarin inhibition of vitamin K and vitamin K 2,3-epoxide reductase activities in the rat, *J. Biol. Chem.*, 257, 4894, 1982.
6. **Wu, S.-M., Morris, D. P., and Stafford, D. W.**, Identification and purification to near homogeneity of the vitamin K-dependent carboxylase, *Proc. Natl. Acad. Sci. U.S.A.*, 88, 2236, 1991.
7. **Esmon, C. T., Sadowski, J. A., and Suttie, J. W.**, A new carboxylation reaction: the vitamin K-dependent incorporation of $H^{14}CO_3^-$ into prothrombin, *J. Biol. Chem.*, 250, 4744, 1975.
8. **De Metz, M., Vermeer, C., Soute, B. A. M., van Scharrenburg, G. J. M., Slotboom, A. J., and Hemker, H. C.**, Partial purification of bovine liver vitamin K-dependent carboxylase by immunospecific adsorption onto antifactor X, *FEBS Lett.*, 123, 215, 1981.
9. **Vermeer, C., Hendrix, H., and Daemen, M.**, Vitamin K-dependent carboxylases in nonhepatic tissues, *FEBS Lett.*, 148, 317, 1982.
10. **De Boer-van den Berg, M. A. G. and Vermeer, C.**, The in vivo effects of oral anticoagulants in man: comparison between liver and non-hepatic tissues, *Thrombos. Haemostas.*, 59, 147, 1988.
11. **De Boer-van den Berg, M. A. G., Uitendaal, M. P., and Vermeer, C.**, Direct measurement of vitamin K-dependent enzymes in various isolated and cultured tumor and non-tumor cells, *Mol. Cell. Biochem.*, 5, 71, 1987.
12. **Price, P. A.**, Role of vitamin K-dependent proteins in bone metabolism, *Annu. Rev. Nutr.*, 8, 565, 1988.
13. **Soute, B. A. M., Müller-Esterl, W., de Boer-van den Berg, M. A. G., Ulrich, M. M. W., and Vermeer, C.**, Discovery of a gammacarboxyglutamic acid-containing protein in human spermatozoa, *FEBS Lett.*, 190, 137, 1985.
14. **Nakagawa, Y., Abram, V., Kézdy, F. J., Kaiser, E. T., and Coe, F. L.**, Purification and characterization of the principal inhibitor of calcium oxalate monohydrate crystal growth in human urine, *J. Biol. Chem.*, 258, 12,594, 1983.

15. **Gijsbers, B. L. M. G., van Haarlem, L. J. M., Soute, B. A. M., Ebberink, R. H. M., and Vermeer, C.**, Characterization of a Gla-containing protein from calcified human atherosclerotic plaques, *Arteriosclerosis,* 10, 991, 1990.

16. **Roncaglioni, M. C., Soute, B. A. M., de Boer-van den Berg, M. A. G., and Vermeer, C.**, Warfarin-induced accumulation of vitamin K-dependent proteins: comparison between hepatic and non-hepatic tissues, *Biochem. Biophys. Res. Commun.,* 114, 991, 1983.

17. **Pettifor, J. M. and Benson, R.**, Congenital malformations associated with the administration of oral anticoagulants during pregnancy, *J. Pediatr.,* 86, 459, 1975.

18. **Price, P. A., Williamson, M. K., Haba, T., Dell, R. B., and Jee, W. S. S.**, Excessive mineralization with growth plate closure in rats on chronic warfarin treatment, *Proc. Natl. Acad. Sci. U.S.A.,* 79, 7734, 1982.

19. **Patterson-Allen, P., Brautigam, C. E., Grindeland, R. E., Asling, C. W., and Callahan, P. X.**, A specific radioimmunoassay for osteocalcin with advantageous species crossreactivity, *Analyt. Biochem.,* 120, 1, 1982.

20. **Soute, B. A. M., Ulrich, M. M. W., Knapen, M. H. J., van Haarlem, L. J. M., and Vermeer, C.**, The quantification of gammacarboxyglutamic acid residues in plasma-osteocalcin, *Calcif. Tissue Int.,* 43, 184, 1988.

21. **Knapen, M. H. J., Hamulyák, K., and Vermeer, C.**, The effect of vitamin K supplementation on circulating osteocalcin (bone Gla-protein) and urinary calcium excretion, *Ann. Int. Med.,* 111, 1001, 1989.

22. **Van Haarlem, L. J. M., Knapen, M. H. J., Hamulyák, K., and Vermeer, C.**, Circulating osteocalcin during oral anticoagulant therapy, *Thrombos. Haemostas.,* 60, 79, 1988.

23. **Hart, J. R., Catterall, A., Dodds, R. A., Klenerman, L., Shearer, M. J., Bitensky, L., and Chayen, J.**, Circulating vitamin K_1 levels in fractured neck of femur, *Lancet,* 2, 283, 1984.

24. **Delmas, P. D., Stenner, D., Wahner, H. W., Mann, K. G., and Riggs, B. L.**, Increase in serum bone gammacarboxyglutamic acid protein with aging women, *J. Clin. Invest.,* 71, 1316, 1983.

25. **Hauschka, P. V., Friedman, P. A., Traverso, H. P., and Gallop, P. M.**, Vitamin K-dependent γ-carboxyglutamic acid formation by kidney microsomes in vitro, *Biochem. Biophys. Res. Commun.,* 71, 1207, 1976.

26. **Van Haarlem, L. J. M.**, Biosynthesis, occurrence and characterization of Gla-containing proteins with a potential importance for cardiovascular diseases, Ph.D. thesis, University of Limburg Maastricht, The Netherlands, 1989.

INDEX

L

R

Rabbit brain thromboplastin, 198
Rabbit lung and brain, 169
Radioimmunoassay (RIA), 168
Recombinant technology, FVIIa prepared by, 97
Recruitment localization, 11, 12
Redox couple, 43
Redox mode, HPLC-ECD using, 45, 46
Reduced clearance, cardiovascular risk due to, 97
Regulatory processes, 17
Restriction fragment length polymorphisms (RFLPs), 165, 177, 182, 197
 extragenic, 182
 intragenic, 177, 180
RFLPs, see Restriction fragment length polymorphisms
RIA, see Radioimmunoassay

S

Salakta, 175
San Juan, 175
SBTI, see Soya bean tripsin inhibitor
SDS-page electrophoresis, 168
Secondary hemorrhagic disease, 233
Secondary hypercoagulability, 20
Secondary hypercoagulable state, 20
Serine protease(s), 16, 138
 activation constant of, 16
 activity, 164
 circulating half-life of active forms of, 16
 inhibitors, 15
Serpins, 15
Sickle cell patients, 138
Skin necrosis, 148
Solid matrix heparin, 127
Soya bean tripsin inhibitor (SBTI), 127
Splenic hematomas, 167
Splice junction, 180
Splicing defects, 196
Square wave voltammetry, 50
Staphylocoagulase, 168
Steric hindrance, 16
Structural fitness, 16
Stuart, 174
Stypven, 168
Stypven clotting time, 172
Subarachnoid hemorrhage, 167
Sulfated polysaccharides, 127

Synthetic peptides, 19
Synthetic vitamin K, 230

T

Taipan venom, 199
*Taq*I, 177
TAT, see Thrombin/antithrombin
Tenase, 17, 106
 complexes, 94
 cleavage of prothrombin by, 19
Termination, of coagulation, 10
Ternary complexes, 14, 15, 92, 94
TF, see Tissue factor
TFPI, see Tissue factor pathway inhibition
Thin-layer voltammetry, 35
Thrombin, 11, 16, 200
 activity, 19, 93
 commercially available, 131
 conversion of prothrombin to, 14
 generation, 15, 135
  association of FVII with, 92
  burst of, 93
  marker of, 18–19
Thrombin/antithrombin (TAT), 20, 139
Thrombin-like activity (TLA), 95
Thrombin-thrombomodulin complex, 20
β-Thromboglobulin, 19
Thrombocytopenia, 97
Thrombocytosis, 21
Thromboembolic complications, 97
Thromboembolic events, incidence of in patients with lupus anticoagulant problems, 138
Thrombogenesis
 factor VII-induced, 92
 hypercoagulability related to, 92
Thrombogenic potential, 130
Thrombogenic stimulus, 139
Thrombo-hemorrhagic balance, 112
Thrombomodulin, 212
 -protein S/protein C inhibitor pathway, 213
 thrombin bound to, 15
Thromboplastin, 14
Thrombosis, patients at risk for, 17
Thrombotest, 167, 169, 236
Thrombotic tendency, 127
Thrombovascular diseases, 137
Thrombus, 97
Tiger snake, 168
Tissue factor (TF), 14, 94, 105, 211, 212, 214, 216, 218